evolve

To access your Student Resources, visit:

http://evolve.elsevier.com/Buck/cpc/

Evolve® Student Resources for *Buck: CPC Coding Exam Review 2007: The Certification Step* offer the following features:

Student Resources

- **Study Tips**
  Thoughts and advice from the author to help medical coding students.

- **Content Updates**
  The latest content updates from the author to keep you current with recent developments in this area.

- **WebLinks**
  Links to places of interest on the web specific to your needs.

- **Links to Related Products**
  See what else Elsevier has to offer in your specific field of interest.

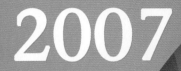

CPC CODING EXAM REVIEW

The Certification Step

2007

CPC CODING EXAM REVIEW

The Certification Step

CAROL J. BUCK, MS, CPC, CPC-H, CCS-P
Program Director, Retired
Medical Secretary Programs
Northwest Technical College
East Grand Forks, Minnesota

Technical Research Assistants

Cynthia Stahl, CPC, CCS-P
Reimbursement and Coding Specialist
Lebanon, Indiana

Deborah Neville, RHIA
HIM Business Manager
MC Strategies, Inc.
Atlanta, Georgia

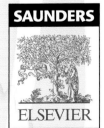

SAUNDERS
ELSEVIER

11830 Westline Industrial Drive
St. Louis, Missouri 63146

Publisher: Michael S. Ledbetter
Associate Developmental Editor: Josh Rapplean
Publishing Services Manager: Melissa Lastarria
Senior Project Manager: Kelly E. M. Steinmann
Designer: Andrea Lutes

Printed in the United States of America

Last digit is the print number: 9 8 7 6 5 4 3 2 1

Dedication

To coding instructors,
who each day strive to enhance the lives
of their students and provide the next generation
of knowledgeable medical coders.

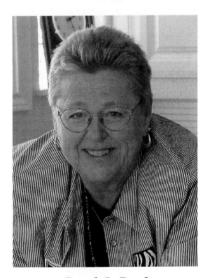

Carol J. Buck

Acknowledgments

There are so many, many people who participated in the development of this text, and only through the effort of all of the team members has it been possible to publish this text. **Jackie Grass,** who lent her technical coding knowledge and enthusiasm to this project. **Nancy Hart,** whose exceptional knowledge of medical terminology improved the terminology material.

    Sally Schrefer, Executive Vice President, Nursing and Health Professions, who possesses great listening skills and the ability to ensure the publication of high-quality educational materials. **Andrew Allen,** Publishing Director, Health Professions, who sees the bigger picture and shares the vision. **Michael Ledbetter,** Publisher, who maintains an excellent sense of humor and is a valued member of the team who can always be depended upon for reasoned judgment. **Josh Rapplean,** Associate Developmental Editor, who has taken over the developmental duties of this text with calm, confidence, and tremendous efficiency. **Julie Louis,** Production Editor, Graphic World, who assumed responsibility for many projects while maintaining a high degree of professionalism. The employees of Elsevier have participated in the publication of this text and demonstrated the highest levels of professionalism and competence.

Preface

Thank you for purchasing *CPC Coding Exam Review 2007: The Certification Step,* the latest guide to the outpatient physician coding certification exam. This 2007 edition has been carefully reviewed and updated with the latest content, making it the most current guide for your review. The author and publishers have made every effort to equip you with skills and tools you will need to succeed on the exam. To this end, this review guide presents essential information about all health care coding systems, anatomy, terminology, and pathophysiology, as well as sample examinations for practice, both in print and on CD-ROM. No other review guide on the market brings together such thorough coverage of all necessary examination material in one source.

ORGANIZATION OF THIS TEXTBOOK

Following a basic outline approach, *CPC Coding Exam Review 2007* takes a practical approach to assisting you with your examination preparations. The text is divided into four units—Anatomy, Terminology, and Pathophysiology; Reimbursement Issues; Overview of CPT, ICD-9-CM, and HCPCS Coding; and Coding Challenge—and there are seven appendices for your reference. Additionally, there is a bound-in CD-ROM with examinations to help your progress.

Unit I, Anatomy, Terminology, and Pathophysiology

Covers all the essential body systems and terms you'll need to get certified. Organized by body systems to follow the CPT codes, the sections also include illustrations to review each major anatomical area and quizzes to check your understanding and recall.

74   UNIT I   Anatomy, Terminology, and Pathophysiology

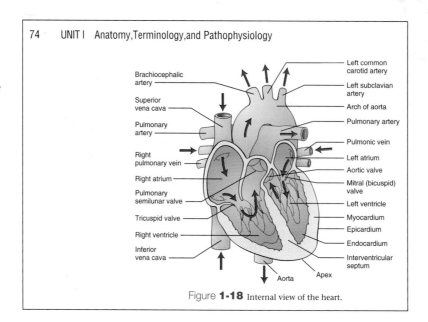

Figure **1-18** Internal view of the heart.

Unit II, Reimbursement Issues

Provides a review of important insurance and billing information to help you review the connections between medical coding, insurance, billing, and reimbursement.

- Accepting assignment
Block 27 on CMS-1500 (Figure 2-1)

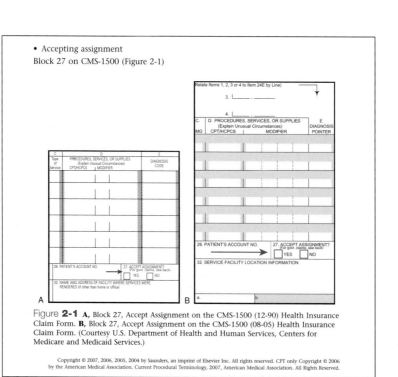

Figure **2-1** **A**, Block 27, Accept Assignment on the CMS-1500 (12-90) Health Insurance Claim Form. **B**, Block 27, Accept Assignment on the CMS-1500 (08-05) Health Insurance Claim Form. (Courtesy U.S. Department of Health and Human Services, Centers for Medicare and Medicaid Services.)

**Unit III,
Overview of
CPT, ICD-9-CM,
and HCPCS
Coding**
Contains comprehensive coverage of the different coding systems and their applications, making other references unnecessary! Simplified text and clear examples are the highlights of this unit, and illustrations are included to clarify difficult concepts.

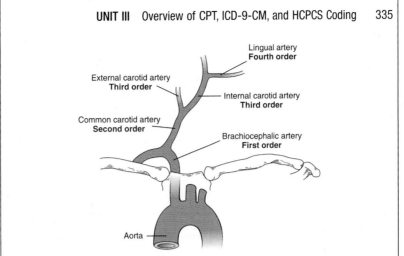

UNIT III   Overview of CPT, ICD-9-CM, and HCPCS Coding   335

Figure **3-12** Brachiocephalic vascular family with first-, second-, third-, and fourth-order vessels.

Balloon Removal: Threaded into vessel, inflated under mass, pulled out with mass

• Codes are divided by site of incision and whether artery or vein

Venous Reconstruction—CV Repairs (34501-34530)
Types of repairs
• Valve of the femoral vein

• Vena Cava

• Saphenopopliteal vein anastomosis

Aneurysm

**Unit IV,
Coding
Challenge**
Contains a Pre-Examination modeled after the CPC examination, to be completed at the start of your review. To help you quantify the examination, this is meant to be taken using paper and pencil.

UNIT IV   Coding Challenge   413

■ PRE-EXAMINATION
SECTION 1

Questions 1-43

Medical Terminology

1. The cup-shaped depression on the hip joint that receives the head of the femur is the:
   A. acetabulum
   B. calcaneus
   C. trochlea
   D. medial malleolus

2. The lower third of the small intestine is the:
   A. jejunum
   B. tenue
   C. ileum
   D. duodenum

ABOUT THE CD-ROM

The companion CD-ROM included in the back of this review guide contains valuable software to assist you with your preparation for the CPC coding certification examination. It includes two timed and scored 150-question practice examinations, each modeled after the actual CPC examination, which contains three major sections. The Pre-Examination in the textbook should be completed at the start of your study, and the Post-Examination on the CD-ROM should be taken after your study is complete. By comparing the results of both examinations, you can see your improvement after using the review guide! Once you check your scores, your are ready to take the Final Examination CD-ROM.

Summary Screen

When using the program, the Summary screen serves as home base. Here you can find information relating to your progress and performance in different examination sections and subject areas. From this screen, you can choose an examination mode, submit an examination section, check your progress, or review your results.

In addition to displaying your scores for completed sections and tracking the total elapsed time, this screen also shows the answered, unanswered, and flagged questions in each subsection. You can return to the Summary screen at any point while taking or reviewing an examination, and all information related to your answers and position is saved.

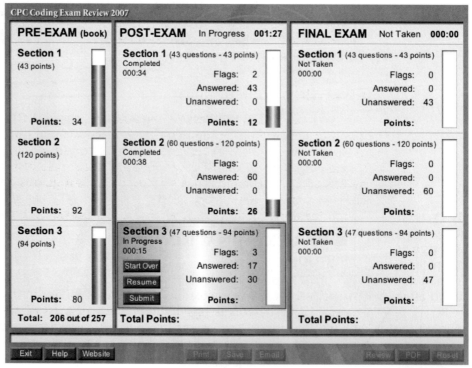

Summary screen.

Taking the Examination

While taking the examination, click on the letter of your answer choice, and the answer will be highlighted in red. You can also use the corresponding letter keys and arrows on the keyboard to answer and navigate. The Question screen displays the current question number, which doubles as a pull-down menu that allows you jump to any question in the current section. Additionally, the Flag button at the bottom of the screen allows you to mark questions for later reference.

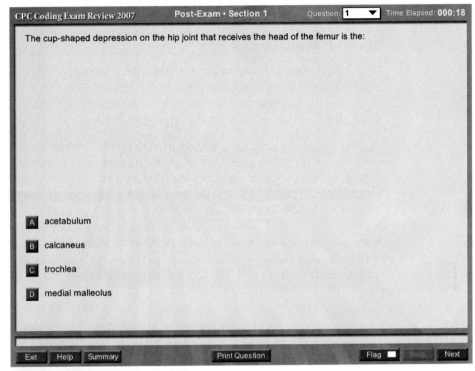

Question screen.

Reviewing Your Results

Once you have taken the Post-Examination on the CD-ROM, you have the option to review all the examination questions with rationales, even the ones you answered correctly. The correct answer is shown for each question, and a rationale is given for each answer option. You can also compare your results on the Pre- and Post-Examinations by viewing the bar graphs on the Summary screen or printing out a score sheet.

Additional instructions and help files are included on the CD-ROM to assist you in using the software.

SUPPLEMENTAL RESOURCES

However you decide to prepare for the certification examination, we have developed supplements designed to complement the *CPC Coding Exam Review 2007*. Each of these supplements has been developed with the needs of both students and instructors in mind.

Instructor's Electronic Resource

No matter what your level of teaching experience, this total-teaching solution will help you plan your lessons with ease, and the author has developed all the curriculum materials necessary to use the textbook in the classroom. This CD-ROM includes all answers to the textbook and workbook exercises, a course calendar and syllabus, lesson plans, and ready-made tests for easy assessment. Also included is a comprehensive PowerPoint collection for the entire text, and ExamView test banks. The PowerPoint slides can be easily customized to support your lectures or formatted as overhead transparencies or handouts for student note-taking. The ExamView test generator will help you quickly and easily prepare quizzes and exams, and the test banks can be customized to your specific teaching methods.

Evolve Resources

The Evolve companion website offers many resources that will extend your studies beyond the classroom. Related WebLinks and industry news offer you the opportunity to expand your knowledge base and stay current with this ever-changing field, and additional material is available for help and practice. Instructors can also download all materials from the Instructor's Electronic Resource, as well as content updates and industry news.

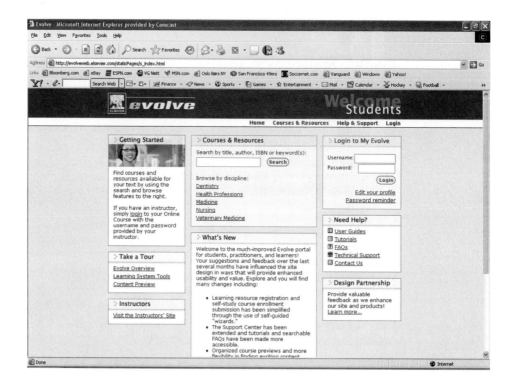

A Course Management System (CMS) is also available free to instructors who adopt this textbook. This web-based platform gives instructors yet another resource to facilitate learning and to make medical coding content accessible to students. In addition to the Evolve Resources available to both faculty and students, there is an entire suite of tools available that allows for communication between instructors and students. Students can log on through the Evolve portal to take online quizzes, participate in threaded discussions, post assignments to instructors, or chat with other classmates, while instructors can use the online grade book to follow class progress.

To access this comprehensive online resource, simply go to the Evolve home page at http://evolve.elsevier.com and enter the user name and password provided by your instructor. If your instructor has not set up a Course Management System, you can still access the free Evolve resources at http://evolve.elsevier.com/Buck/cpc/.

Development of This Edition

This book would not have been possible without a team of educators and professionals, including practicing coders and technical consultants. The combined efforts of the team members have made this text an incredible learning tool.

CODING SPECIALISTS

Cynthia Stahl, CPC, CCS-P
Reimbursement and Coding Specialist
Lebanon, Indiana

Jacqueline Klitz Grass, MA, CPC
Business Manager/Reimbursement
   Coding
The Kidney and Hypertension Center
Grand Forks, North Dakota

Russell D. Robbins, MD, MBA, CPC
Medical Director
iHealth Technologies
Atlanta, Georgia

TERMINOLOGY SPECIALIST

Nancy Hart, RN, BS
Registered Nurse
Plano, Texas

REVIEWERS

Karen Drummond, CPC, CPC-H, CMC
Medical Billing/Coding Instructor and
   Consultant
Stark State College, Canton City
   Schools Adult Education
Canton, Ohio
American Academy of Professional
   Coders
Salt Lake City, Utah

Andrea Potteiger, CPC, CMAA, CBCS, NR-CMA, NR-CAHA, NR-CPT, NR-CEKG, CHI
Lead Healthcare Instructor
New Horizons, Harrisburg
Harrisburg, Pennsylvania

Contents

CPC CODING EXAM REVIEW
The Certification Step

2007

Success Strategies

This review was developed to help you as you prepare for your certification examination. First, congratulations on your initiative. Preparing for a certification examination can seem like a daunting and formidable task. You have already taken the first and hardest step: you have made a commitment. Your steely determination and organizational skills are your best tools as you prepare to complete this exciting journey successfully.

How do you prepare for a certification examination? The answers to that question are as varied as the persons preparing for it. Each person comes to the preparation with different educational, coding, and personal experiences. Therefore, each must develop a plan that meets his or her individual needs and preferences. Success Strategies will help you to develop your individual plan.

THE CERTIFICATION EXAMINATION

This text has been developed to serve as a tool in your preparation for the outpatient (physician-based) **CPC** (Certified Professional Coder) certification examination offered by the American Academy of Professional Coders (AAPC). The CPC certification examination consists of Sections 1, 2, and 3 covering medical terminology, anatomy, pathophysiology, CPT, ICD-9-CM, HCPCS, and coding concepts. You have 5 hours to complete the examination. Visit the AAPC website (www.aapc.com) for the latest information on computer-based testing that may be implemented soon.

To be successful on the CPC certification examination, you will have to know how to assign medical codes to patient services and diagnoses. This textbook focuses on providing you with that coding practice as well as anatomy, terminology, pathophysiology, reimbursement, and coding concepts in preparation for the CPC examination.

Date and Location

Although every journey begins with the first step, you have to know where you are going to make a plan to get there.

- Choose the **date and location** for taking the certification examination. The AAPC's website contains detailed information about the examination sites and dates.

- The American Academy of Professional Coders has information that can be downloaded from their website at www.aapc.com or sent for by contacting:

  American Academy of Professional Coders
  2480 South 3850 West, Suite B
  Salt Lake City, UT 84120
  Telephone: 800-626-2633

- After you have obtained the examination materials, read all the information carefully. Review all competencies outlined in the material to ensure that your study plan contains strategies to address each of these competencies.

- The questions within this textbook are not the same questions that are in the certification examination, but the skill and knowledge that you gain through analysis, coding, and recall will increase your ability to be successful on examination day.

- The AAPC's examination information will indicate the coding specifics. For example, the levels of the evaluation and management key components (history, examination, and medical decision making complexity) are stated in the certification questions. Do not challenge the levels.

MANAGING YOUR TIME

Role strain! That is what you get when you have so many different roles in your life and you cannot find time for all of them! Know that feeling? Are you a daughter/son, mother/father, wife/husband, student, friend, worker, volunteer, hobbyist—the list is endless. Each takes time from your schedule, and somehow you now need to fit into the role of successful learner. Because you have only 24 hours in your day, being a successful learner requires a time-balancing act. Maybe you will have to be satisfied with dust bunnies under your bed, dishes in your kitchen sink, or fewer visits with your friends. Whatever you have to do to juggle the time around to give yourself ample time to devote to this important task of examination preparation, you must do and make a plan for in advance; otherwise, life just takes over and you find you do not have adequate study time.

If you are planning a big event in your life—moving, a trip, and so on, think about postponing it until after the examination. Your focus right now has to be on yourself. Make your motto **"It's All About Me!"** Sounds self-centered, I know, and most likely very different from who you are, but just this once, you need to carve out the time you need to accomplish this important goal. This time is for yourself. Make it happen for yourself. Move everything you can out of the way, focus on this preparation, and give this preparation your best effort.

SCHEDULE

Each person has an individual learning style. The coding profession seems to attract those most influenced by logic and facts. The best way for a logical and factual person to learn is to problem-solve and apply the information. Hands-on practice is how you will build your skill and confidence for the examination.

- Choose a location to be your Study Central.

- Gather into Study Central the following study resources:

  - Certification packet or handbook from the certifying organization

  - CPT, current edition

- ICD-9-CM, current edition

- HCPCS, current edition

- ICD-9-CM Official Guidelines for Coding and Reporting (Appendix A)

- Medical dictionary

- Coding textbooks, professional journals, and magazines

- Terminology, anatomy, or pathology text, as needed

- See Appendix G for Further Text Resources

Make Study Central your special place where you can get away from all other responsibilities. Make it a quiet, calm getaway, even if it is a corner of your bedroom. In this quiet place have a comfortable chair, adequate lighting, supplies, and sufficient desktop surface to use all your coding books. This is your place to focus all your attention on preparation for the examination, without distractions.

- Plan your **schedule** from now until the certification examination using a calendar. Make weekly goals so that you have definite tasks to accomplish each week and you can check the tasks off—a great feeling of accomplishment comes from being able to check off a task. In this way, you can see your progress on your countdown to success.

- Choose a specific **time** each day or several times a week when you are going to study and mark them on your calendar. Make this commitment in writing. After each study session, you should check off that date on the calendar as a visual reminder that you are sticking to your plan and are one step closer to your goal.

- You should plan your study time in advance, know what you are going to be studying the next session, and **be prepared** for that upcoming study session. This will greatly increase the amount of material you are able to cover during the session. At the end of each session, decide what you are going to study next session and ensure that you have all the material and references you will need readily available. At the end of each session, you should be ready for the next study session.

- Your plan should include those areas where you know you will need improvement. For example, when is the last time you read, not referenced or reviewed, but really read, the CPT Anesthesia Guidelines? You probably do not code anesthesia services often, if ever, and as such are not familiar with the information in these guidelines. That is an area of improvement, and your plan should include a thorough reading of all the CPT section guidelines.

- **DO THIS BEFORE YOU BEGIN YOUR STUDY: Assess** your strengths and weaknesses. By making this assessment, you will know where to concentrate your efforts and where to focus your study schedule. You know those areas where you already have strong skills and knowledge and will not need to spend as much time preparing in these areas. The **Pre-Examination** is an examination that you can use as a tool to assess your current skill level. This examination should be taken before you begin your study and then again immediately after you have completed your entire study schedule. Do not analyze the questions by reviewing the rationales provided; rather, wait until after you have completed your studies and have taken this same examination a second time. If you review the rationales after the first time you take the examination, you will know the answers too well to provide a valid comparison between examinations. See Unit IV of this textbook for further information and directions on the Pre-Examination.

- After you have completed your course of study, take the **Post-Examination** on CD. You should plan to cover the examination in the same amount of time as will be given for the certification examination you are going to take. Compare your scores to those from the first time you took this examination. Note the areas where you did not demonstrate sufficient skills and knowledge.

- Develop a **second plan** to improve the specific areas where you believe you need further study.

- You are now ready to take the **Final Examination** that is on the accompanying CD. Take the examination in the same amount of time that will be allocated for the certification examination. It is best if you do this final in one sitting, thereby mimicking the actual examination. If your schedule does not allow for taking the examination in one sitting, plan to take it in several sessions, but always keep track of the time used to ensure that you take the examination in the same amount of time allowed for the official examination. Learning to work within the time allocated is part of the skill you are developing. Remember the certification examinations assess not only your coding knowledge but also your efficiency in completing the examination within the allocated time.

USING THIS TEXT

This text is divided into:

- Success Strategies
- Unit I, Anatomy, Terminology, and Pathophysiology
- Unit II, Reimbursement Issues
- Unit III, Overview of CPT, ICD-9-CM, and HCPCS Coding
- Unit IV, Coding Challenge
- Appendix A, ICD-9-CM Official Guidelines for Coding and Reporting
- Appendix B, Medical Terminology
- Appendix C, Combining Forms
- Appendix D, Prefixes
- Appendix E, Suffixes
- Appendix F, Abbreviations
- Appendix G, Further Text Resources

Appendices B-F are combined lists of Medical Terminology, Combining Forms, Prefixes, Suffixes, and Abbreviations used within Unit I, Anatomy, Terminology, and Pathophysiology.

The material in this review features the following:

- Comprehensive guide in outline format
- Photos and drawings to illustrate key points
- Pre-/Post-Examination (Pre-Examination in text, Post-Examination on CD)— 150 questions

- Final Examination (CD)—150 questions

- **Unit I** is a review of the anatomy, terminology, and pathophysiology by organ systems designed to provide you with a quick review of that organ system. In addition, there is a list of combining forms, prefixes, suffixes, and abbreviations that are often used in that organ system. At the end of each organ system, there is a quiz that will give you an opportunity to assess your knowledge.

- **Unit II** is a review of reimbursement issues and terminology. A quiz is located at the end of the unit to assess your knowledge.

- **Unit III** is a review of CPT, HCPCS, and ICD-9-CM. The CPT and ICD-9-CM material follows the order of the manuals. There is no quiz at the end of this unit because you will be applying this material in the practice examinations and in the Final Examination.

- **Unit IV** contains the examinations. The Pre-/Post-Examination is a 150-question examination located as a pre-examination in the textbook and as a post-examination on the **CD.** This same exam should be taken twice—once before you begin your study and the second time after you have completed your study. You should allow 5 hours (300 minutes) to complete each examination because this is the amount of time you will have for the CPC examination. You will enter your Pre-Examination results into the computer software, which stores your scores and compares the results from the first and second time you took the examination; so you can see not only your score on each section but also the improvement from the first to the second examination. The Final Examination is also a 150-question examination on CD, and you should allow 5 hours (300 minutes) to complete the examination. All examinations are divided into the following sections:

  - **Section 1—43 questions**
    - Medical Terminology (13)
    - Anatomy (9)
    - ICD-9-CM (11)
    - HCPCS (5)
    - Concepts of Coding (5)

  - **Section 2—60 questions**
    - Integumentary System (10000 range) (9)
    - Musculoskeletal System (20000 range) (10)
    - Respiratory and Cardiovascular Systems (30000 range) (10)
    - Digestive System (40000 range) (10)
    - Urinary, Male Genital System, Female Genital System, and Maternity Care and Delivery (50000 range) (11)
    - Endocrine and Nervous Systems, and Eye/Ocular Adnexa (60000 range) (10)

  - **Section 3—47 questions**
    - Evaluation and Management (99201-99499 range) (12)
    - Anesthesia (00100-01999, 99100-99140 range) (6)

· Radiology (70000 range) (9)

· Pathology and Laboratory (80000 range) (10)

· Medicine (90281-99199, 99500-99602 range) (10)

A passing score for this test is as follows:

- **Section I 63% or 27 of the 43 questions correct**

- **Section II 72% or 44 of the 60 questions correct**

- **Section III 60% or 28 of the 47 questions correct**

There are many ways you could use this text. However you decide to prepare, you should take the examination before you begin your study to ensure that you develop a study plan that includes time and activities that will increase your knowledge in those areas where your test scores indicate areas of weakness. You could then take the units in the order they are presented, or you may want to review the anatomy, terminology, and pathophysiology for a body system and then review the CPT material for that body system. There is no one best way to approach the use of this text because each individual will have a personal learning style and preferences that will direct how the material is used. Your skills may be very strong in one or more coding or knowledge areas, and you will want to delete those areas from your individual study plan.

This text is not meant to be the only study source, but only one tool of many that you will use. For example, if your terminology skills need a complete overhaul, the brief overview in this text may not meet your needs. You may want to supplement this text with a terminology text and an in-depth study of terminology.

- **Appendices** are a resource for you as you prepare your study plan.

  · **Appendix A,** ICD-9-CM Official Guidelines for Coding and Reporting, is the rules for use of ICD-9-CM codes and will be referenced in Unit III when reviewing the use of ICD-9-CM codes.

  · **Appendix B,** Medical Terminology, is a complete alphabetic list of all the medical terms listed in the Medical Terminology portion of the organ system reviews used in Unit I.

  · **Appendix C,** Combining Forms, is a complete alphabetic list of the combining forms used in Unit I.

  · **Appendix D,** Prefixes, is a complete alphabetic list of the prefixes used in Unit I.

  · **Appendix E,** Suffixes, is a complete alphabetic list of the suffixes used in Unit I.

  · **Appendix F,** Abbreviations, is a complete list of the abbreviations referenced in Unit I.

  · **Appendix G,** Further Text Resources, is a list of texts that you may want to obtain to supplement your study plan.

DAY BEFORE THE EXAMINATION

- No cramming! Your study time is now over, and cramming the day before the test is not a good idea because it just increases your anxiety level. This day is your day to prepare yourself. Do some things you enjoy this day. Take your mind off the examination. Pamper yourself: you deserve it.

- Prepare pencils (no. 2), erasers, picture identification, CPT, ICD-9-CM (Vols. 1 and 2), HCPCS code books, and examination admission card. For a paper/pencil examination, take a ruler so that if you skip a question and want to mark that question to return to later, you can use the ruler to make certain you return to the correct question. Contact the AAPC to be certain that the examination is paper/pencil. There has been discussion that in the future the examination may be computer-based.

- You cannot have excessive writing, sticky notes, labels, etc. in your code books. Check the examination information to ensure that your books meet the specifications identified by the testing organization.

- Review the certification packet information one last time to ensure that you have all the required material.

- Listen to the weather and traffic reports. Plan your route to the examination site. If it is in a new location, drive to the location before the big day.

- Eat a light supper and get to bed early. Set the alarm in plenty of time to arrive at the site early. It is a good idea to have a friend or family member give you an early wake-up call to ensure that you do not oversleep.

DAY OF THE EXAMINATION

- Wear comfortable clothes and be prepared for any room temperature. A short-sleeved shirt with a sweater is a good plan. Dress in layers so you can ensure that you will be comfortable in any environment.

- Take a watch with you.

- Eat a good breakfast. Avoid caffeine because it initially stimulates you, but in the long run will decrease your concentration.

- Arrive early. The doors are locked to those who arrive late. This is a day to be early.

- Ensure that you have the correct room for your examination. Often there are several examinations being administered at one time, so be certain you are in the correct room for your examination.

THE CERTIFICATION EXAMINATION

You are ready for this! You have planned your work and have worked your plan. Now it is time to reap the rewards for all that hard work.

- Choose a good location in which to sit. Choose a location that will not get a lot of traffic from those leaving the room.

- Place all your supplies on the table.

- Take several deep breaths before you begin to help relax you.

- Some prefer to take the parts of the examination out of order, taking those questions they are most confident of first. Others prefer to start at the beginning and work through all questions in order. The approach that you use will depend on your individual test-taking style.

- When you come to a question for which you are unsure of the answer, you may wish to skip over and come back to all those ones you were unsure of at the end of the examination, depending on the time available. Or you may want to attempt each question and note those you are unsure of to return to when you have finished the exam section. Again, the approach you will use depends on your individual style.

- Read the directions. This may sound too simple, but many persons do not completely read the directions, only to find that the directions gave specific directions about what or what not to code on a certain case (for example, "code only this certain portion of the procedure"). Yet the choices for answers included the full coding of the case as a selection; if you did not read all the directions, you would choose the response with codes for all the items listed in the report. For example, the question may have directed you to code the service only, not the diagnosis, and yet one of the choices would be the correct service and diagnosis codes, which of course would be an incorrect answer based on the directions. So read all of the directions.

- Your speed and accuracy are being tested. You do not have time to labor over each question for a long time if you intend to complete all the questions. Read the directions, read the question, put down your best assessment of the answer, and then move on to the next question.

- Words such as *always, every, never,* and *all* generally indicate broad terms that, with true/false questions, usually indicate a false question.

- If you do not know the answer to the question, try eliminating those that you know are incorrect first and then select that answer that seems more likely to be correct.

- Judge the time as you are moving through the examination. Keep assessing whether you are making sufficient progress or whether you can slow down or need to speed up.

- Answer all questions. Even if you have to guess quickly, at least fill in an answer. The best situation is that you answer all questions and have time left over to go back over the questions about which you are in doubt.

- Be certain to carefully complete the information sheet that accompanies the examination. This sheet will include your name, address, and other information that ensures that your test results are accurately recorded.

- Use every minute of the test time, but it is not a good idea to begin second-guessing yourself. Do not return to those questions for which you did not have serious doubts about the correct answer. Usually, your first answer is the best.

- When the time is finished, hand in your examination, and pat yourself on the back! You have done an excellent job. Now it is time to go get a good supper and a good night's sleep.

DAYS AFTER THE EXAMINATION

- You will miss the preparation! Okay, maybe not miss it exactly, but your life will be different now without that constant preparation.

- Relax and await the results in confidence. You have done your best. That is always good enough!

- Be proud of yourself; this was no small undertaking, and you did it.

My personal best wishes to you as you prepare for your certification. You can do this!

Best regards
Carol J. Buck, MS, CPC, CPC-H, CCS-P

Our goals can only be reached through a vehicle of a plan, in which we must fervently believe, and upon which we must vigorously act. There is no other route to success.

Stephen A. Brennen

Course Syllabus and Student Calendar

The following documents are the syllabus and the course calendar that would be used in a classroom setting. It is suggested that these documents be used in development of your personal educational plan. Note that *The Extra Step: Physician-Based Coding Practice* is suggested for supplemental practice. This product can be purchased at www.elsevier-health.com or other textbook retailers.

COURSE SYLLABUS

Course Description

The focus of this class is a review of terminology, anatomy, pathophysiology, and reimbursement as a preparation to take the coding certification examination. A review of CPT, ICD-9-CM, and HCPCS coding will be an integral part of this review course. Two practice certification review examinations will be taken under timed conditions. The course assists the learner in establishing a personal plan for continued development in preparation for a certification examination.

Texts

CPC Coding Exam Review 2007: The Certification Step, by Carol J. Buck, Elsevier.

Saunders 2007 ICD-9-CM, Volumes 1 & 2, by Carol J. Buck, Elsevier.

Saunders 2007 HCPCS Level II, by Carol J. Buck, Elsevier.

2007 CPT, American Medical Association

Medical dictionary

Optional Text

The Extra Step: Physician-Based Coding Practice, by Carol J. Buck, Elsevier.

Performance Objectives

1. Write a personal plan for preparation for a certification examination.

2. Review the structure, function, terminology, pathophysiology, and abbreviations of the integumentary system.

3. Review the structure, function, terminology, pathophysiology, and abbreviations of the musculoskeletal system.

4. Review the structure, function, terminology, pathophysiology, and abbreviations of the respiratory system.

5. Review the structure, function, terminology, pathophysiology, and abbreviations of the cardiovascular system.

6. Review the structure, function, terminology, pathophysiology, and abbreviations of the female genital system and pregnancy.

7. Review the structure, function, terminology, pathophysiology, and abbreviations of the male genital system.

8. Review the structure, function, terminology, pathophysiology, and abbreviations of the urinary system.

9. Review the structure, function, terminology, pathophysiology, and abbreviations of the digestive system.

10. Review the structure, function, terminology, pathophysiology, and abbreviations of the mediastinum and diaphragm.

11. Review the structure, function, terminology, pathophysiology, and abbreviations of the hemic and lymphatic systems.

12. Review the structure, function, terminology, pathophysiology, and abbreviations of the endocrine system.

13. Review the structure, function, terminology, pathophysiology, and abbreviations of the nervous system.

14. Review the structure, function, terminology, pathophysiology, and abbreviations of the senses of the body.

15. Demonstrate knowledge of organ system structure, function, terminology, pathophysiology, and abbreviations.

16. Review medical reimbursement issues.

17. Demonstrate knowledge of medical reimbursement issues.

18. Review CPT E/M section.

19. Review CPT Anesthesia section.

20. Review CPT Surgery section.

21. Review CPT Radiology section.

22. Review CPT Pathology and Laboratory section.

23. Review CPT Medicine section.

24. Review HCPCS.

25. Review format and conventions of ICD-9-CM.

26. Review assignment of ICD-9-CM codes.

27. Review ICD-9-CM Official Guidelines for Coding and Reporting.

28. Demonstrate coding ability by assigning CPT codes.

29. Demonstrate coding ability by assigning HCPCS codes.

30. Demonstrate coding ability by assigning ICD-9-CM codes.

Personal Objectives

The student will:

- Attend class sessions.

- Prepare for class sessions.

- Complete assignments in a timely manner.

- Demonstrate a high level of responsibility.

- Display respect for other members of the class.

- Participate in class discussions.

Evaluation and Grading

- Evaluation is directly related to the performance objectives.

- Performance is measured by examination, assignments, and/or quizzes.

- The letter grade is based on the percentage of the total points earned throughout the semester based on the following scale:

  - A = 93% to 100%

  - B = 85% to 92%

  - C = 79% to 84%

  - D = 70% to 78%

  - F = 69% and below

- Examinations are scheduled in advance. To qualify for the total points on the examinations, the student must take the examination at the scheduled time. Five points will be deducted from each examination if the examination is not taken at the scheduled time. This rule reinforces the need for on-time performance. Any make-up examination must be completed within 3 days of the scheduled examination or no points will be awarded for the examination.

- Assignments are scheduled in advance. To qualify for the total points on the assignment, the student must submit the completed assignment at the scheduled time. Five points are deducted from each assignment if the assignment is not submitted at the scheduled time. This rule reinforces the need for on-time performance. Any late assignment must be completed within 3 days from the date the assignment was due or no points will be awarded for the assignment.

- Quizzes are scheduled in advance. Quizzes cannot be made up, and no points are awarded for missed quizzes.

Methods of Instruction

The instructional methods used include lecture, class discussion, and assignments.

COURSE CALENDAR

Lesson 1

Reading assignment(s):	Success Strategies, pages S1-S10
Assignment(s):	Complete the Pre-Examination located in the text, and at **Lesson 3** class period, hand in your answer sheet with your scores (NOT the examination, just the answer sheet with your scores calculated) on the two sections for 128 points. The Pre-Examination is NOT graded if each question has been attempted. 2 points will be deducted for each question not attempted.
Optional assignment(s):	Download certification examination information at http://www.aapc.com/
	Print one page to hand in at **Lesson 2** to demonstrate successful access to certification information from web (10 points—nongraded)
	The Extra Step: Physician-Based Coding Practice, Integumentary, Cases 1-4 (8 points)

Lesson 2

Student hand in:	One printed page to demonstrate successful access to certifying organization's information from web (10 points—nongraded)
	The Extra Step: Physician-Based Coding Practice, Integumentary, Cases 1-4 (8 points)
Reading assignment(s):	Unit 1, pages 1-54 (through Musculoskeletal System)
Assignment(s):	Develop a personal plan for preparation for Certification Review (20 points—graded) to be submitted at **Lesson 6** class period
	Integumentary Anatomy/Terminology (10 points) and Pathophysiology Quizzes (10 points)
	Musculoskeletal Anatomy/Terminology (10 points) and Pathophysiology Quizzes (10 points)
Optional assignment(s):	*The Extra Step: Physician-Based Coding Practice,* Orthopedics, Cases 1-4 (8 points)

Lesson 3

Student hand in:	Integumentary System Quizzes (20 points)
	Musculoskeletal Quizzes (20 points)
	Pre-Examination (128 points, nongraded if each question attempted, deduct 2 points for each question not attempted)
	The Extra Step: Physician-Based Coding Practice, Orthopedics, Cases 1-4 (8 points)
Reading assignment(s):	Unit 1, pages 55-116 (through Female Genital System and Pregnancy)
Optional assignment(s):	Respiratory Anatomy/Terminology (10 points) and Pathophysiology Quizzes (10 points)
	Cardiovascular Anatomy/Terminology (10 points) and Pathophysiology Quizzes (10 points)

Female Genital System and Pregnancy Anatomy/Terminology (10 points) and Pathophysiology Quizzes (10 points)

The Extra Step: Physician-Based Coding Practice,
Emergency Medicine, Cases 11-12 (4 points)
Cardiology, Cases 1-6 (12 points)
Obstetrics and Gynecology, Cases 1-4 (8 points)
Pediatrics, Neonatology, and Adolescent Medicine, Cases 1-4 (8 points)

Lesson 4

Student hand in:

Respiratory Quizzes (20 points)
Cardiovascular Quizzes (20 points)
Female Genital System and Pregnancy Quizzes (20 points)
The Extra Step: Physician-Based Coding Practice,
Emergency Medicine, Cases 11-12 (4 points)
Cardiology, Cases 1-6 (12 points)
Obstetrics and Gynecology, Cases 1-4 (8 points)
Pediatrics, Neonatology, and Adolescent Medicine, Cases 1-4 (8 points)

Reading assignment(s):

Unit 1, pages 117-184 (through Mediastinum and Diaphragm)

Optional assignment(s):

Male Genital System Anatomy/Terminology (10 points) and Pathophysiology Quizzes (10 points)
Urinary System Anatomy/Terminology (10 points) and Pathophysiology Quizzes (10 points)
Digestive System Anatomy/Terminology (10 points) and Pathophysiology Quizzes (10 points)
Mediastinum and Diaphragm Quiz (10 points) (There is NO pathophysiology quiz for Mediastinum and Diaphragm.)
The Extra Step: Physician-Based Coding Practice, Urology, Cases 1-4 (8 points)
Gastroenterology, Cases 1-4 (8 points)
Nephrology, Cases 1-4 (8 points)
Pediatrics, Neonatology, and Adolescent Medicine, Cases 5-9 (10 points)

Lesson 5

Student hand in:

Male Genital System Quizzes (20 points)
Urinary System Quizzes (20 points)
Digestive System Quizzes (20 points)
Mediastinum and Diaphragm Quiz (10 points)
(There is no pathophysiology quiz for Mediastinum and Diaphragm.)
The Extra Step: Physician-Based Coding Practice, Urology, Cases 1-4 (8 points)
Gastroenterology, Cases 1-4 (8 points)
Nephrology, Cases 1-4 (8 points)
Pediatrics, Neonatology, and Adolescent Medicine, Cases 5-9 (10 points)

Reading assignment(s):   Unit 1, pages 185-212 (through Endocrine System)

Optional assignment(s):   Hemic and Lymphatic Anatomy/Terminology (10 points) and Pathophysiology Quizzes (10 points)
Endocrine Anatomy/Terminology (10 points) and Pathophysiology Quizzes (10 points)
Prepare to submit Personal Plan for Preparation for Certification Examination (20 points—graded)
The Extra Step: Physician-Based Coding Practice, Nephrology, Cases 5-8 (8 points)

Lesson 6

Student hand in: Hemic and Lymphatic Quizzes (20 points)
Endocrine Quizzes (20 points)
Submit Personal Plan for Preparation for Certification Examination
The Extra Step: Physician-Based Coding Practice, Nephrology, Cases 5-8 (8 points)

Reading assignment(s):   Unit 1, pages 213-260 (through end of Unit 1)

Optional assignment(s):   Nervous System Anatomy/Terminology (10 points) and Pathophysiology Quizzes (10 points)
Senses Anatomy/Terminology (10 points) and Pathophysiology Quizzes (10 points)
Prepare for Unit 1, Anatomy, Terminology, and Pathophysiology, Test 1 (50 points, 25 questions, 15 minutes)
The Extra Step: Physician-Based Coding Practice, Neurology and Ophthalmology, Cases 1-4 (8 points)

Lesson 7

UNIT 1: ANATOMY, TERMINOLOGY, AND PATHOPHYSIOLOGY, TEST 1
Timed Test: 15 Minutes

Student hand in: Nervous System Quizzes (20 points)
Senses Quizzes (20 points)
The Extra Step: Physician-Based Coding Practice, Neurology and Ophthalmology, Cases 1-4 (8 points)

Reading assignment(s):   Unit 2, pages 261-276 (through end of Unit 2)

Optional assignment(s):   None

Lesson 8

Student hand in: Reimbursement Quiz (10 points)

Reading assignment(s):   Unit 3, pages 277-284 (up to E/M section)

Optional assignment(s):   Prepare for Reimbursement, Test 2 (20 points, 10 questions, 10 minutes)

Lesson 9

UNIT 2: REIMBURSEMENT, TEST 2
Timed Test: 10 Minutes

Student hand in: None

Reading assignment(s):	Unit 3, pages 285-293 (up to Contributing Factors) Read E/M Guidelines
Optional assignment(s):	*The Extra Step: Physician-Based Coding Practice,* Evaluation and Management, Cases 1-8 (16 points) Emergency Medicine, Cases 1-6 (12 points)

Lesson 10

Student hand in:	*The Extra Step: Physician-Based Coding Practice,* Evaluation and Management, Cases 1-8 (16 points) Emergency Medicine, Cases 1-6 (12 points)
Reading assignment(s):	Unit 3, pages 294-301 (up to Anesthesia section)
Optional assignment(s):	*The Extra Step: Physician-Based Coding Practice,* Evaluation and Management, Cases 9-19 (22 points) Emergency Medicine, Cases 7-10 (8 points)

Lesson 11

Student hand in:	*The Extra Step: Physician-Based Coding Practice,* Evaluation and Management, Cases 9-19 (22 points) Emergency Medicine, Cases 7-10 (8 points)
Reading assignment(s):	Unit 3, pages 301-303 (up to CPT/HCPCS Level I Modifiers) Read Anesthesia Guidelines
Optional assignment(s):	Prepare for E/M, Test 3 (25 points, 5 Guidelines questions [10 points] and 3 cases [15 points], 15 minutes) *The Extra Step: Physician-Based Coding Practice,* Anesthesiology, Cases 1-6 (12 points)

Lesson 12

E/M, TEST 3
Timed Test: 15 Minutes

Student hand in:	*The Extra Step: Physician-Based Coding Practice,* Anesthesiology, Cases 1-16 (12 points)
Reading assignment(s):	Unit 3, pages 303-310 (up to Surgery section)
Optional assignment(s):	Prepare for Anesthesia, Test 4 (20 points, 5 Guidelines questions [10 points], 2 cases [10 points], 15 minutes) *The Extra Step: Physician-Based Coding Practice,* Anesthesiology, Cases 7-11 (10 points)

Lesson 13

ANESTHESIA, TEST 4
Timed Test: 15 Minutes

Student hand in:	*The Extra Step: Physician-Based Coding Practice,* Anesthesiology, Cases 7-11 (10 points)
Reading assignment(s):	Unit 3, pages 310-312 (up to Integumentary System Subsection) Read Surgery Guidelines
Optional assignment(s):	None

Lesson 14

Student hand in: None

Reading assignment(s):   Unit 3, pages 312-321 (up to Musculoskeletal System
                            Subsection)

Optional assignment(s):   *The Extra Step: Physician-Based Coding Practice*,
                            Integumentary, Cases 5-9 (10 points)

Lesson 15

Student hand in: *The Extra Step: Physician-Based Coding Practice*,
                            Integumentary, Cases 5-9 (10 points)

Reading assignment(s):   Unit 3, pages 321-326 (up to Respiratory System
                            Subsection)

Optional assignment(s):   *The Extra Step: Physician-Based Coding Practice*,
                            Orthopedics, Cases 5-13 (18 points)

Lesson 16

Student hand in: *The Extra Step: Physician-Based Coding Practice*,
                            Orthopedics, Cases 5-13 (18 points)

Reading assignment(s):   Unit 3, pages 326-330 (up to Cardiovascular [CV]
                            System Subsection)

Optional assignment(s):   *The Extra Step: Physician-Based Coding Practice*,
                            Cardiology, Case 7 (Respiratory case) (2 points)
                            Otorhinolaryngology, Cases 2, 8, 11, and 12 (8 points)

Lesson 17

Student hand in: *The Extra Step: Physician-Based Coding Practice*,
                            Cardiology, Case 7 (Respiratory case) (2 points)
                            Otorhinolaryngology, Cases 2, 8, 11, and 12 (8 points)

Reading assignment(s):   Unit 3, pages 330-335 (up to Venous Reconstruction—
                            CV Repairs)

Optional assignment(s):   *The Extra Step: Physician-Based Coding Practice*,
                            Cardiology, Cases 8-10 (Cardiology cases) (6 points)

Lesson 18

Student hand in: *The Extra Step: Physician-Based Coding Practice*,
                            Cardiology, Cases 8-10 (Cardiology cases) (6 points)

Reading assignment(s):   Unit 3, pages 335-341 (up to Hemic and Lymphatic
                            System Subsection)

Optional assignment(s):   None

Lesson 19

Student hand in: None

Reading assignment(s):   Unit 3, pages 341-346 (up to Female Genital System
                            Subsection)

Optional assignment(s):   *The Extra Step: Physician-Based Coding Practice,*
                           Gastroenterology, Cases 5-8 (8 points)
                           Urology, Cases 5-10 (12 points)

Lesson 20

Student hand in: *The Extra Step: Physician-Based Coding Practice,*
                    Gastroenterology, Cases 5-8 (8 points)
                    Urology, Cases 5-10 (12 points)

Reading assignment(s):   Unit 3, pages 346-356 (through Auditory System
                          Subsection)

Optional assignment(s):   *The Extra Step: Physician-Based Coding Practice,*
                           Obstetrics and Gynecology, Cases 5-10 (12 points)
                           General Surgery, Cases 1-10 (20 points)

Lesson 21

Student hand in: *The Extra Step: Physician-Based Coding Practice,*
                    Obstetrics and Gynecology, Cases 5-10 (12 points)
                    General Surgery, Cases 1-10 (20 points)

Reading assignment(s):   None

Optional assignment(s):   *The Extra Step: Physician-Based Coding Practice,*
                           Neurology and Ophthalmology, Cases 5-11
                           (14 points)
                           Otorhinolaryngology, Cases 1, 3-7, 9, and 10 (16
                           points)
                           Diagnostic Radiology, Cases 1-10 (20 points)

Lesson 22

Student hand in: *The Extra Step: Physician-Based Coding Practice,*
                    Neurology and Ophthalmology, Cases 5-11
                    (14 points)
                    Otorhinolaryngology, Cases 1, 3-7, 9, and 10 (16
                    points)
                    Diagnostic Radiology, Cases 1-10 (20 points)

Reading assignment(s):   Unit 3, pages 356-363 (up to Nuclear Medicine
                          Subsection)

Optional assignment(s):   Prepare for Surgery, Test 5 (30 points, 9 questions,
                           5 Guidelines questions [10 points], 4 cases
                           [20 points], 20 minutes)
                           The Extra Step: Physician-Based Coding Practice,
                           Interventional Radiology and Radiation Oncology,
                           Cases 1-7 (14 points)

Lesson 23

SURGERY, TEST 5
Timed Test: 20 Minutes

Student hand in: *The Extra Step: Physician-Based Coding Practice,*
                    Interventional Radiology and Radiation Oncology,
                    Cases 1-7 (14 points)

Reading assignment(s):   Unit 3, pages 363-368 (up to Medicine Section)

Optional assignment(s):   Prepare for Radiology, Test 6 (22 points, 5 Guidelines questions, 1 non-Guidelines question [12 points], 2 cases [10 points], 15 minutes)
The Extra Step: Physician-Based Coding Practice, Interventional Radiology and Radiation Oncology, Cases 8-14 (14 points)

Lesson 24

RADIOLOGY, TEST 6
Timed Test: 15 Minutes

Student hand in: *The Extra Step: Physician-Based Coding Practice,* Interventional Radiology and Radiation Oncology, Cases 8-14 (14 points)

Reading assignment(s):   Unit 3, pages 368-374 (up to Ophthalmology)

Optional assignment(s):   Prepare for Pathology and Laboratory, Test 7 (47 points, 5 Guidelines questions, 1 non-Guidelines question [12 points], 7 cases [35 points], 20 minutes)
The Extra Step: Physician-Based Coding Practice, Pathology, Cases 1-10 (20 points)

Lesson 25

PATHOLOGY AND LABORATORY, TEST 7
Timed Test: 20 Minutes

Student hand in: *The Extra Step: Physician-Based Coding Practice,* Pathology, Cases 1-10 (20 points)

Reading assignment(s):   Unit 3, pages 374-379 (up to HCPCS Coding)

Optional assignment(s):   *The Extra Step: Physician-Based Coding Practice,* Medicine, Cases 1-5 (10 points)

Lesson 26

Student hand in: *The Extra Step: Physician-Based Coding Practice,* Medicine, Cases 1-5 (10 points)

Reading assignment(s):   Unit 3, pages 379-387 (up to Using the ICD-9-CM)

Optional assignment(s):   Prepare for Medicine/HCPCS, Test 8 (41 points, 5 Guidelines questions, 3 non-Guidelines questions [16 points], 5 cases [25 points], 10 minutes)
The Extra Step: Physician-Based Coding Practice, Medicine, Cases 6-10 (10 points)

Lesson 27

MEDICINE/HCPCS, TEST 8
Timed Test: 10 Minutes

Student hand in: *The Extra Step: Physician-Based Coding Practice,* Medicine, Cases 6-10 (10 points)

Reading assignment(s):   Unit 3, pages 387-388 (up to Selection of Primary Diagnosis)

Optional assignment(s):   None

Lesson 28

Student hand in: None

Reading assignment(s):   Unit 3, pages 388-399 (up to Chapter 8, Diseases of Respiratory System)

Optional assignment(s):   Post-Examination (to hand in results at Lesson 30 class period)

Lesson 29

Student hand in: None

Reading assignment(s):   Unit 3, pages 399-406 (through end of Unit 3)

Optional assignment(s):   None

Lesson 30

Student hand in: Post-Examination results (129 points, nongraded if each question attempted, deduct 2 points for each question not attempted; hand in printed copy of summary of your score)

Reading assignment(s):   None

Optional assignment(s):   Prepare for ICD-9-CM, Test 9 (25 points, 5 cases, 20 minutes)
Bring ICD-9-CM, CPT, and HCPCS to class to begin Final Examination

Lesson 31

ICD-9-CM, TEST 9
Timed Test: 20 Minutes

Final Examination beginning

Student hand in: None

Reading assignment(s):   None

Optional assignment(s):   Complete Final Examination

Lesson 32

Final grade calculation
Course evaluation

Anatomy, Terminology, and Pathophysiology

■ INTEGUMENTARY SYSTEM

INTEGUMENTARY SYSTEM—ANATOMY AND TERMINOLOGY

The skin and accessory organs (nails, hair, and glands)

Layers (Figure 1-1)

Epidermis. Outermost layer

Basal layer, deepest region of epidermis (stratum germinativum)

Stratum corneum is the outermost layer of epidermis

Dermis. Middle layer, also known as corium, meaning true skin

Two layers of stratum

Subcutaneous Tissue or Hypodermis. Innermost layer contains fat tissue

Nails

Keratin plates covering the dorsal surface of each finger and toe

Lunula—semilunar or half-moon: white area at base of nail plate

Cuticle: narrow band of epidermis at base and sides of nail

Paronychium: soft tissue around nail border

Glands

Sebaceous glands located in dermal layer

Secrete sebum, which lubricates skin and hair

Sweat glands (sudoriferous) originate in dermis (subcutaneous tissue, see Figure 1-1) and extend up through epidermis

Openings are pores

COMBINING FORMS

1.	aden/o	in relationship to a gland
2.	adip/o	fat
3.	albin/o	white
4.	aut/o	self
5.	bi/o	life
6.	cauter/o	burn
7.	crypt/o	hidden
8.	cutane/o	skin
9.	cyan/o	blue
10.	derm/o, dermat/o	skin
11.	eosin/o	rosy
12.	erythem/o	red

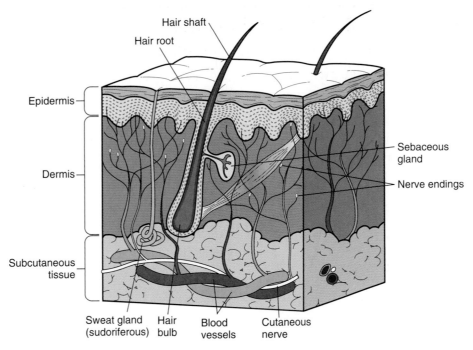

Figure **1-1** Integumentary system.

13.	erythr/o	red
14.	heter/o	different
15.	hidr/o	sweat
16.	ichthy/o	dry/scaly
17.	jaund/o	yellow
18.	kerat/o	hard
19.	lip/o	fat
20.	lute/o	yellow
21.	melan/o	black
22.	myc/o	fungus
23.	necr/o	death
24.	onych/o	nail
25.	pachy/o	thick
26.	pil/o	hair
27.	poli/o	gray matter
28.	rhytid/o	wrinkle
29.	rube/o	red
30.	seb/o	sebum/oil
31.	staphyl/o	clusters
32.	steat/o	fat
33.	strept/o	twisted chain

34.	trich/o	hair
35.	ungu/o	nail
36.	xanth/o	yellow
37.	xer/o	dry

PREFIXES

1.	epi-	on/upon
2.	hyper-	over
3.	hypo-	under
4.	intra-	within
5.	para-	beside
6.	per-	through
7.	peri-	surrounding
8.	sub-	under

SUFFIXES

1.	-coccus	spherical bacterium
2.	-ectomy	removal
3.	-ia	condition
4.	-malacia	softening
5.	-opsy	view of
6.	-plasty	surgical repair
7.	-rrhea	discharge
8.	-tome	an instrument to cut
9.	-tomy	to cut

MEDICAL ABBREVIATIONS

1.	bx	biopsy
2.	ca	cancer
3.	derm	dermatology
4.	I&D	incision and drainage
5.	subcu, subq, SC, SQ	subcutaneous

MEDICAL TERMS

Absence	Without
Adipose	Fatty
Albinism	Lack of color pigment
Allograft	Homograft, same species graft

Alopecia	Condition in which hair falls out
Anhidrosis	Deficiency of sweat
Autograft	From patient's own body
Avulsion	Ripping or tearing away of part either surgically or accidentally
Biopsy	Removal of a small piece of living tissue for diagnostic purposes
Causalgia	Burning pain
Collagen	Protein substance of skin
Debridement	Cleansing of or removal of dead tissue from a wound
Delayed flap	Pedicle of skin with blood supply that is separated from origin over time
Dermabrasion	Planing of the skin by means of sander, brush, or sandpaper
Dermatologist	Physician who treats conditions of the skin
Dermatoplasty	Surgical repair of skin
Electrocautery	Cauterization by means of heated instrument
Epidermolysis	Loosening of the epidermis
Epidermomycosis	Superficial fungal infection
Epithelium	Surface covering of internal and external organs of the body
Erythema	Redness of skin
Escharotomy	Surgical incision into necrotic (dead) tissue
Fissure	Cleft or groove
Free full-thickness graft	Graft of epidermis and dermis that is completely removed from donor area
Furuncle	Nodule in the skin caused by *Staphylococci* entering through hair follicle
Hematoma	A localized collection of blood, usually the result of a break in a blood vessel
Hemograft	Allograft, same species graft
Ichthyosis	Skin disorder characterized by scaling
Incise	To cut into
Island pedicle flap	Contains a single artery and vein that remains attached to origin temporarily or permanently
Leukoderma	Depigmentation of skin
Leukoplakia	White patch on mucous membrane
Lipocyte	Fat cell
Lipoma	Fatty tumor
Melanin	Dark pigment of skin
Melanoma	Tumor of epidermis, malignant and black in color
Mohs' surgery or Mohs' micrographic surgery	Removal of skin cancer in layers by a surgeon who also acts as a pathologist during surgery
Muscle flap	Transfer of muscle from origin to recipient site
Neurovascular flap	Contains artery, vein, and nerve

Pedicle	Growth attached with a stem
Pilosebaceous	Pertains to hair follicles and sebaceous glands
Sebaceous gland	Secretes sebum
Seborrhea	Excess sebum secretion
Sebum	Oily substance
Split-thickness graft	All epidermis and some of dermis
Steatoma	Fat mass in sebaceous gland
Stratified	Layered
Stratum (strata)	Layer
Subungual	Beneath the nail
Xanthoma	Tumor composed of cells containing lipid material, yellow in color
Xenograft	Different species graft
Xeroderma	Dry, discolored, scaly skin

INTEGUMENTARY SYSTEM ANATOMY AND TERMINOLOGY QUIZ

1. This is the outermost layer of the skin:
   a. basal
   b. dermis
   c. epidermis
   d. subcutaneous

2. Which of the following is NOT a part of the skin or accessory organs:
   a. hair
   b. sebaceous gland
   c. nail
   d. haversian

3. This prefix means beside:
   a. para-
   b. intra-
   c. per-
   d. epi-

4. This combining form means hair:
   a. xanth/o
   b. trich/o
   c. ichthy/o
   d. kerat/o

5. The lunula is the:
   a. narrow band of epidermis at the base of the nail
   b. opening of the pores
   c. outermost layer of epidermis
   d. white area at the base of the nail plate

6. The subcutaneous tissue is also known as:
   a. dermal
   b. adipose
   c. hypodermis
   d. stratum corneum

7. Which of the following combining forms does not refer to a color?
   a. cyan/o
   b. jaund/o
   c. eosin/o
   d. pachy/o

8. This medical term means the surgical incision into dead tissue:
   a. onychomycosis
   b. escharotomy
   c. keratotomy
   d. curettage

9. This suffix means surgical repair:
   a. -opsy
   b. -rrhea
   c. -plasty
   d. -tome

10. The soft tissue around the nail border is the:
    a. cuticle
    b. lunula
    c. paronychium
    d. corium

INTEGUMENTARY SYSTEM—PATHOPHYSIOLOGY

Lesions and Other Abnormalities (Figure 1-2)

Macule
Flat area of color change

No elevation or depression

> ***Example:*** flat moles (nevi), measles, freckles

Papule
Solid elevation

Less than 0.5 cm in diameter

> ***Example:*** warts, lichen planus, elevated mole

Nodule
Solid elevation 0.5 to 1 cm in diameter

Extends deeper into dermis than papule

> ***Example:*** lipoma

Pustule
Elevated area

Filled with purulent fluid

> ***Example:*** pimple

Tumor
Solid mass

Larger than 1 cm

> ***Example:*** hemangioma, neoplasm

Plaque
Flat, elevated surface

Equal or greater than 1.0 cm

> ***Example:*** psoriasis, seborrheic keratosis

Wheal
Temporary localized elevation of the skin

Results in transient edema in dermis

> ***Example:*** insect bite, allergic reaction

Vesicle
Small blister

Fluid within or under epidermis

> ***Example:*** herpes zoster (shingles), varicella (chickenpox)

Bulla
Large blister

Greater than 0.5 cm

> ***Example:*** blister

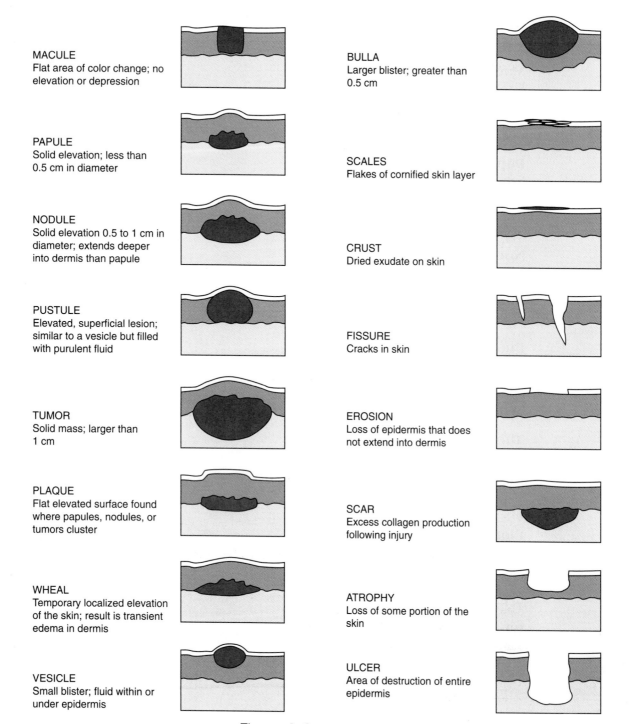

MACULE
Flat area of color change; no elevation or depression

PAPULE
Solid elevation; less than 0.5 cm in diameter

NODULE
Solid elevation 0.5 to 1 cm in diameter; extends deeper into dermis than papule

PUSTULE
Elevated, superficial lesion; similar to a vesicle but filled with purulent fluid

TUMOR
Solid mass; larger than 1 cm

PLAQUE
Flat elevated surface found where papules, nodules, or tumors cluster

WHEAL
Temporary localized elevation of the skin; result is transient edema in dermis

VESICLE
Small blister; fluid within or under epidermis

BULLA
Larger blister; greater than 0.5 cm

SCALES
Flakes of cornified skin layer

CRUST
Dried exudate on skin

FISSURE
Cracks in skin

EROSION
Loss of epidermis that does not extend into dermis

SCAR
Excess collagen production following injury

ATROPHY
Loss of some portion of the skin

ULCER
Area of destruction of entire epidermis

Figure **1-2** Lesions of the skin.

Scales
Flakes of cornified skin layer

> *Example:* dry skin

Crust
Dried exudate on skin

> *Example:* scab

Fissure
Cracks in skin

> *Example:* athlete's foot

Erosion
Loss of epidermis

Does not extend into the dermis

> *Example:* blisters

Scar
Excess collagen production following surgery or trauma

> *Example:* healed surgical wound

Atrophy
Loss of some portion of skin

> *Example:* aged skin

- Not a lesion, but a physiologic response in aging process

Ulcer
Area of destruction of entire epidermis

> *Example:* missing tissue on heel, decubitus bedsore (pressure sore)

Pressure Ulcer (Decubitis Ulcer) (Figure 1-3)
Result of pressure or force
Occludes blood flow, causing ischemia

Develops over bony prominence

Locations
Coccygeal (end of spine)

Sacral (between hips)

Heel

Elbow

Ischial (lower hip)

Trochanteric (outer hip)

Staging or classification system
Stage I: erythema of skin

Stage II: partial loss of skin (epidermis or dermis)

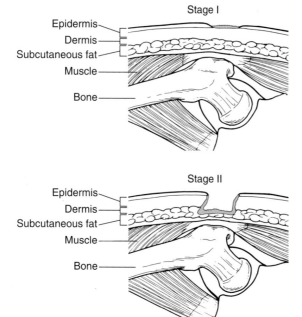

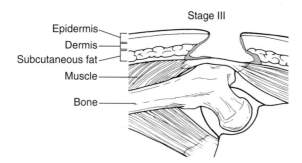

Figure **1-3** Stage I, II, III, and IV of pressure ulcers.

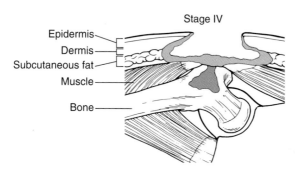

Stage III: full thickness loss of skin (up to but not through fascia)

Stage IV: full thickness loss (extensive destruction and necrosis)

• Deep ulcers may require surgical debridement

Keloids

Sharply elevated, irregularly shaped scars that progressively enlarge

Due to excessive collagen in corneum

Result of tissue repair or trauma

Familial tendency for formation

Inflammatory Disorders

Atopic Dermatitis
Unknown etiology

Exogenous (external causes) include
Irritant dermatitis

Allergic contact dermatitis

Endogenous (internal cause) includes
Seborrheic dermatitis

Results in activation of
Mast cells

Eosinophils

T lymphocytes

Monocytes

Greater in those with family history of
Asthma

Dry skin

Eczema

Allergic rhinitis

Common in
Children

Infants

Results in
Chronic inflammation

Scratching

Erythema

Thickened leathery skin (lichenification)

Secondary *Staphylococcus aureus* infection

Treatment
Topical steroid

Antibiotic for secondary infection

Antihistamines

Allergic Contact Dermatitis
Most common in infants and children

Hypersensitivity to sensitizing antigens
Microorganisms

Drugs

Foreign proteins

Chemicals

Latex

Metals

Plants

Manifestations
Scaling

Lichenification (leathery, thickened skin)

Erythema

Itching (pruritus)

Vesicular lesions

Edema

Diagnosis and treatment
Check medical history

Patch test

Avoidance of irritant

Skin lubrication and hydration

Steroids

- Topical

- Systemic

Topical tacrolimus (immunosuppressive agent)

Irritant Contact Dermatitis
Response to
Chemical

Exposure to irritant

Treatment
Removal of irritant

Topical agents

Stasis Dermatitis
Usually on the legs

Associated with
Phlebitis

Vascular trauma

Varicosities

Progress
Begins with erythema and pruritus

Progresses to scaling, hyperpigmentation, petechia (small hemorrhagic areas)

Lesion becomes ulcerated

Treatment

Elevate legs

Reduce standing

No constricting clothes

External compression

Antibiotics for acute lesions

Silver nitrate or Burow's solution for chronic lesions

Seborrheic Dermatitis

Common chronic inflammation of the sebaceous glands

Periods of remission and exacerbation

Commonly occurs on

Scalp (cradle cap in infants)

Ears

Eyelids

Eyebrow

Nose

Axillae

Chest

Groin

Lesions are

Scaly (dry or greasy)

White or yellowish

Mildly pruritic

Treatment

Mild cases

- Soap/shampoo of
  - Coal tar
  - Sulfur
  - Salicylic acid

More severe cases

- Corticosteroid

Papulosquamous Disorders

Conditions associated with

Scales

Papules

Plaque

Erythema

Three types

Psoriasis

Pityriasis

Lichen planus

Psoriasis

Chronic, relapsing, proliferating disorder

Usually begins by age 20

Cause unknown, suggested to be

Genetic

Immunologic

Biochemical alterations

Triggering agent

Commonly occurs on

Face

Scalp

Elbows

Knees

Results in

Thickened dermis and epidermis

Well-demarcated plaque

Cell hyperproliferation

Inflammation (pruritus)

Treatment

Only palliative (treatment of symptoms)

Mild cases

• Keratolytic agents

• Corticosteroids

• Emollients

Moderate cases

• Interleukin-2 inhibitors

• Ultraviolet light

• Coal tar

• Cyclosporin

• Vitamin D analogs

Severe cases

• Topical agents

• Corticosteroids

- Antimetabolic

- Hospitalization

Pityriasis Rosea (*P. rosea*)
Unknown cause

Self-limiting inflammatory disorder

Type of pityriasis

Occurs most often in young adults

Primary lesions
Begin with herald patch

3 to 4 cm

Salmon-pink colored

Circular

Well-defined lesions

Secondary lesions
14 to 21 days

Trunk and upper extremities

Oval lesions

Severe itching

Diagnosis
May be confused with

- Secondary syphilis

- Seborrheic dermatitis

- Psoriasis

Treatment
Antipruritics

Antihistamines

Corticosteroids

Ultraviolet light

Sunlight

Lichen Planus
Occurs on skin and mucous membranes

Unknown cause (idiopathic)

Autoimmune inflammatory disorder

Onset ages 30 to 70

Lesions
Begin as pink lesions that turn into violet-colored pruritic papules

Results in hyperpigmentation

2- to 10-mm flat lesions with central depression

Last 12 to 18 months

Tend to reoccur

Treatment
Antihistamines

Corticosteroids

- Topical

- Systemic

Acne Vulgaris
Site of lesion is sebaceous (pilosebaceous) follicles

Primarily on face and upper trunk

Usually occur in patients between the ages of 12 and 25

Types
Noninflammatory acne

- Whiteheads

- Blackheads

Inflammatory acne

- Follicle walls rupture

- Sebum expels into dermis

- Inflammation begins

Cause
Unknown

Treatment
Topical

- Antibiotics

- Benzoyl peroxide

- Tretinoin

Systemic

- Antibiotic

- Hormones

- Corticosteroids

- Isotretinoin

Diaper Dermatitis
Variety of disorders

Causes
Urine

Feces

Plastic diaper cover

Allergic reaction

Secondary *Candida albicans* infection

Treatment
Clean, dry area

Expose to air

Topical antifungal medications

Topical steroids

Pruritus (Itching)

Symptom of skin disorder

Can be localized or generalized

Causes
Primary skin disorder

> ***Example:*** eczema or lice

Systemic disease

> ***Example:*** chronic renal failure

Opiates

Treatment is for underlying condition
Antihistamines

Minor tranquilizers

Application of emollients (lotions)

Topical steroids

Skin Infections

■ Bacterial
Impetigo

Most common in infants and children

Usually on face and begins as small vesicles

Caused primarily by *Staphylococcus*

• Sometimes by group A beta-hemolytic *Streptococcus*

Treatment in mild cases
Topical antibiotics

Topical antiseptics

Treatment in moderate cases
Systemic antibiotics

Local compresses

Analgesics

Cellulitis
Caused primarily by *Staphylococcus*

Often secondary to an injury

Results in
Erythema, usually of lower trunk and legs

Fever

Localized pain

Lymphangitis

Treatment
Systemic antibiotics

Burow's soaks for pain relief

Furuncles (Boils)
Infected hair follicle

Usually caused by *Staphylococcus*

Developed boil drains pus and necrotic tissue

Squeezing spreads infection

Collection of furuncles that have merged is a carbuncle

Folliculitis
Infection of hair follicles

Results in
Erythema

Pustules

Causes
Skin trauma, such as irritation or friction

Poor hygiene

Excessive skin moisture

Treatment
Cleansing of area

Topical antibiotics

Erysipelas
Infection of skin

Cause
Group A beta-hemolytic *Streptococci*

Prior to outbreak, presents with

- Fever
- Malaise
- Chills

Lesions appear as
Red, firm spots

- Develops raised borders

- Itching

- Burning

- Tenderness

Acute Necrotizing Fasciitis

Flesh-eating disease
Virulent strain of gram-positive, group A beta-hemolytic *Streptococcus*

Mortality rate of over 40%

Causes
Skin trauma

Skin infection

Areas secrete tissue-destroying enzyme, proteases
Extreme inflammation and pain

Rapidly increasing

Dermal gangrene develops

Systemic toxicity may develop with
Fever

Disorientation

Hypotension

Tachycardia (fast heart rate)

May lead to organ failure

Treatment
Antimicrobial therapy

Fluid replacement

Removal of areas of infection

■ Viral
Herpes Simplex (Cold Sores)

Causes
Herpes simplex virus type 1 (HSV-1)

- Most common type

- Results in fever blisters or cold sores on or near lips

Herpes simplex virus type 2 (HSV-2)

- Genital and oral type

- Prominent sexually transmitted disease

Primary infections may show no symptoms (asymptomatic)

Virus remains in nerve tissue to later reactivate

Reactivation may be triggered by
Stress

Common cold

Exposure to sun

Presents with
Burning or tingling

Develops painful vesicles that rupture
Causes spreading

May cause secondary infection of the eye

- Episode lasts several weeks

- Treatment may include antiviral medication

  • No permanent cure exists

Herpes Zoster (Shingles)
Usually older adult

Caused by varicella-zoster virus (VZV)
Virus was dormant and then reactivates

Result of varicella or chickenpox, usually in childhood

Affects
One cranial nerve or one dermatome (an area of skin served by one nerve or one side of the body)

Results in
Pain

Rash (unilateral)

Paresthesia (abnormal touch sensation, such as burning)

Course
Several weeks

Pain may continue even after lesion disappears

Treatment
Clears spontaneously

Antiviral medications provide symptomatic relief

Sedatives

Analgesic

Antipruritics

Warts (Verrucae)
Caused by human papillomavirus (HPV)

- Numerous types of HPV

Spread by contact

Appear anywhere on body

Present with a grayish appearance

Variety of shapes and sizes

Plantar warts are located on pressure points of the body (such as feet; *plantar* means the bottom surface of the foot)

Painful when pressure is applied

Treatment
Liquid nitrogen

Topical keratolytics

Laser

Often persist even with treatment

Fungal (Mycoses)
Usually superficial

Fungus lives off dead cells

Tinea
Superficial skin infections

Tinea capitis

- Infection of scalp

- Common in children

- Treatment with oral antifungal medication

Tinea corporis (ringworm)

- Infection of the body

- Presents as a red ring

- Produces burning sensation and pruritus

- Treatment with topical antifungal medication

Tinea pedis (athlete's foot)

- Involves feet and toes

- Produces pain, inflammation, fissures, and foul odor

- Treatment with topical antifungal medication

Tinea unguium (onychomycosis)

- Nail infection

  - Usually toenails

- Nail turns white then brown, thickens and cracks

- Spreads to other nails

Candidiasis
Caused by *Candida albicans*

Normally on mucous membranes of the gastrointestinal tract and vagina

Poor health and certain conditions predispose individuals to overarching infection by candidiasis

• Such as antibiotic therapy, which changes the balance of the normal flora in the body

Treatment is topical or oral antifungal medications

Tumors of the Skin

■ Benign Tumors
Keratosis(es)
Seborrheic keratosis
Proliferation of basal cells

Dark colored lesion

Found on trunk and face

Actinic keratosis
Pigmented, scaly patch

Often caused by exposure to sun

Often in fair-skinned individuals

Pre-malignant lesion

May develop into squamous cell carcinoma

Treatment with cryosurgery (freezing area) or excision

Keratoacanthoma
Occurs in hair follicles

Usually in those over 60

Often of face, neck, back of hands, and other locations exposed to the sun

Resolve spontaneously or are excised

Moles (Nevi)
Located on any body part

Various shapes and sizes

May become malignant

• Especially if located in area of continual irritation

■ Malignant Tumors
Squamous Cell Carcinoma
Similar to basal cell carcinoma

Most often appears in areas exposed to the sun

Scaly appearance

Rarely metastatic (spreading)

Easily treated with good prognosis

Basal Cell Carcinoma
Common type of skin cancer

Developed in deeper skin layers (basal cells) than squamous cell carcinoma

Often occurs with sun exposure in fair-skinned individuals

Shiny appearance

Easily treated with good prognosis

Malignant Melanoma
Originates in cells that produce pigment (melanocytes) or a mole

Increased incidence with
Sun exposure

Genetic predisposition

Often multicolored with irregular borders

Grow downward into tissues

• Metastasize quickly

Treatment is removal with extensive border excision

• Depending on extent, chemotherapy or radiation therapy may be used

Kaposi's Sarcoma
Rare form of skin cancer

Associated with
Human immunodeficiency virus (HIV)

Acquired immunodeficiency syndrome (AIDS)

Herpes virus may be found in lesions

Cells originate from the endothelium in small blood vessels

Painful lesions develop rapidly, appearing as purple macules

Radiation and chemotherapy are common treatments

INTEGUMENTARY SYSTEM PATHOPHYSIOLOGY QUIZ

1. A pimple is an example of a:
   a. papule
   b. vesicle
   c. pustule
   d. nodule

2. A Stage III pressure ulcer involves:
   a. erythema of skin
   b. partial loss of epidermis and dermis
   c. full thickness loss of skin up to but not through fascia
   d. full thickness loss of skin with extensive destruction and necrosis

3. This type of dermatitis may be exogenous or endogenous and is common in children and infants:
   a. atopic
   b. irritant contact
   c. stasis
   d. seborrheic

4. Psoriasis, pityriasis, and lichen planus are three types of this disorder:
   a. dermatitis
   b. inflammatory
   c. acne
   d. papulosquamous

5. This condition begins with a herald spot:
   a. psoriasis
   b. pityriasis
   c. lichen planus
   d. dermatitis

6. This skin infection is caused by group A beta hemolytic *Streptococci*, and the lesions appear as firm red spots with itching, burning, and tenderness:
   a. furuncles
   b. folliculitis
   c. erysipelas
   d. fasciitis

7. This type of herpes produces cold sores:
   a. herpes zoster
   b. shingles
   c. VZV
   d. herpes simplex

8. This condition is caused by the human papillomavirus:
   a. mycoses
   b. verrucae
   c. shingles
   d. folliculitis

9. This type of tumor occurs in the hair follicles:
   a. keratoses
   b. nevi
   c. Kaposi's
   d. keratoacanthoma

10. This type of superficial carcinoma is rarely metastatic:
    a. squamous cell
    b. basal cell
    c. melanoma
    d. Kaposi's sarcoma

■ MUSCULOSKELETAL SYSTEM

MUSCULOSKELETAL SYSTEM—ANATOMY AND TERMINOLOGY

Skeletal System

Comprises 206 bones, cartilage, and ligaments

Provides organ protection, movement, framework, stores calcium, hematopoiesis (formation of blood cells)

Classification of Bones

Long bones (tubular)
Length exceeds width of bone

Broad at ends, such as the thigh, lower leg, upper arm, and lower arm

Short bones (cuboidal)
Larger ends on short bones, such as the wrist and ankle

Flat
Thin

Cover body parts, such as the skull

Irregular
Varied shapes, such as zygoma of face or vertebrae

Sesamoid
Rounded

Found near joint, such as the kneecap

Structure

Long Bones (Figure 1-4)
Diaphysis: shaft

Epiphysis: ends

• Articular cartilage covers epiphyses and serves as a cushion

Epiphyseal line or plate: growth plate that disappears when fully grown

Metaphysis: flared portion of bone near epiphyseal plate

Periosteum: outer covering

Cortical or compact bone: hard bone beneath periosteum mainly found in shaft

• Medullary cavity contains yellow marrow (fatty bone marrow)

Cancellous bones: spongy or trabecular

• Contains red bone marrow (blood cell development)

Two Skeletal Divisions

Axial (trunk)

Appendicular (appendages)

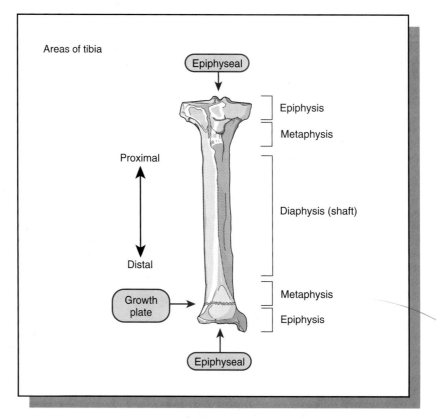

Figure **1-4** Structure of bones.

Axial Skeleton, 80
Skull (Figure 1-5)
Cranial
Frontal (forehead)

Parietal (sides and top)

Temporal (lower sides)

Occipital (posterior of cranium)

Sphenoid (floor of cranium)

Ethmoid (area between orbits and nasal cavity)

Styloid process (below ear)

Zygomatic process (cheek)

Middle ear bones (Figure 1-6)
Malleus

Incus

Stapes

Face (Figure 1-7)
Nasal (bridge of nose)

Maxilla (upper jaw)

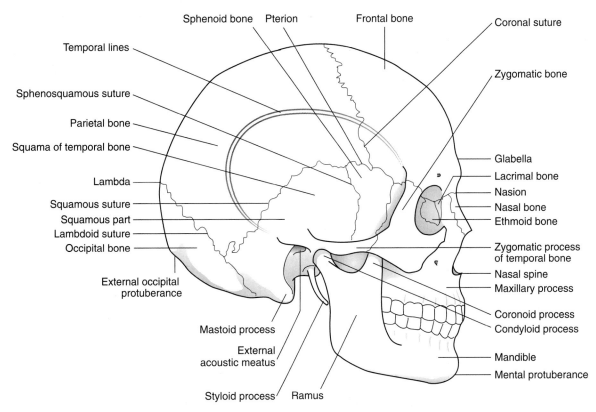

Figure **1-5** Lateral view of the skull.

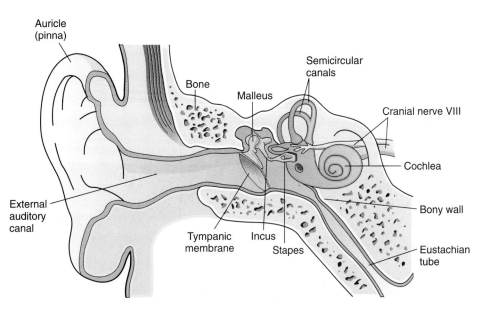

Figure **1-6** Structure of the ear and three divisions of external, middle, and inner ear.

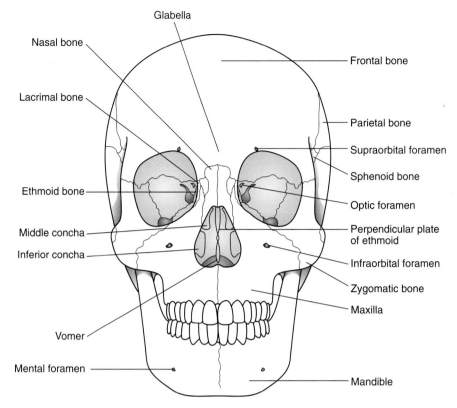

Figure **1-7** Frontal view of the skull.

Zygomatic (arch of cheekbone)

Mandible (lower jawbone)

Lacrimal (near orbits)

Palate (separates oral and nasal cavities)

Vomer (base, nasal septum)

Hyoid
Supports tongue

U shaped

Attached by ligaments and muscles to larynx and skull

Spine (Figure 1-8)
Cervical vertebrae

- C1-7

- First atlas (C1)

- Second axis (C2)

Thoracic vertebrae (T1-12)

Lumbar vertebrae (L1-5)

Sacrum

Coccyx

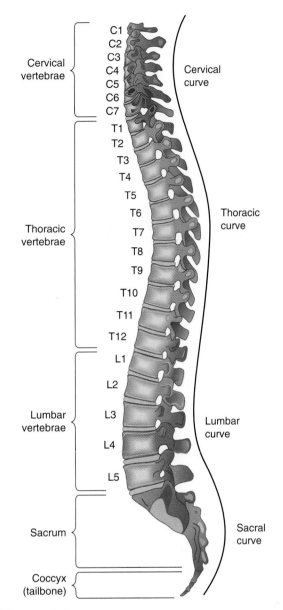

Figure **1-8** Anterior view of the vertebral column.

Thorax (Figure 1-9)
Ribs, 12 pairs

- True ribs, 1-7

- False ribs, 8-10

- Floating ribs, 11 and 12

Sternum

Appendicular Skeleton, 126 (Figure 1-10)
Lower extremities
Pelvis
Ilium (uppermost part) wing shaped

- Acetabulum, depression on lateral hip surface into which head of femur fits

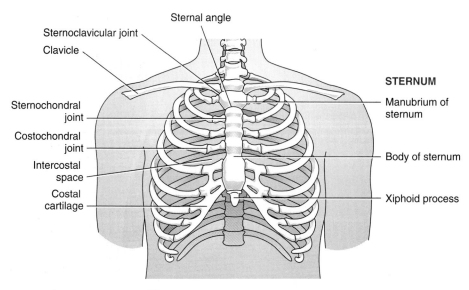

Figure **1-9** The thoracic cage.

Ischium (posterior part)

Pubis (anterior part)

Pubis symphysis (cartilage between pubic bones)

Femur (thighbone)
Trochanter (processes at neck of femur)

Head fits into the acetabulum

Patella (kneecap)

Tibia (shinbone)

Fibula (smaller bone in lower leg)

Talus (ankle bone)

Calcaneus (heel bone)

Metatarsals (foot instep)

Phalanges (toes)

Lateral malleolus (lower part of fibula)

Medial malleolus (lower part of tibia)

Upper extremities
Clavicle (collarbone)

Scapula (shoulder blade)

Humerus (upper arm)

Radius (forearm, thumb side)

Ulna (forearm, little finger side)

Carpals (wrist)

Metacarpals (hand)

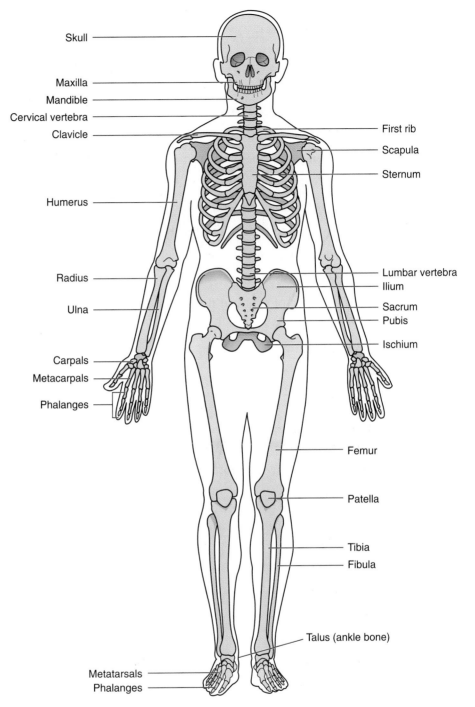

Figure **1-10** Skeletal system.

Phalanges (finger)

Olecranon (tip of elbow)

Joints (Articulations)
Condyle, rounded end of bone

Classified by degree of movement

- Synarthrosis (immovable)

  Example: joint between cranial bones

- Amphiarthrosis (slightly movable)

  Example: intervertebral (joint between bodies of the vertebra)

- Diarthrosis (considerably movable)

  • Types, hinge or ball and socket

  Example: elbow, hip

  • Bursa, sac of synovial fluid located near joints

Muscular System

Functions
Heat production

Movement

Posture

Protection

Shape

Muscle Tissue Types

Skeletal
Striated (cross stripes) (Figures 1-11 and 1-12)

Move body

Voluntary

Attaches to bones

- Most attach to two bones with a joint in between

- Origin, point where muscle attaches to stationary bone

- Insertion, where muscle attaches to movable bone

- Body of muscle, main part of muscle

Cardiac/Heart Muscle
Striated

Involuntary

Moves blood by means of contractions

Smooth/Visceral
Linings such as bowel, urethra, blood vessels

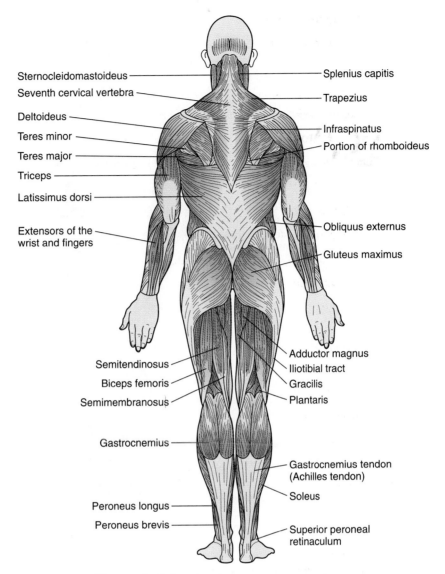

Sternocleidomastoideus

Seventh cervical vertebra

Deltoideus

Teres minor

Teres major

Triceps

Latissimus dorsi

Extensors of the
wrist and fingers

Splenius capitis

Trapezius

Infraspinatus

Portion of rhomboideus

Obliquus externus

Gluteus maximus

Semitendinosus

Biceps femoris

Semimembranosus

Adductor magnus

Iliotibial tract

Gracilis

Plantaris

Gastrocnemius

Gastrocnemius tendon
(Achilles tendon)

Soleus

Peroneus longus

Peroneus brevis

Superior peroneal
retinaculum

Figure **1-11** Muscular system, posterior view.

Nonstriated

Involuntary

Tendons Anchor Muscle to Bone

Ligaments Anchor Bones to Bones

Muscle Action

Muscle Capabilities

Stretches

Contracts

Receives and responds to stimulus

Returns to original shape and length

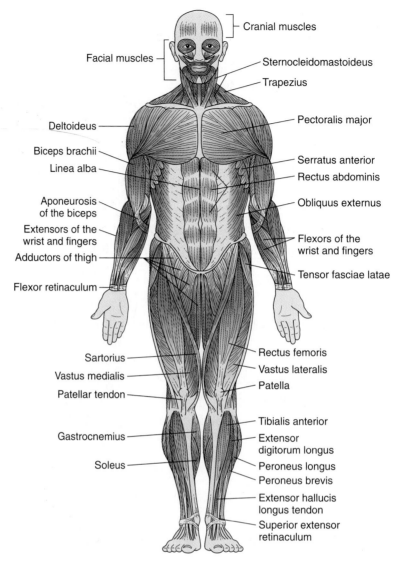

Figure **1-12** Muscular system, anterior view.

Muscle Movement

Prime mover, responsible for movement

Synergist, assists prime mover

Antagonist, relaxes as prime mover and synergists contract, resulting in movement

Terms of Movement

Flexion (bend)

Extension (straighten)

Abduction (away)

Adduction (toward)

Rotation (turn on axis)

Circumduction (circular)

Supination (upward)

Pronation (downward)

Hyperextension (overextension)

Inversion (inward)

Eversion (outward)

Names of Muscles
Head and neck
Facial

- Orbicularis oris (opens mouth)

- Zygomaticus (elevates corners of mouth)

- Orbicularis oculi (opens and closes eyelid)

Mastication (chewing)

- Masseter (used to chew)

- Temporal (closes jaw)

Sternocleidomastoid (rotates head and neck)

Trapezius (extends head)

Upper extremities
Biceps (flexes elbow)

Triceps brachii (extends elbow)

Deltoid (abducts upper arm)

Latissimus dorsi (extends upper arm)

Pectoralis major (flexes upper arm)

Trunk
External oblique (compresses abdomen)

Internal oblique (compresses abdomen)

Transversus abdominis (compresses abdomen)

Rectus abdominis (flexes trunk)

Respiratory
Diaphragm (separates thorax from abdomen)

Intercostal (between ribs)

Lower extremities
Thigh

- Gluteus maximus (abducts thigh)

- Abductor brevis (abducts thigh)

- Iliopsoas (flexes thigh)

Hamstring (flexes lower leg)

Quadriceps (extends lower leg)

Sartorius (flexes and rotates leg)

Tibialis anterior (dorsiflexes foot)

Peroneus longus (everts foot)

Gastrocnemius (calf, with soleus flexes foot, also flexes knee)

Soleus (calf, flexes foot)

Achilles tendon (largest tendon)

COMBINING FORMS

1.	acetabul/o	hip socket
2.	ankyl/o	bent, fused
3.	aponeur/o	tendon type
4.	arthr/o	joint
5.	burs/o	fluid-filled sac in a joint
6.	calc/o, calci/o	calcium
7.	carp/o	carpals (wrist bones)
8.	chondr/o	cartilage
9.	clavic/o, clavicul/o	clavicle (collar bone)
10.	cost/o	rib
11.	crani/o	cranium (skull)
12.	disk/o	intervertebral disk
13.	femor/o	thighbone
14.	fibul/o	fibula
15.	humer/o	humerus (upper arm bone)
16.	ili/o	ilium (upper pelvic bone)
17.	ischi/o	ischium (posterior pelvic bone)
18.	kinesi/o	movement
19.	kyph/o	hump
20.	lamin/o	lamina
21.	lord/o	curve
22.	lumb/o	lower back
23.	mandibul/o	mandible (lower jawbone)
24.	maxill/o	maxilla (upper jawbone)
25.	menisc/o	meniscus
26.	menisci/o	meniscus
27.	metacarp/o	metacarpals (hand)
28.	metatars/o	metatarsals (foot)
29.	myel/o	bone marrow
30.	my/o, muscul/o	muscle

31. olecran/o	olecranon (elbow)
32. orth/o	straight
33. oste/o	bone
34. patell/o	patella (kneecap)
35. pelv/i	pelvis (hip)
36. petr/o	stone
37. phalang/o	phalanges (finger or toe)
38. pub/o	pubis
39. rachi/o	spine
40. radi/o	radius (lower arm)
41. sacr/o	sacrum
42. scapul/o	scapula (shoulder)
43. scoli/o	bent
44. spondyl/o	vertebra
45. stern/o	sternum (breast bone)
46. synovi/o	synovial joint membrane
47. tars/o	tarsal (ankle/foot)
48. ten/o	tendon
49. tend/o	tendon (connective tissue)
50. tendin/o	tendon (connective tissue)
51. tibi/o	shin bone
52. uln/o	ulna (lower arm bone)
53. vertebr/o	vertebra

PREFIXES

1. inter-	between
2. supra-	above
3. sym-	together
4. syn-	together

SUFFIXES

1. -asthenia	weakness
2. -blast	embryonic
3. -clast, -clasia, -clasis	break
4. -desis	fusion
5. -listhesis	slipping
6. -malacia	softening

7.	-physis	to grow
8.	-porosis	passage
9.	-schisis	split
10.	-tome	instrument that cuts
11.	-tomy	incision

MEDICAL ABBREVIATIONS

1.	ACL	anterior cruciate ligament
2.	AKA	above-knee amputation
3.	BKA	below-knee amputation
4.	C1-C7	cervical vertebrae
5.	CTS	carpal tunnel syndrome
6.	fx	fracture
7.	L1-L5	lumbar vertebrae
8.	OA	osteoarthritis
9.	RA	rheumatoid arthritis
10.	T1-T12	thoracic vertebrae
11.	TMJ	temporomandibular joint

MEDICAL TERMS

Arthrocentesis	Injection and/or aspiration of joint
Arthrodesis	Surgical immobilization of a joint
Arthrography	Radiography of joint
Arthroplasty	Reshaping or reconstruction of a joint
Arthroscopy	Use of scope to view inside joint
Arthrotomy	Incision into a joint
Articular	Pertains to a joint
Aspiration	Use of a needle and a syringe to withdraw fluid
Atrophy	Wasting away
Bunion	Hallux valgus, abnormal increase in size of metatarsal head that results in displacement of the great toe
Bursitis	Inflammation of bursa (joint sac)
Chondral	Referring to the cartilage
Closed fracture repair	Not surgically opened with/without manipulation and with/without traction
Closed treatment	Fracture site that is not surgically opened and visualized
Colles' fracture	Fracture at lower end of radius that displaces the bone posteriorly

Dislocation	Placement in a location other than the original location
Endoscopy	Inspection of body organs or cavities using a lighted scope that may be inserted through an existing opening or through a small incision
Fasciectomy	Removal of the band of fibrous tissue
Fissure	Groove
Fracture	Break in a bone
Ganglion	Knot
Internal/External fixation	Application of pins, wires, screws, placed externally or internally to immobilize a body part
Kyphosis	Humpback
Lamina	Flat plate
Ligament	Fibrous band of tissue that connects cartilage or bone
Lordosis	Anterior curve of spine
Lumbodynia	Pain in the lumbar area
Lysis	Releasing
Manipulation or reduction	Alignment of a fracture or joint dislocation to normal position
Open fracture repair	Surgical opening (incision) over or remote opening as access to a fracture site
Osteoarthritis	Degenerative condition of articular cartilage
Osteoclast	Absorbs or removes bone
Osteotomy	Cutting into bone
Percutaneous	Through the skin
Percutaneous fracture repair	Repair of a fracture by means of pins and wires inserted through the fracture site
Percutaneous skeletal fixation	Considered neither open nor closed; the fracture is not visualized, but fixation is placed across the fracture site under x-ray imaging
Reduction	Replacement to normal position
Scoliosis	Lateral curve of the spine
Skeletal traction	Application of pressure to bone by means of pins and/or wires inserted into the bone
Skin traction	Application of pressure to bone by means of tape applied to the skin
Spondylitis	Inflammation of vertebrae
Subluxation	Partial dislocation
Supination	Supine position
Synchondrosis	Union between two bones (connected by cartilage)
Tendon	Attaches a muscle to a bone
Tenodesis	Suturing of a tendon to a bone

Tenorrhaphy	Suture repair of tendon
Traction	Application of pressure to maintain normal alignment
Trocar needle	Needle with a tube on the end; used to puncture and withdraw fluid from a cavity

MUSCULOSKELETAL SYSTEM ANATOMY AND TERMINOLOGY QUIZ

1. Tubular is another name for these bones:
   a. short
   b. long
   c. flat
   d. irregular

2. These bones are found near joints:
   a. irregular
   b. flat
   c. sesamoid
   d. broad

3. The zygoma is an example of this type of bone:
   a. irregular
   b. flat
   c. sesamoid
   d. broad

4. The diaphysis is this part of the bone:
   a. end
   b. surface
   c. shaft
   d. marrow

5. Which is NOT a part of the cranium?
   a. condyle
   b. sphenoid
   c. ethmoid
   d. parietal

6. This is NOT an ear bone:
   a. malleus
   b. stapes
   c. incus
   d. styloid

7. This term describes the growth plate:
   a. endosteum
   b. epiphyseal
   c. metaphysis
   d. periosteum

8. This is a depression on the lateral hip surface into which the head of the femur fits:
   a. ilium
   b. ischium
   c. patella
   d. acetabulum

9. The tip of the elbow is the:
   a. olecranon
   b. trapezium
   c. humerus
   d. tarsal

10. This term describes an immovable joint:
    a. amphiarthrosis
    b. diarthrosis
    c. synarthrosis
    d. ischium

MUSCULOSKELETAL SYSTEM—PATHOPHYSIOLOGY

Injuries

■ Fractures

Classification of fractures

Open/closed

Open (compound): broken bone penetrates skin

Closed (simple): broken bone does not penetrate skin

Complete/incomplete

Complete: bone is broken all the way through

   Example: oblique, linear, and transverse

Incomplete: bone is not broken all the way through

   Example: greenstick, torus, stress, and transchondral

Treatment

Reduction (realignment of bone fragments by manipulation)

Immobilization (returns to normal alignment and holds in place)

Traction (application of pulling force to hold bone in alignment)

- Skeletal traction uses internal devices (pins, screws, wires, etc.) inserted into bone with ends sticking out through skin for attachment of traction device (Figure 1-13)

- Skin traction is the use of strapping, elastic wrap, or tape attached to skin to which weights are attached (Figure 1-14)

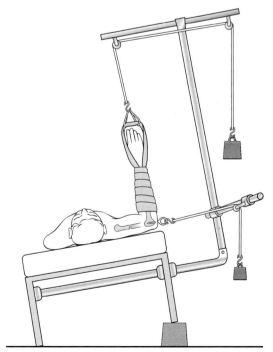

Figure **1-13** Skeletal traction uses the patient's bones to secure internal devices to which traction is attached.

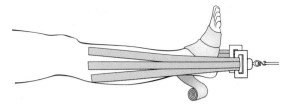

Figure **1-14** Skin traction utilizes strapping, wraps, or tape to which traction is attached.

Improper union
Nonunion: failure of bone ends to grow together

Malunion: incorrect alignment of bone ends

Delayed union: union only after delay of many months

Dislocations
Soft tissue damage usually caused by trauma

May cause fracture of bone due to displacement

Can result in nerve and tissue damage

Treatment is reduction and immobilization

Sprains and strains
Soft tissue damage usually caused by trauma to tendons and ligaments

Strain partial tear of muscle or ligament

Sprain results from overuse or overextension of a ligament

Bone Disorders

Osteomyelitis
Bone infection

Usually caused by bacteria

- Exogenous osteomyelitis is caused by bacteria that enter from outside the body

- Hematogenous osteomyelitis is from infection within the body

Osteoporosis
Common disorder in postmenopausal women

- Lower levels of calcium and phosphate

Decreased bone mass and density

- Fractures more common due to decrease in strength of bone

Treatment
Increased intake of calcium and vitamin D

Increased weight-bearing activity

Osteomalacia and Rickets
Caused by vitamin D and phosphate deficiency

Osteitis Deformans (Paget's Disease)

Abnormal enlarging and softening of bone

Unknown cause

Treatment

Increased intake of protein, calcium, and vitamin D

Spinal Curvatures

Lordosis: swayback

• Inward curvature of the spine

Kyphosis: humpback

• Outward curvature of the spine

Scoliosis

• Lateral curvature of the spine

Spina Bifida

Congenital abnormality in which vertebrae do not close correctly around the spinal cord

Joint Disorders

Bursitis: inflammation of the bursa (joint sac)

Arthritis: inflammation of the joints

Osteoarthritis (OA)

This is degenerative or wear/tear arthritis

• DJD, degenerative joint disease

Chronic inflammation of joint

Increased pain on weight-bearing or movement

Affects weight-bearing joints

• Leads to loss of articular cartilage

• Sclerosis of bone

• Osteophytes (bone spurs)

Symptoms

Pain and stiffness

Crepitation (bone on bone creates characteristic grinding sound)

Classifications

Primary (idiopathic)

• No known cause

Secondary

• Associated with joint instability, joint stress, or congenital abnormalities

Treatment

Symptomatic

Arthroplasty

Rheumatoid Arthritis (RA)
Inflammatory disease that is progressive

Systemic autoimmune disease

• Can invade arteries, lung, skin, and other organs with nodules

Affects small joints

• Destroys the synovial membrane, articular cartilage, and surrounding tissues

Leads to loss of function due to fixation and deformity

Treatment
Symptomatic

Arthroplasty

Infectious and Septic Arthritis
Infectious process

Usually affects single joint

Without antimicrobial intervention, permanent joint damage results

> ***Example:*** Lyme disease

Gout (Gouty Arthritis)
Inflammatory arthritis

Often affects the joint of the great toe

Caused by excessive amounts of uric acid that crystallizes in connective tissue of joints

Leads to inflammation and destruction of joint

Ankylosing Spondylitis (AS)
Inflammatory disease that is progressive

Affects vertebral joints

Leads to rigid spinal column and sacroiliac joints

Tendon, Muscle, and Ligament Disorders

Muscular Dystrophy
Progressive degenerative muscle disorder

Most often affects boys

• Genetic predisposition

Primary Fibromyalgia Syndrome
Symptoms
Generalized aching and pain

Tender points

Fatigue

Depression

Usually appears in
Middle-aged women

Polymyositis

General muscle inflammation causing weakness

- With skin rash = dermatomyositis

Tumors

Bone Tumors

Origin of bone tumors

Osteogenic (bone cells)

Chondrogenic (cartilage cell)

Collagenic (fibrous tissue cell)

Myelogenic (marrow cell)

Osteoma

Benign

Abnormal outgrowth of bone

Chondroblastoma

Rare

Usually benign

Osteosarcoma

Malignant tumor of long bones

Usually in young adults

Typically causes bone pain

Multiple myeloma

Malignant

Progressive and generally fatal

Usually in those over 40

Chondrosarcoma

Malignant cartilage tumor

Usually in middle-aged and older individuals

In late stages, symptoms include local swelling and pain

- Worsens with time

Surgical excision is usually treatment of choice

Muscle Tumors

Rare

Rhabdomyosarcoma is an aggressive, invasive carcinoma with widespread metastasis

MUSCULOSKELETAL SYSTEM PATHOPHYSIOLOGY QUIZ

1. A compound fracture is also known as:
   a. complete
   b. incomplete
   c. closed
   d. open

2. This is a common bone disorder in postmenopausal women resulting from lower levels of calcium and potassium:
   a. Paget's disease
   b. lordosis
   c. osteoporosis
   d. rheumatoid arthritis

3. This inflammatory disease is progressive and leads to a rigid spinal column:
   a. polymyositis
   b. ankylosing spondylitis
   c. primary fibromyalgia syndrome
   d. septic arthritis of the spine

4. This type of tumor arises from the bone cells:
   a. osteogenic
   b. chondrogenic
   c. collagenic
   d. myelogenic

5. This type of tumor is the most common type of malignant bone tumor that occurs in those over 40:
   a. rhabdomyosarcoma
   b. chondrosarcoma
   c. osteosarcoma
   d. multiple myeloma

6. A general muscle inflammation with an accompanying skin rash is:
   a. muscular dystrophy
   b. dermatologic arthritis
   c. ankylosing spondylitis
   d. dermatomyositis

7. A cartilage tumor that usually occurs in middle-aged and older individuals:
   a. chondrosarcoma
   b. osteosarcoma
   c. chondroblastoma
   d. rhabdomyosarcoma

8. The returning of the bone to normal alignment is:
   a. immobilization
   b. traction
   c. reduction
   d. manipulation

9. The result of overuse or overextension of a ligament is:
   a. strain
   b. sprain
   c. fracture
   d. displacement

10. Primary osteoarthritis is also known as:
    a. secondary
    b. functional
    c. congenital
    d. idiopathic

■ RESPIRATORY SYSTEM

RESPIRATORY SYSTEM—ANATOMY AND TERMINOLOGY

Supplies oxygen to body and helps clean body of waste

Two tracts (Figure 1-15A)

- Upper respiratory tract (nose, sinuses, pharynx, and larynx)
- Lower respiratory tract (trachea, bronchial tree, and lungs)

Lined with specialized membranes

- Purifies air by trapping irritants
- Covered with cilia that move mucus upward

Upper Respiratory Tract (URT)

Nose

Sense of smell (olfactory)

Moistens and warms air

Nasal septum divides interior

Sinuses

Frontal

Ethmoidal

Maxillary

Sphenoidal

Turbinates

Bones on inside of nose

Divided into inferior, middle, and superior (Figure 1-15B)

Warms and humidifies the air

Pharynx (Throat)

Passageway for both food and air

Nasopharynx contains adenoids

Oropharynx contains tonsils

Laryngopharynx leads to larynx

Larynx (Voice Box)

Contains vocal cords

Lower Respiratory Tract (LRT)

Trachea (Windpipe)

Mucus-lined tube with C-shaped cartilage rings to hold windpipe open

Air passageway

Bronchi

Trachea divides into branches—right branch and left branch

Branches divide into smaller bronchioles that are tipped with alveoli (air sacs that exchange gases)

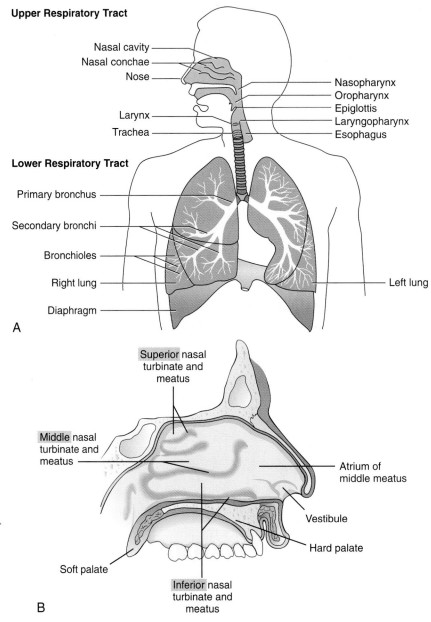

Figure **1-15** **A,** Upper and lower respiratory system. **B,** Superior, inferior, and middle nasal turbinates.

Lungs

Covered by pleura

Cone-shaped organs

Base rests on diaphragm

Left lung contains two lobes

Right lung contains three lobes

Respiration

Inspiration—oxygen moves in

Expiration—carbon dioxide moves out

COMBINING FORMS

1.	adenoid/o	adenoid
2.	alveol/o	alveolus
3.	atel/o	incomplete
4.	bronch/o	bronchus
5.	bronchi/o	bronchus
6.	bronchiol/o	bronchiole
7.	coni/o	dust
8.	diaphragmat/o	diaphragm
9.	epiglott/o	epiglottis
10.	laryng/o	larynx
11.	lob/o	lobe
12.	muc/o	mucus
13.	nas/o	nose
14.	orth/o	straight
15.	ox/i	oxygen
16.	oxy/o	oxygen
17.	pharyng/o	pharynx
18.	phren/o	diaphragm
19.	pleur/o	pleura
20.	pneum/o	lung/air
21.	pneumat/o	air
22.	pneumon/o	lung/air
23.	pulmon/o	lung
24.	py/o	pus
25.	rhin/o	nose
26.	sept/o	septum
27.	sinus/o	sinus
28.	spir/o	breath
29.	thorac/o	thorax
30.	tonsill/o	tonsil
31.	trache/o	trachea

PREFIXES

1.	a-	not
2.	an-	not
3.	endo-	within

4. eu-	good
5. pan-	all
6. poly-	many

SUFFIXES

1. -algia	pain
2. -ar	pertaining to
3. -ary	pertaining to
4. -capnia	carbon dioxide
5. -centesis	puncture to remove (drain)
6. -dynia	pain
7. -eal	pertaining to
8. -ectasis	stretching
9. -emia	blood
10. -gram	record
11. -graph	recording instrument
12. -graphy	recording process
13. -itis	inflammation
14. -meter	measurement or instrument that measures
15. -metry	measurement of
16. -oxia	oxygen
17. -pexy	fixation
18. -phonia	sound
19. -pnea	breathing
20. -rrhage, -rrhagia	bursting of blood
21. -scopy	to examine
22. -spasm	contraction of muscle
23. -stenosis	blockage, narrowing
24. -stomy	opening
25. -thorax	chest
26. -tomy	cutting, incision

MEDICAL ABBREVIATIONS

1. ABG	arterial blood gas
2. AFB	acid-fast bacillus
3. ARDS	adult respiratory distress syndrome
4. BiPAP	bi-level positive airway pressure
5. COPD	chronic obstructive pulmonary disease

6.	CPAP	continuous positive airway pressure
7.	DLCO	diffuse capacity of lungs for carbon monoxide
8.	FEF	forced expiratory flow
9.	FEV_1	forced expiratory volume in one second
10.	FEV_1:FVC	ratio of forced expiratory volume in one second to forced vital capacity
11.	FRC	functional residual capacity
12.	FVC	forced vital capacity
13.	HHN	hand-held nebulizer
14.	IPAP	inspiratory positive airway pressure
15.	IRDS	infant respiratory distress syndrome
16.	MDI	metered dose inhaler
17.	MVV	maximum voluntary ventilation
18.	PAWP	pulmonary artery wedge pressure
19.	PCWP	pulmonary capillary wedge pressure
20.	PEAP	positive end-airway pressure
21.	PEEP	positive end-expiratory pressure
22.	PFT	pulmonary function test
23.	PND	paroxysmal nocturnal dyspnea
24.	RDS	respiratory distress syndrome
25.	RV	respiratory volume
26.	RV:TLC	ratio of respiratory volume to total lung capacity
27.	TLC	total lung capacity
28.	TLV	total lung volume
29.	URI	upper respiratory infection
30.	V/Q	ventilation/perfusion scan

MEDICAL TERMS

Ablation	Removal or destruction by cutting, chemicals, or electrocautery
Adenoidectomy	Removal of adenoids
Apnea	Cessation of breathing
Asphyxia	Lack of oxygen
Asthma	Shortage of breath caused by contraction of bronchi
Atelectasis	Incomplete expansion of lung, collapse
Auscultation	Listening to sounds, such as to lung sounds
Bacilli	Plural of bacillus, a rod-shaped bacteria

Bilobectomy	Surgical removal of two lobes of a lung
Bronchiole	Smaller division of bronchial tree
Bronchoplasty	Surgical repair of the bronchi
Bronchoscopy	Inspection of the bronchial tree using a bronchoscope
Catheter	Tube placed into the body to put fluid in or take fluid out
Cauterization	Destruction of tissue by the use of cautery
Cordectomy	Surgical removal of the vocal cord(s)
Crackle	Abnormal sound when breathing (heard on auscultation)
Cyanosis	Bluish discoloration
Drainage	Free flow or withdrawal of fluids from a wound or cavity
Dysphonia	Speech impairment
Dyspnea	Shortage of breath, difficult breathing
Emphysema	Air accumulated in organ or tissue
Epiglottidectomy	Excision of the covering of the larynx
Epistaxis	Nose bleed
Glottis	True vocal cords
Hemoptysis	Bloody sputum
Intramural	Within the organ wall
Intubation	Insertion of a tube
Laryngeal web	Congenital abnormality of connective tissue between the vocal cords
Laryngectomy	Surgical removal of the larynx
Laryngoplasty	Surgical repair of the larynx
Laryngoscope	Fiberoptic scope used to view the inside of the larynx
Laryngoscopy	Direct visualization and examination of the interior of larynx with a laryngoscope
Laryngotomy	Incision into the larynx
Lavage	Washing out
Lobectomy	Surgical excision of a lobe of the lung
Nasal button	Synthetic circular disk used to cover a hole in the nasal septum
Orthopnea	Difficulty in breathing, needing to be in erect position to breathe
Percussion	Tapping with sharp blows as a diagnostic technique
Pharyngolaryngectomy	Surgical removal of the pharynx and larynx
Pleura	Covers the lungs and lines the thoracic cavity
Pleurectomy	Surgical excision of the pleura
Pleuritis	Inflammation of the pleura
Pneumocentesis	Surgical puncturing of a lung to withdraw fluid
Pneumonolysis	Surgical separation of the lung from the chest wall to allow the lung to collapse

Pneumonotomy	Incision of the lung
Rales	Coarse sound on inspiration, also known as crackle (heard on auscultation)
Rhinoplasty	Surgical repair of nose
Rhinorrhea	Nasal mucous discharge
Segmentectomy	Surgical removal of a portion of a lung
Septoplasty	Surgical repair of the nasal septum
Sinusotomy	Surgical incision into a sinus
Spirometry	Measuring breathing capacity
Tachypnea	Quick, shallow breathing
Thoracentesis	Surgical puncture of the thoracic cavity, usually using a needle, to remove fluids
Thoracoplasty	Surgical procedure that removes rib(s) and thereby allows the collapse of a lung
Thoracoscopy	Use of a lighted endoscope to view the pleural spaces and thoracic cavity or to perform surgical procedures
Thoracostomy	Surgical incision into the chest wall and insertion of a chest tube
Thoracotomy	Surgical incision into the chest wall
Total pneumonectomy	Surgical removal of an entire lung
Tracheostomy	Creation of an opening into the trachea
Tracheotomy	Incision into the trachea
Transtracheal	Across the trachea

RESPIRATORY SYSTEM ANATOMY AND TERMINOLOGY QUIZ

1. This is NOT a part of the lower respiratory tract:
   a. trachea
   b. larynx
   c. bronchi
   d. lungs

2. Another name for the voice box is:
   a. oropharynx
   b. pharynx
   c. laryngopharynx
   d. larynx

3. This is the windpipe:
   a. pharynx
   b. larynx
   c. trachea
   d. sphenoid

4. The interior of the nose is divided by the:
   a. septum
   b. sphenoid
   c. oropharynx
   d. apical

5. This combining form means incomplete:
   a. atel/o
   b. alveol/o
   c. ox/i
   d. pneumat/o

6. This prefix means breathe:
   a. py/o
   b. lob/o
   c. spir/o
   d. pleur/o

7. This prefix means all:
   a. a-
   b. an-
   c. pan-
   d. poly-

8. This abbreviation refers to a syndrome that involves difficulty in breathing:
   a. ABG
   b. ARDS
   c. BiPAP
   d. FEF

9. This abbreviation refers to the amount of air the patient can expel from the lungs in 1 second:
   a. PFT
   b. PND
   c. RDS
   d. FEV_1

10. This suffix means breathing:
    a. -stenosis
    b. -spasm
    c. -pexy
    d. -pnea

RESPIRATORY SYSTEM—PATHOPHYSIOLOGY

Signs and Symptoms of Disorders

Dyspnea
Difficult or painful breathing

Increased respiratory effort

Hypoventilation
Decreased alveolar ventilation

Hyperventilation
Increased alveolar ventilation

Hemoptysis
Bloody sputum

Hypoxia
Reduced oxygenation of tissue cells

Cough
Caused by irritant

Protective reflex

Acute cough is up to 3 weeks

Chronic cough is over 3 weeks

Tachypnea
Rapid breathing

Apnea
Lack of breathing

Orthopnea
Requiring sitting upright to facilitate breathing

Pulmonary Diseases and Disorders

Hypercapnia
Increased carbon dioxide in arterial blood

Decreased ability to breathe

Can result in respiratory acidosis

Hypoxemia
Reduced oxygenation of arterial blood

Acute Respiratory Failure
Inadequate gas exchange

Hypoxemia

Can result from trauma or disease

Adult Respiratory Distress Syndrome (ARDS)
Acute injury to alveolocapillary membrane

Results in edema and atelectasis

In infants, infant respiratory distress syndrome (IRDS)

Pulmonary Edema
Accumulation of fluid in lung tissue

Most common cause is heart disease

Aspiration
Passage of fluid and solid particles into the lung

Can cause severe pneumonitis

- Localized inflammation of the lung

Atelectasis
Compression atelectasis
Collapse of alveoli

May be caused by external pressure on lung from abdominal distention, pleural effusion, or pneumothorax

Absorption Atelectasis
Most common type

Mucus blocks airways

Excess gas absorbed into alveoli causes collapse

Bronchiectasis
Chronic, irreversible dilation of bronchi

Examples:
- Capillary

- Cystic

- Follicular

- Varicose

Respiratory Acidosis
Decreased level of pH

Bronchiolitis
Inflammation of bronchioles

Usually in children less than 2

Viral infection (respiratory syncytial virus, or RSV)

Examples:
- Constrictive

- Proliferative

- Obliterative

Pneumothorax

Air collected in pleural cavity

Can lead to lung collapse

Spontaneous pneumothorax is spontaneous rupture of visceral pleura

Secondary pneumothorax is a result of trauma to the chest

Pneumoconiosis

Dust particles in the lung

Examples:

- Coal

- Asbestos

- Fiberglass

Empyema

Infectious pleural effusion
Pus in pleural space

May be a complication of pneumonia

Treatment is that for pneumonia

Pulmonary Embolism

Air, tissue, or embolus occlusion

Lodges in pulmonary artery or branch of artery

Risk with congestive heart failure

Most clots originate in leg veins

Cor Pulmonale

Hypertrophy or failure of right ventricle

Result of lung, pulmonary vessels, or chest wall disorders

Acute is secondary to pulmonary embolus

Chronic is secondary to obstructive lung disease

Pleurisy (Pleuritis)

Inflammation of the pleura

Often preceded by an upper respiratory infection

Infectious Disease

Upper respiratory infection (URI)
Acute inflammatory process of mucous membranes in trachea and above

Examples:

- Common cold

- Croup

- Sinusitis

- Laryngitis

Lower Respiratory Infection (LRI)

Pneumonia

Inflammation of the lungs with consolidation

Categorized according to causative organism

Can be caused by bacteria, protozoa, fungi, or virus

Examples:

- Lobar pneumonia

- Legionnaires' disease

- Bronchitis

- Bronchiolitis

Tuberculosis
Communicable lung disease

Caused by *Mycobacterium tuberculosis*

Chronic Obstructive Pulmonary Disease (COPD)
Irreversible airway obstruction that decreases expiration

Includes
Asthma

- Bronchial spasms

- Dyspnea

- Wheezing

Chronic bronchitis

- Constant inflammation of bronchial tubes

Emphysema

- Loss of elasticity and enlargement of alveoli

RESPIRATORY SYSTEM PATHOPHYSIOLOGY QUIZ

1. Acute injury to the alveolocapillary membrane that results in edema and atelectasis:
   a. hypoxemia
   b. acute respiratory distress syndrome
   c. bronchiolitis
   d. pneumoconiosis

2. The condition in which pus is in the pleural space and is often a complication of pneumonia:
   a. empyema
   b. cor pulmonale
   c. pneumothorax
   d. atelectasis

3. The most common type of atelectasis is:
   a. compression
   b. inflammation
   c. chronic
   d. absorption

4. This condition is a result of the accumulation of dust particles in the lung:
   a. pleurisy
   b. tuberculosis
   c. chronic obstructive pulmonary disease
   d. pneumoconiosis

5. An irreversible airway obstructive disease in which the symptoms are bronchial spasm, dyspnea, and wheezing:
   a. pleurisy
   b. empyema
   c. bronchiolitis
   d. asthma

6. Capillary, cystic, follicular, and varicose are examples of:
   a. bronchiectasis
   b. cor pulmonale
   c. pneumothorax
   d. atelectasis

7. The condition in which there is a loss of elasticity and enlargement of alveoli:
   a. chronic bronchitis
   b. asthma
   c. emphysema
   d. empyema

8. The definition of a chronic cough is one that lasts for over this number of weeks:
   a. 2
   b. 3
   c. 4
   d. 5

9. A condition marked by an increase in the carbon dioxide in the arterial blood and decreased ability to breathe that can result in respiratory acidosis:
   a. hypercapnia
   b. hypoxemia
   c. acute respiratory failure
   d. pulmonary edema

10. This condition often follows a viral infection and occurs in children under 2 years of age. Examples of the various types of the condition are constrictive, proliferating, and obliterative.
    a. pneumoconiosis
    b. pulmonary edema
    c. bronchiolitis
    d. bronchiectasis

■ CARDIOVASCULAR SYSTEM

CARDIOVASCULAR SYSTEM—ANATOMY AND TERMINOLOGY

Consists of blood, blood vessels, and heart

Blood

Carries

Oxygen and nutrients to cells

Waste and carbon dioxide to kidneys, liver, and lungs

Hormones from endocrine system

Regulates

Temperature by circulating blood

Protection

White cells produce antibodies

Composed of Two Parts

Liquid part (extracellular) is plasma
Water 91%

Protein 1%, albumin, globulins, fibrinogen

2% ions, nutrients, waste products, gases, regulating substances

Formed part
Leukocytes (WBCs)

- Neutrophils
- Lymphocytes
- Monocytes
- Eosinophils
- Basophils

Erythrocytes (RBCs)

Platelets/thrombocytes

Vessels

Function

To carry nutrients and oxygen (blood)

Types

Arteries (Figure 1-16)
Inner layer, endothelium

Lead away from heart

Branches are arterioles

Capillaries
Carry blood from arterioles to venules

Exchange vessels

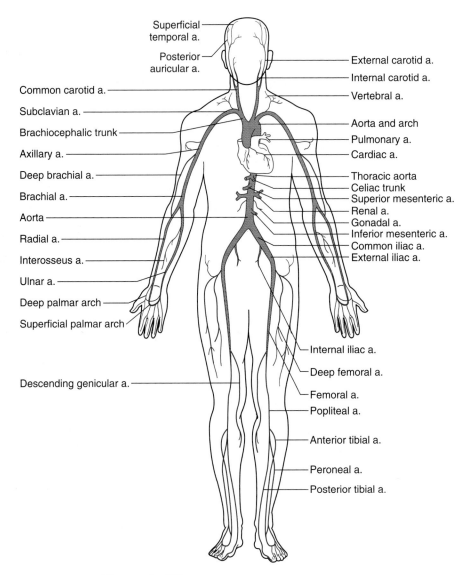

Superficial temporal a.
Posterior auricular a.
External carotid a.
Internal carotid a.
Vertebral a.
Common carotid a.
Subclavian a.
Brachiocephalic trunk
Axillary a.
Deep brachial a.
Brachial a.
Aorta
Radial a.
Interosseus a.
Ulnar a.
Deep palmar arch
Superficial palmar arch
Aorta and arch
Pulmonary a.
Cardiac a.
Thoracic aorta
Celiac trunk
Superior mesenteric a.
Renal a.
Gonadal a.
Inferior mesenteric a.
Common iliac a.
External iliac a.
Internal iliac a.
Deep femoral a.
Descending genicular a.
Femoral a.
Popliteal a.
Anterior tibial a.
Peroneal a.
Posterior tibial a.

Figure **1-16** Arteries of the circulatory system.

Veins (Figure 1-17)
Carry blood to heart

Venules are small branches

Heart

Circulates blood

Four Chambers (Figure 1-18)
Two upper
Right and left atria (singular atrium) receive blood

Two lower
Right and left ventricles discharge blood (pump)

Chamber Walls
Composed of three layers

• Endocardium: smooth inner layer

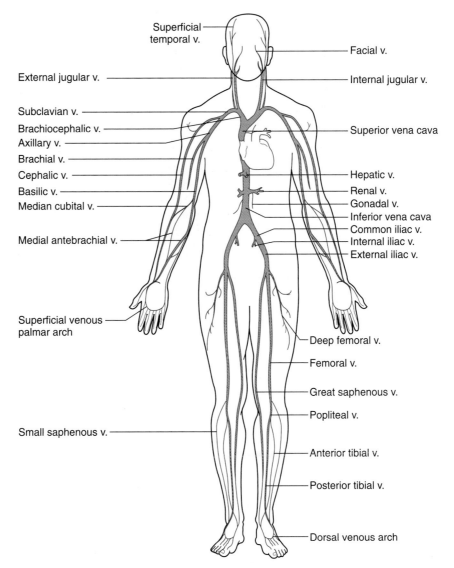

Figure **1-17** Veins of the circulatory system.

- Myocardium: middle muscular layer

- Epicardium: outer layer

Septa (Singular Septum)
Divide chambers

- Interatrial septum: separates two upper chambers

- Interventricular septum: separates two lower chambers

Pericardium
Sac that covers heart in two layers

- Parietal pericardium: outermost covering

- Visceral pericardium: innermost (epicardium)

- Pericardial cavity: contains fluid

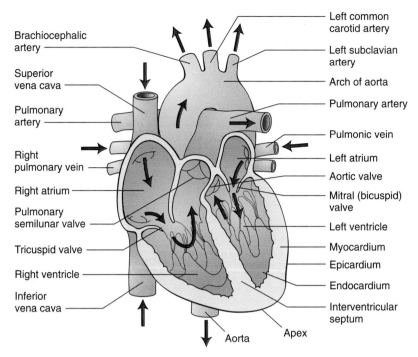

Figure **1-18** Internal view of the heart.

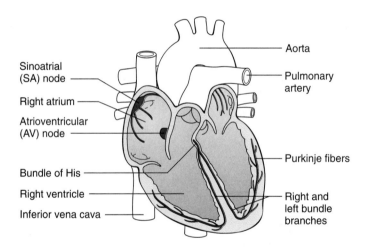

Figure **1-19** Electrical system of the heart.

Valves

Tricuspid: right atrium to right ventricle

Pulmonary: at entrance of pulmonary artery

Aortic: at entrance of aorta

Bicuspid (mitral): left atrium to left ventricle

Conduction System (Figure 1-19)

Sinoatrial node: SAN, nature's pacemaker, sends impulses to atrioventricular node

Atrioventricular node: AVN, located on interatrial septum and sends impulses to bundle of His

Purkinje fibers: located at the base of the heart

Bundle of His: divides into right bundle branch (RBB) and left bundle branch (LBB) in septum

Heartbeat

Two Phases
Diastole: relaxation

Systole: contraction

COMBINING FORMS

1.	angi/o	vessel
2.	aort/o	aorta
3.	ather/o	plaque
4.	arter/o	artery
5.	arteri/o	artery
6.	atri/o	atrium
7.	brachi/o	arm
8.	cardi/o	heart
9.	cholester/o	cholesterol
10.	coron/o	heart
11.	cyan/o	blue
12.	my/o, muscul/o	muscle
13.	ox/o	oxygen
14.	pericardi/o	pericardium
15.	phleb/o	vein
16.	sphygm/o	pulse
17.	steth/o	chest
18.	thromb/o	clot
19.	valv/o	valve
20.	valvul/o	valve
21.	vascul/o	vessel
22.	vas/o	vessel
23.	ven/o	vein
24.	ventricul/o	ventricle

PREFIXES

1.	a-	not
2.	an-	not
3.	bi-	two

4.	brady-	slow
5.	de-	lack of
6.	dys-	bad, difficult, painful
7.	endo-	in
8.	hyper-	over
9.	hypo-	under
10.	inter-	between
11.	intra-	within
12.	meta-	change, after
13.	peri-	surrounding
14.	tachy-	fast
15.	tetra-	four
16.	tri-	three

SUFFIXES

1.	-dilation	widening, expanding
2.	-emia	blood
3.	-graphy	recording process
4.	-lysis	separation
5.	-megaly	enlargement
6.	-oma	tumor
7.	-osis	condition
8.	-plasty	repair
9.	-sclerosis	hardening
10.	-stenosis	blockage, narrowing
11.	-tomy	cutting, incision

MEDICAL ABBREVIATIONS

1.	ASCVD	arteriosclerotic cardiovascular disease
2.	ASD	atrial septal defect
3.	ASHD	arteriosclerotic heart disease
4.	AV	atrioventricular
5.	CABG	coronary artery bypass graft
6.	CHF	congestive heart failure
7.	CK	creatine kinase
8.	CPK	creatine phosphokinase
9.	CVI	cerebrovascular insufficiency

10.	DSE	dobutamine stress echocardiography
11.	HCVD	hypertensive cardiovascular disease
12.	LBBB	left bundle branch block
13.	LVH	left ventricular hypertrophy
14.	MAT	multifocal atrial tachycardia
15.	MI	myocardial infarction
16.	NSR	normal sinus rhythm
17.	PAC	premature atrial contraction
18.	PAT	paroxysmal atrial tachycardia
19.	PST/PSVT	paroxysmal supraventricular tachycardia
20.	PTCA	percutaneous transluminal coronary angioplasty
21.	PVC	premature ventricular contraction
22.	RBBB	right bundle branch block
23.	RSR	regular sinus rhythm
24.	RVH	right ventricular hypertrophy
25.	SVT	supraventricular tachycardia
26.	TEE	transesophageal echocardiography
27.	TST	treadmill stress test

MEDICAL TERMS

Anastomosis	Surgical connection of two tubular structures, such as two pieces of the intestine
Aneurysm	Abnormal dilation of vessels, usually an artery
Angina	Sudden pain
Angiography	Radiography of the blood vessels
Angioplasty	Procedure in a vessel to dilate the vessel opening
Atherectomy	Removal of plaque by percutaneous method
Auscultation	Listening for sounds within the body
Bundle of His	Muscular cardiac fibers that provide the heart rhythm to the ventricles
Bypass	To go around
Cardiopulmonary	Refers to the heart and lungs
Cardiopulmonary bypass	Blood bypasses the heart through a heart-lung machine
Cardioverter-defibrillator	Surgically placed device that directs an electric shock to the heart to restore rhythm
Circumflex	A coronary artery that circles the heart
Cutdown	Incision into a vessel for placement of a catheter
Edema	Swelling due to abnormal fluid collection in the tissue spaces

Electrode	Lead attached to a generator that carries the electric current from the generator to the atria or ventricles
Electrophysiology	Study of the electrical system of the heart, including study of arrhythmias
Embolectomy	Removal of blockage (embolism) from vessel
Endarterectomy	Incision into an artery to remove inner lining
Epicardial	Over the heart
False aneurysm	Sac of clotted blood that has completely destroyed the vessel and is being contained by the tissue that surrounds the vessel
Fistula	Abnormal opening from one area to another area or to the outside of the body
Hematoma	Mass of blood that forms outside the vessel
Hemolysis	Breakdown of red blood cells
Hypoxemia	Low level of oxygen in the blood
Hypoxia	Low level of oxygen in the tissue
Intracardiac	Inside the heart
Invasive	Entering the body, breaking skin
Noninvasive	Not entering the body, not breaking skin
Nuclear cardiology	Diagnostic specialty that uses radiologic procedures to aid in diagnosis of cardiologic conditions
Order	Shows subordination of one thing to another; family or class
Pericardiocentesis	Procedure in which a surgeon withdraws fluid from the pericardial space by means of a needle inserted percutaneously
Pericardium	Membranous sac enclosing heart and ends of great vessels
Swan Ganz catheter	A catheter that measures pressure in the heart
Thoracostomy	Incision into the chest wall and insertion of a chest tube
Thromboendarterectomy	Procedure to remove plaque or clot formations from a vessel by percutaneous method
Transvenous	Through a vein

CARDIOVASCULAR SYSTEM ANATOMY AND TERMINOLOGY QUIZ

1. Carry blood to the heart:
   a. capillaries
   b. arteries
   c. arterioles
   d. veins

2. The relaxation phase of the heartbeat:
   a. diastole
   b. systole

3. Nature's pacemaker is this node:
   a. atrioventricular
   b. Bundle of His
   c. sinoatrial
   d. mitral

4. Node located on the interatrial septum:
   a. atrioventricular
   b. Bundle of His
   c. sinoatrial
   d. Purkinje

5. Which of the following is NOT one of the three layers of the chamber walls of the heart:
   a. endocardium
   b. myocardium
   c. epicardium
   d. parietal

6. Septum that divides the upper two chambers of the heart:
   a. intraventricular
   b. interatrial
   c. tricuspid
   d. myocardium

7. This is the valve between the right atrium and right ventricle:
   a. pulmonary
   b. aortic
   c. bicuspid
   d. tricuspid

8. The outer two-layer covering of the heart:
   a. pericardium
   b. mitral
   c. myocardium
   d. epicardium

9. These are the chambers that receive blood:
   a. right and left ventricle
   b. left ventricle and right atrium
   c. right atrium and right ventricle
   d. right and left atria

10. This combining form means plaque:
    a. atri/o
    b. brachi/o
    c. cyan/o
    d. ather/o

CARDIOVASCULAR SYSTEM—PATHOPHYSIOLOGY

Vascular Disorders

Coronary Artery Disease (CAD)/Ischemic Heart Disease (IHD)
Thickening of the arterial intima (innermost layer) and accumulation of lipid

- Produces narrowing and stiffening of vessel

Location of lesions leads to various vascular diseases

- Femoral and popliteal arteries = peripheral vascular disease
- Carotid arteries = stroke
- Aorta = aneurysmal disease
- Coronary arteries = ischemic heart disease or myocardial infarction

Result of decreased oxygen supply

Risk factors increased by:

- Age
- Family history of CAD
- Hyperlipidemia
- Low HDL-C (good cholesterol)
- Hypertension
- Cigarette smoking
- Diabetes mellitus
- Obesity, particularly abdominal

Ischemia
Deficiency of blood

- Often due to constriction or obstruction of blood vessel

Localized myocardial ischemia
Oxygen demand in excess of ability of the vessel

Presenting symptoms

- Chest pain (angina pectoris)
- Hypotension
- Changes in ECG

Transient ischemia
Heart muscle begins to perform at a low level due to lack of oxygen (reversible ischemia)

Irreversible ischemia
Heart muscle dies—necrosis (myocardial infarction)

- Prolonged ischemia of 30 minutes or more
- Reestablishment of blood flow reduces the residual necrosis
  - Thrombolytic agents to dissolve or split up thrombus
  - Primary percutaneous transluminal coronary angioplasty (PTCA)

Cardiac enzymes are released from the damaged cells

- Blood test reveals elevation of enzymes confirming myocardial infarction

Hypertension
Normal is less than 120/80 for adults

- Figure 1-20 illustrates the new hypertension classifications

Leading cause of death in United States due to damage to brain, heart, and kidneys

Cause is unknown in 95% of cases

- Known as
  - Primary hypertension
  - Essential hypertension

5% of cases are secondary to underlying disease

Increased resistance damages heart and blood vessels

- Retinal vascular changes are monitored to assess therapy and disease progression

Chronic hypertension often leads to end-stage renal disease

- Result of progressive sclerosis of renal vessels

Treatment
Medications

- ACE (angiotensin-converting enzyme) inhibitor
- Alpha-adrenergic or beta-adrenergic receptor blocker
- Diuretic
- Calcium channel blocker

Lifestyle changes

Classification of blood pressure for adults aged 18 years or older[1]

Category	Systolic (mm Hg)	Diastolic (mm Hg)
Normal	<120	<80
Prehypertension (stays between)	120–139	80–89
Hypertension[2]		
Stage 1 (mild)	140–159	90–99
Stage 2 (moderate)	160–179	100–109
Stage 3 (severe)	≥180	≥110

[1] Not taking antihypertensive drugs and not acutely ill. When systolic and diastolic pressures fall into different categories, the higher category should be selected.

[2] Based on the average of two or more readings taken at each of two or more visits after an initial screening.

Figure **1-20** Classification of blood pressure.

Hypotension

Abnormally low blood pressure

Types

Orthostatic (postural) hypotension

- Fall in both systolic and diastolic arterial blood pressure on standing

- Associated with

  - Dizziness

  - Blurred vision

  - Possibly fainting (syncope)

- Caused by insufficient blood flow through brain

- Can be acute (temporary) or chronic

Chronic orthostatic hypotension

- Secondary to a disease

- Such as:

  - Endocrine

  - Metabolic

  - Central nervous system disorders

- Idiopathic or primary

  - No known cause

- Treatment for secondary hypotension is correction of underlying disease

Aneurysm

Dilation of a vessel wall or cardiac chamber

- Danger is rupture of the aneurysm

Atherosclerosis is common cause

Arteriosclerosis and hypertension also common in persons with aneurysms

True aneurysm

Involves all three layers of arterial wall

Causes weakening in arterial wall

Weakness allows ballooning effect along artery wall

False aneurysm

Usually result of trauma

Also known as pseudoaneurysm

Tear or cut in artery wall

Bleeds into and is contained by connective tissue around artery

Thrombus

Blood clot that remains attached to vessel wall and occludes the vessel

Dislodged thrombus is a thromboembolus

Causes
Trauma

Infection

Low blood pressure

Obstruction

Atherosclerosis

Risks that thrombus can
Dislodge

Grow to occlude blood flow

Pharmacologic treatment with anticoagulants
Heparin

Warfarin derivatives

Invasive intervention
Balloon-tipped catheter to remove or compress thrombus

Thrombophlebitis Caused by Inflammation (Phlebitis)
Causes
Trauma

Infection

Immobility

Commonly associated with
Endocarditis

Rheumatic heart disease

Embolism
Mass that is present and circulating in the blood

Can be a(n)
Air bubble

Fat

Bacterial

Cancer cells

Foreign substances

Dislodged thrombus

Obstructs vessel
Pulmonary emboli goes through the venous side or right side of the heart on the way to the pulmonary artery

Systemic or arterial emboli originates in left side of the heart

Associated with

• Myocardial infarction

• Left-side heart failure

- Endocarditis

- Valvular disease

- Dysrhythmias

Peripheral Arterial Disease

Thromboangiitis obliterans (Buerger disease)
Occurs most often in young men who are heavy smokers

Inflammatory disease of the peripheral arteries

Involves small or medium arteries of feet

- Sometimes involves hands

- May necessitate amputation

Raynaud disease and phenomenon
Spasms of small arteries of hands

- Sometimes involves feet

Fingertips thicken and nails become brittle

Raynaud phenomenon is secondary to primary disease, such as

- Scleroderma

- Pulmonary hypertension

Treatment of underlying condition
No known origin or treatment

Smoking aggravates the condition

Varicose Veins

Blood pools in vessel

Tends to be progressive

Often in legs

Leads to
Swelling

Fatigue

Possible ulcerations

Heart Disorders

Congestive Heart Failure

Can be left-sided or right-sided heart failure

Heart cannot generate adequate output

Acute onset often a result of acute myocardial ischemia

Congenital Heart Defects

Valvular defects

Tetralogy of Fallot

Septal defect

Infection and Inflammation of the Heart

Infective endocarditis

Leads to destruction and permanent damage to heart valves

Caused by bacteria (most common), virus, fungi, parasites

Patients with heart defects or damage usually take antibacterial medication prior to invasive procedures

Pericarditis

Inflammation of pericardium of heart

Rheumatic Fever

Results in formation of scar tissue of the myocardium and heart valves

In 10% of cases leads to rheumatic heart disease

Family tendency to develop

Begins as carditis (inflammation of heart)

Cardiac Dysrhythmias

Includes abnormal heart rate of

- Slow (bradyarrhythmia or bradycardia, <60bpm)

- Fast (tachyarrhythmia or tachycardia, >100bpm)

- Extrasystoles (intermittent additional heart contractions)

- Heart blocks (missed contractions)

May result from myocardial infarction or systemic abnormalities

Valvular Heart Disease

Valves are made of endocardial tissue

Endocardial damage can be congenital or acquired

Damage leads to stenosis and/or incompetent valve

Includes

- Valvular stenosis creates increased resistance, resulting in increased pressure in cardiac chamber behind valve

- Valvular regurgitation is failure of valve leaflet to close tightly, allowing back-flow of blood

  - Result of lesion that shrinks

  - Functional valvular regurgitation is a result of increased chamber size (cardiomegaly)

Stenosis

Aortic stenosis

Caused by congenital malformation, degeneration, or infection such as rheumatic fever

Results in a decreased blood flow

Symptoms are bradycardia and faint pulse

May lead to heart murmur and hypertrophy

Mitral stenosis
Impaired flow from left atrium to left ventricle

Caused by rheumatic fever, bacterial infections

Symptom is decreased cardiac output

May lead to

- Pulmonary hypertension

- Right ventricular heart failure

- And/or edema

Regurgitation
Flow in the opposite direction from normal

Types of valves
Mitral regurgitation (MR): backflow of blood from left ventricle into left atrium

Aortic regurgitation (AR): backflow of blood from aorta into the left ventricle

Pulmonic regurgitation (PR): backflow of blood from pulmonary artery into right ventricle

Tricuspid regurgitation (TR): backflow of blood from right ventricle into the right atrium

Heart Wall Disorders

Acute Pericarditis
Roughening and inflammation of pericardium (sac around heart)

Constrictive Pericarditis (Restrictive Pericarditis)
Forms fibrous lesions that encase heart
Compresses heart

Reduces output

Pericardial Effusion
Accumulation of fluid in pericardial cavity

Results in pressure on the heart

- Sudden development of pressure on the heart is tamponade

Cardiomyopathies

Myocardium: muscular walls of heart

Group of diseases that affect myocardium

Cause can be idiopathic (most common) or caused by an underlying condition

Types of Cardiomyopathy
Dilated cardiomyopathy (congestive cardiomyopathy)

- Ventricular distention and impaired systolic function

Hypertrophic cardiomyopathy

- Cause is often hypertensive or valvular heart disease
- Results in thickened interventricular septum (septum between the ventricle chambers)

Restrictive cardiomyopathy

- Myocardium becomes stiffened
- Heart enlarges (cardiomegaly)
- Dysrhythmias common
- Caused by infiltrative diseases such as amyloidosis

CARDIOVASCULAR SYSTEM PATHOPHYSIOLOGY QUIZ

1. Lesion of the carotid artery may lead to:
   a. heart attack
   b. stroke
   c. peripheral vascular disease
   d. ischemic heart disease

2. This blood pressure is hypertension:
   a. 120/80
   b. 130/70
   c. 140/90
   d. 110/70

3. Tachyarrhythmia or fast heart rate is that in excess of _____ bpm.
   a. 60
   b. 80
   c. 90
   d. 100

4. Angina pectoris is
   a. heart block
   b. heart murmur
   c. chest pain
   d. barrel chest

5. In this type of regurgitation there is a backflow of blood from the left ventricle into the left atrium:
   a. aortic
   b. pulmonic
   c. tricuspid
   d. mitral

6. In this type of heart wall disorder, fibrous lesions form and encase the heart:
   a. constrictive pericarditis
   b. acute pericarditis
   c. pericardial effusion
   d. cardiomyopathy

7. Which of the following terms means "of unknown cause"?
   a. etiology
   b. manifestation
   c. idiopathic
   d. late effect

8. This condition is also known as congestive cardiomyopathy:
   a. hypertrophic
   b. valvular
   c. dilated
   d. restrictive

9. This peripheral arterial disease most often occurs in young men who are heavy smokers:
   a. Buerger's
   b. Pick's
   c. Addison's
   d. Glasser's

10. This cardiomyopathy results in a thickened interventricular septum:
    a. restrictive
    b. congestive
    c. dilated
    d. hypertrophic

■ MALE GENITAL SYSTEM

MALE GENITAL SYSTEM—ANATOMY AND TERMINOLOGY

Function, reproduction

Structure, essential organs, and accessory organs (Figure 1-27)

Essential Organs

Testes (Gonads)

Produce sperm (male gamete)

Covered by tunica albuginea, located in scrotum

Produce testosterone

Vas Deferens

Is a tube

End of epididymis

Accessory Organs

Ducts (carry sperm from testes to exterior), sex glands (produce solutions that mix with sperm), and external genitalia

Seminal vesicles produce most seminal fluid

Prostate gland produces some seminal fluid and activates sperm

Bulbourethral gland (Cowper's glands) secretes a very small amount of seminal fluid

External genitalia: penis and scrotum

• Penis contains three columns of erectile tissue: two corpora cavernosa and one spongiosum

• Scrotum encloses testes

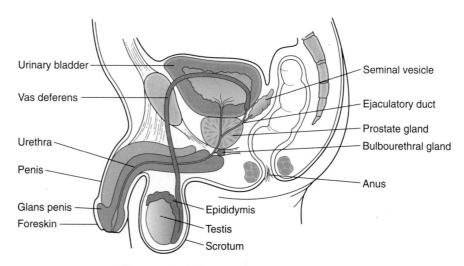

Figure **1-27** Male reproductive system.

COMBINING FORMS

1.	andr/o	male
2.	balan/o	glans penis
3.	epididym/o	epididymis
4.	orch/i	testicle
5.	orch/o	testicle
6.	orchi/o	testicle
7.	orchid/o	testicle
8.	prostat/o	prostate gland
9.	semin/i	semen
10.	sperm/o	sperm
11.	spermat/o	sperm
12.	test/o	testicle
13.	vas/o	vessel, vas deferens
14.	vesicul/o	seminal vesicles

SUFFIXES

1.	-one	hormone
2.	-pexy	fixation

MEDICAL ABBREVIATIONS

1.	BPH	benign prostatic hypertrophy
2.	PSA	prostate-specific antigen
3.	TURBT	transurethral resection of bladder tumor
4.	TURP	transurethral resection of prostate

MEDICAL TERMS

Cavernosa	Connection between the cavity of the penis and a vein
Cavernosography	Radiographic recording of a cavity, e.g., the pulmonary cavity or the main part of the penis
Cavernosometry	Measurement of the pressure in a cavity, e.g., the penis
Chordee	Condition resulting in the penis being bent downward
Corpora cavernosa	The two cavities of the penis
Epididymectomy	Surgical removal of the epididymis
Epididymis	Tube located at the top of the testes that stores sperm
Epididymovasostomy	Creation of a new connection between the vas deferens and epididymis
Meatotomy	Surgical enlargement of the opening of the urinary meatus

Orchiectomy	Castration, removal of the testes
Orchiopexy	Surgical procedure to release undescended testis and fixate within the scrotum
Penoscrotal	Referring to the penis and scrotum
Plethysmography	Determining the changes in volume of an organ part or body
Priapism	Painful condition in which the penis is constantly erect
Prostatotomy	Incision into the prostate
Transurethral resection, prostate	Procedure performed through the urethra by means of a cystoscopy to remove part or all of the prostate
Tumescence	State of being swollen
Tunica vaginalis	Covering of testes
Varicocele	Swelling of a scrotal vein
Vas deferens	Tube that carries sperm from the epididymis to the urethra
Vasogram	Recording of the flow in the vas deferens
Vasotomy	Incision in the vas deferens
Vasorrhaphy	Suturing of the vas deferens
Vasovasostomy	Reversal of a vasectomy
Vesiculectomy	Excision of the seminal vesicle
Vesiculotomy	Incision into the seminal vesicle

MALE GENITAL SYSTEM ANATOMY AND TERMINOLOGY QUIZ

1. This gland activates the sperm and produces some seminal fluid:
   a. seminal vesicle
   b. bulbourethral gland
   c. prostate gland
   d. scrotum

2. Carries the sperm from the testes to the exterior:
   a. duct
   b. sex gland
   c. tunica
   d. seminal

3. The penis contains these erectile tissues:
   a. one corpora cavernosa and two spongiosa
   b. two corpora cavernosa and two spongiosa
   c. one corpora cavernosa and one spongiosum
   d. two corpora cavernosa and one spongiosum

4. Also known as Cowper's gland:
   a. seminal vesicles
   b. bulbourethral gland
   c. prostate gland
   d. scrotum

5. Which of the following is NOT an accessory organ?
   a. gonads
   b. seminal vesicles
   c. prostate
   d. penis

6. Combining form meaning male:
   a. andr/o
   b. balan/o
   c. orchi/o
   d. test/o

7. Combining form meaning glans penis:
   a. balan/o
   b. vas/o
   c. vesicul/o
   d. orch/o

8. The testes are covered by the:
   a. seminal vesicles
   b. androgen
   c. chancre
   d. tunica albuginea

9. This abbreviation describes a surgical resection of the prostate that is accomplished by means of an endoscope inserted into the urethra:
   a. TURBT
   b. BPH
   c. UPJ
   d. TURP

10. This abbreviation describes a condition of the prostate in which there is an enlargement that is benign:
    a. TURBT
    b. BPH
    c. UPJ
    d. TURP

MALE GENITAL SYSTEM—PATHOPHYSIOLOGY

Male Genital System Disorders

Disorders of the Scrotum, Testes, and Epididymis

Cryptorchidism

Undescended testes

- Unilateral or bilateral

- Primarily result from obstruction

Treatment

- May descend spontaneously

- Administration of hormone to stimulate testosterone production

- Surgical intervention

Orchitis

Inflammation of testes

Most common cause is virus

- Such as mumps orchitis

May be associated with

- Gonorrhea

- Syphilis

- Tuberculosis

Symptoms

- Mild to severe pain in testes

- Mild to severe edema

- Feeling of weight in testicular area

Treatment

- Depends upon presence of underlying condition

Epididymitis

Inflammation of epididymis

Inflammatory response to trauma or infection

Abscess may form

Types

Sexually transmitted epididymitis

- Gonorrhea

- *T. pallidum*

- *T. vaginalis*

Nonspecific bacterial epididymitis

- *E. coli*

- *Streptococci*

- *Staphylococci*
- Associated with underlying urological disorder

Symptoms

Scrotal pain

Swelling

Erythema

Perhaps hydrocele formation

Treatment

Antibiotic

Bed rest

Ice packs

Scrotal support

Analgesics

Hydrocele (Figure 1-28)

Collection of fluid in membranes of tunica vaginalis

May be congenital or acquired

Congenital hydrocele may reabsorb due to a communication between the scrotal sac and peritoneal cavity and require no intervention

Symptoms

Scrotal enlargement

Usually painless

- Unless infection is present

Varicocele

Abnormal dilation of the plexus of veins in the spermatic cord leading to the scrotum

Decreases sperm production and motility

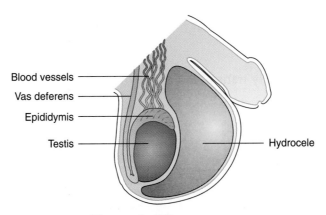

Figure **1-28** Hydrocele.

Symptoms

Usually painless

In elderly, may signal renal tumor

Treatment

Surgical intervention

Torsion of the testes (Figure 1-29)

Twisting of testes

Congenital abnormal development of the tunica vaginalis and spermatic cord

Trauma may precipitate

Symptoms

Sudden onset of severe pain

Nausea

Vomiting

Scrotal edema and tenderness

Fever

Treatment

Immediate surgical intervention

Cancer of testes

Usually occurs in younger men

Two main groups

- Germ cell tumors (GCT)

- Sex cord tumors

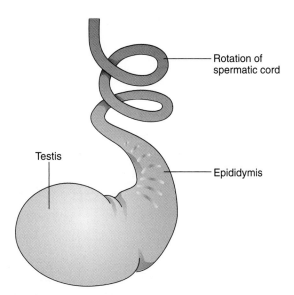

Figure **1-29** Torsion of testis.

Cancer of scrotum
Rare form of cancer

- Squamous cell carcinoma

Symptoms
Asymptomatic in early stages

Ulcerations in later stages

Treatment
Wide local excision

Mohs' microscopic technique

- Precise removal of tumor
- Layers are removed until no further microscopic evidence of abnormal cells is seen

Laser therapy

Lymph nodes are examined for metastasis

Disorders of the Urethra
Epispadias
Congenital anomaly

Urethral meatus is located on dorsal side of penis

Usually occurs in conjunction with other abnormalities

Treatment
Surgical reconstruction

Hypospadias
Most common abnormality of the penis

Urethral opening on the ventral side of penis

Results in curvature of penis

- Due to chordee

Treatment
Surgical reconstruction

Urethritis
Inflammation of urethra

Infectious urethritis can be gonococcal or nongonococcal

Nongonococcal organisms

- *C. trachomatis*
- *U. urealyticum*

Symptoms
Discharge

Inflammation of meatus

Burning

Itching

Urgent and frequent urination

In nongonococcal, symptoms are less

Treatment
Antibiotics based on organism

Disorders of the Penis
Balanitis
Inflammation of the glans

Causes
Syphilis

Trichomoniasis

Gonorrhea

Candida albicans

Tinea

Underlying disease

No circumcision

Symptoms
Irritation

Tenderness

Discharge

Edema

Ulceration

Swelling of lymph nodes

Treatment
Culture of discharge

Saline irrigation

Antibiotics

Phimosis and paraphimosis
Phimosis
Condition in which prepuce (foreskin) is constricted

• Prepuce cannot be retracted over the glans penis

Can occur at any age

Associated with poor hygiene and chronic infection in uncircumcised males

Symptoms
Erythema

Edema

Tenderness

Treatment
Surgical circumcision

Paraphimosis
Condition in which prepuce (foreskin) is constricted

Prepuce is retracted over glans penis and cannot be moved forward

Symptom
Edema

Treatment
Surgical

Peyronie disease
Also known as bent nail syndrome

Fibrotic condition

- Results in lateral curvature of penis during erection

Occurs most often in middle-aged men

Cause is unknown but associated with

- Diabetes

- Keloid development

- Dupuytren contracture (flexion deformity of toes and fingers)

Treatment
Sometimes spontaneous remission

Pharmacologic oxygenation increasing therapies

Surgical resection of fibrous bands

Cancer of penis
Occurs most often in men over 60

Increased risks

- More common in uncircumcised men

- Sexual partner with cervical carcinoma

- Human papillomavirus

Usually begins with small lesion beneath prepuce

Intraepithelial neoplasia is also known as

- Bowen's disease

- Erythroplasia of Queyrat

- Begins as noninvasive

Progresses to invasive if untreated

Metastasis to lymph nodes

Treatment
Excision

Mohs' micrographic technique

Radiation therapy

Laser therapy

Cryosurgery

Advanced tumors are treated with partial or total penectomy and chemotherapy

Disorders of the Prostate Gland
Benign prostatic hyperplasia (BPH)
Multiple fibroadenomatous nodules

• Related to aging

Growth compresses prostate

• Prostate obstructs bladder neck and urethra

• Decreases urine flow

It is thought that increased levels of estrogen/androgen cause BPH

Symptoms
Increased frequency and urgency of urination

Nocturia

Incontinence

Hesitancy

Diminished force

Postvoiding dribble

Screening
Prostate-specific antigen (PSA)

Digital rectal examination (DRE)

Treatment
Partial prostatectomy

Transurethral resection of prostate (TURP)

Excision of nodules

Hormone therapy

Placement of urethral stents

Prostatitis
Inflammation of prostate

• Acute or chronic

Causes
   Bacterial
Escherichia coli

Enterococci

Staphylococci

Streptococci

Chlamydia trachomatis

Ureaplasma urealyticum

Neisseria gonorrhea

Nonbacterial
Spontaneous

Symptoms
Acute prostatitis
Fever and chills

Lower back pain

Perineal pain

Dysuria

Tenderness, suprapubic

Urinary tract infection

Chronic prostatitis
Same as acute only with no infection in urinary tract

Treatment
Acute
Antibiotic based on culture

Chronic
No treatment available

Cancer of prostate
Indications are the cause is related to androgens

Predominately adenocarcinoma (95%)

No relationship between BPH and cancer of prostate

Symptoms
Asymptomatic in early stages

Later symptoms include

- Dysuria

- Back pain

- Hematuria

- Frequent urination

- Urinary retention

- Increased incidence of uremia

Stages

Two systems used to stage prostate cancer

- Whitmore-Jewett stages as indicated in Figure 1-30

- Tumor node metastasis (TNM) as indicated in Figure 1-31

Treatment

Dependent upon stage

WHITMORE-JEWETT STAGES:

Stage A is clinically undetectable tumor confined to
    the gland and is an incidental finding at prostate surgery.
A1: well-differentiated with focal involvement
A2: moderately or poorly differentiated or involves multiple foci in the gland
Stage B is tumor confined to the prostate gland.
B0: nonpalpable, PSA-detected
B1: single nodule in one lobe of the prostate
B2: more extensive involvement of one lobe or involvement of both lobes
Stage C is a tumor clinically localized to the periprostatic area but extending through the prostatic capsule; seminal vesicles may be involved.
C1: clinical extracapsular extension
C2: extracapsular tumor producing bladder outlet or ureteral obstruction
Stage D is metastatic disease.
D0: clinically localized disease (prostate only)
but persistently elevated enzymatic serum acid phosphatase
D1: regional lymph nodes only
D2: distant lymph nodes, metastases to bone or visceral organs
D3: D2 prostate cancer patients who relapse after adequate endocrine therapy

Figure **1-30** Whitmore-Jewett stages.

TNM STAGES:

Primary Tumor (T)

TX: Primary tumor cannot be assessed

T0: No evidence of primary tumor

T1: Clinically inapparent tumor not palpable or visible by imaging

    T1a: Tumor incidental histologic finding in 5% or less of tissue resected

    T1b: Tumor incidental histologic finding in more than 5% of tissue resected

    T1c: Tumor identified by needle biopsy (e.g., because of elevated PSA)

T2: Tumor confined within the prostate

    T2a: Tumor involves half a lobe or less

    T2b: Tumor involves more than half of a lobe, but not both lobes

    T2c: Tumor involves both lobes; extends through the prostatic capsule

T3a: Unilateral extracapsular extension

T3b: Bilateral extracapsular extension

T3c: Tumor invades the seminal vesicle(s)

T4: Tumor is fixed or invades adjacent structures other than the seminal vesicle(s)

    T4a: Tumor invades any of bladder neck, external sphincter, or rectum

    T4b: Tumor invades levator muscles and/or is fixed to the pelvic wall

Regional lymph nodes (N)

NX: Regional lymph nodes cannot be assessed

N0: No regional lymph node metastasis

N1: Metastasis in a single lymph node, 2 cm or less in greatest dimension

N2: Metastasis in a single lymph node, more than 2 cm but not more than 5 cm in greatest dimension; or multiple lymph node metastases, none more than 5 cm in greatest dimension

N3: Metastasis in a single lymph node more than 5 cm in greatest dimension

Distant metastases (M)

MX: Presence of distant metastasis cannot be assessed

M0: No distant metastasis

M1: Distant metastasis

    M1a: Nonregional lymph node(s)

    M1b: Bone(s)

    M1c: Other site(s)

Figure **1-31** TNM stages.

MALE GENITAL SYSTEM PATHOPHYSIOLOGY QUIZ

1. What is the condition in which the testes do not descend?
   a. cryptorchidism
   b. Bowen's disease
   c. torsion
   d. hypospadias

2. Orchitis is most often caused by a:
   a. bacteria
   b. virus
   c. parasite
   d. fungus

3. A condition that can be either congenital or acquired through trauma and that involves twisting of the testes is:
   a. hydrocele
   b. hypospadias
   c. cryptorchidism
   d. torsion

4. Cancer of the _____ is divided into two main groups of germ cell tumors and sex cord tumors.
   a. testes
   b. penis
   c. scrotum
   d. prostate

5. This type of surgical technique involves excision of a lesion in layers until no further evidence of abnormality is seen:
   a. Bowen's
   b. Addison's
   c. Mohs'
   d. laser

6. Epispadias is a disorder of the urethra in which the urethral meatus is located on the _____ side of the penis:
   a. ventral
   b. dorsal
   c. lateral
   d. medial

7. Inflammation of the glans is:
   a. phimosis
   b. paraphimosis
   c. urethritis
   d. balanitis

8. This disease is also known as the bent nail syndrome:
   a. Bowen's
   b. Peyronie
   c. Addison's
   d. Whitmore-Jewett

9. The condition in which multiple fibroadenomatous nodules form and lead to decreased urine flow. The condition is thought to be related to increased levels of estrogen/androgen.
   a. BPH
   b. DRE
   c. GCT
   d. TNM

10. Cancer of the prostate is predominately this type of cancer:
    a. sex cord
    b. adenocarcinoma
    c. squamous cell
    d. seminoma

■ URINARY SYSTEM

URINARY SYSTEM—ANATOMY AND TERMINOLOGY

Removes waste materials

Regulates fluid volume

Maintains electrolytes, water, and acid balance

Assists liver in detoxification

Organs (Figure 1-32)

Kidneys

Ureters

Urinary bladder

Urethra

Kidneys (Figure 1-33)

Electrolytes and fluid balance

Controls pH balance

Two organs located behind peritoneum (retroperitoneal space)

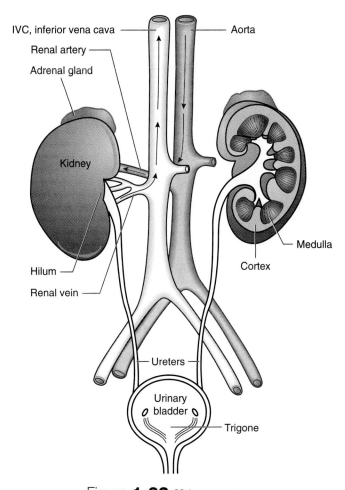

Figure **1-32** Urinary system.

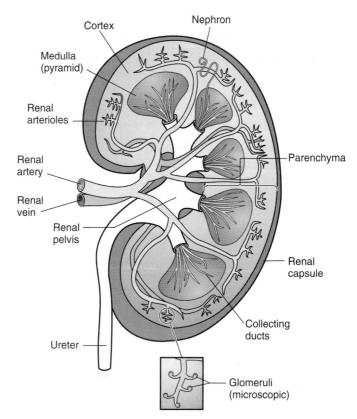

Figure **1-33** Kidney.

Cortex (outer layer)

Medulla (inner portion)

Pyramids (divisions of medulla)

Papilla (inner part of pyramids)

Pelvis (receptacle for urine within the kidney)

Calyces surround top of renal pelvis

Ureters
Narrow tubes connecting kidney and bladder

Urinary Bladder
Reservoir for urine

Shaped like an upside down pear with three surfaces

- Posterior (base)

- Anterior (neck)

- Superior (peritoneum)

Trigone

- Smooth area inside bladder

- Formed by openings of the ureters and urethra

Urethra

Canal from bladder to exterior of body

Urinary meatus, outside opening of the urethra

COMBINING FORMS

1.	albumin/o	albumin
2.	azot/o	urea
3.	cyst/o	bladder
4.	glomerul/o	glomerulus
5.	glyc/o	sugar
6.	glycos/o	sugar
7.	hydr/o	water
8.	lith/o	stone
9.	meat/o	meatus
10.	nephr/o	kidney
11.	noct/i	night
12.	olig/o	scant, few
13.	pyel/o	renal pelvis
14.	ren/o	kidney
15.	son/o	sound
16.	ur/o	urine
17.	ureter/o	ureter
18.	urethr/o	urethra
19.	urin/o	urine
20.	vesic/o	bladder

PREFIXES

1.	dys-	painful
2.	peri-	surrounding
3.	poly-	many
4.	retro-	behind

SUFFIXES

1.	-eal	pertaining to
2.	-lithiasis	condition of stones
3.	-lysis	separation
4.	-plasty	repair
5.	-rrhaphy	suture
6.	-tripsy	crush

MEDICAL ABBREVIATIONS

1.	ARF	acute renal failure
2.	BUN	blood urea nitrogen
3.	ESRD	end-stage renal disease
4.	HD	hemodialysis
5.	IVP	intravenous pyelogram
6.	KUB	kidney, ureter, bladder
7.	pH	symbol for acid/base level
8.	sp gr	specific gravity
9.	UA	urinalysis
10.	UPJ	ureteropelvic junction
11.	UTI	urinary tract infection

MEDICAL TERMS

Bulbocavernosus	Muscle that constricts the vagina in a female and the urethra in a male
Bulbourethral	Gland with duct leading to the urethra
Calculus	Concretion of mineral salts, also called a stone
Calycoplasty	Surgical reconstruction of recess of renal pelvis
Calyx	Recess of renal pelvis
Cystolithectomy	Removal of a calculus (stone) from urinary bladder
Cystometrogram	CMG, measurement of the pressures and capacity of the urinary bladder
Cystoplasty	Surgical reconstruction of the bladder
Cystorrhaphy	Suture of the bladder
Cystoscopy	Use of a scope to view the bladder
Cystostomy	Surgical creation of an opening into the bladder
Cystotomy	Incision into the bladder
Cystourethroplasty	Surgical reconstruction of the bladder and urethra
Cystourethroscopy	Use of a scope to view the bladder and urethra
Dilation	Stretching or expansion
Dysuria	Painful urination
Endopyelotomy	Procedure involving the bladder and ureters, including the insertion of a stent into the renal pelvis
Extracorporeal	Occurring outside of the body
Fundoplasty	Repair of the bottom of the bladder
Hydrocele	Sac of fluid

Kock pouch	Surgical creation of a urinary bladder from a segment of the ileum
Nephrocutaneous fistula	A channel from the kidney to the skin
Nephrolithotomy	Removal of a kidney stone through an incision made into the kidney
Nephrorrhaphy	Suturing of the kidney
Nephrostomy	Creation of a channel into the renal pelvis of the kidney
Transureteroureterostomy	Surgical connection of one ureter to the other ureter
Transvesical ureterolithotomy	Removal of a ureter stone (calculus) through the bladder
Ureterectomy	Surgical removal of a ureter, either totally or partially
Ureterocutaneous fistula	Channel from ureter to exterior skin
Ureteroenterostomy	Creation of a connection between the intestine and the ureter
Ureterolithotomy	Removal of a stone from the ureter
Ureterolysis	Freeing of adhesions of the ureter
Ureteroneocystostomy	Surgical connection of the ureter to a new site on the bladder
Ureteropyelography	Ureter and renal pelvis radiography
Ureterotomy	Incision into the ureter
Urethrocystography	Radiography of the bladder and urethra
Urethromeatoplasty	Surgical repair of the urethra and meatus
Urethropexy	Fixation of the urethra by means of surgery
Urethroplasty	Surgical repair of the urethra
Urethrorrhaphy	Suturing of the urethra
Urethroscopy	Use of a scope to view the urethra
Vesicostomy	Surgical creation of a connection of the viscera of the bladder to the skin

URINARY SYSTEM ANATOMY AND TERMINOLOGY QUIZ

1. The outer covering of the kidney:
   a. medulla
   b. pyramids
   c. cortex
   d. papilla

2. Which is not a division of the kidneys?
   a. pelvis
   b. pyramids
   c. cortex
   d. trigone

3. The inner portion of the kidneys:
   a. medulla
   b. pyramids
   c. cortex
   d. papilla

4. The smooth area inside the bladder:
   a. pyramids
   b. calyces
   c. trigone
   d. cystocele

5. The narrow tube connecting the kidney and bladder:
   a. urethra
   b. ureter
   c. meatus
   d. trigone

6. Which of the following is NOT a surface of the urinary bladder?
   a. posterior
   b. anterior
   c. superior
   d. inferior

7. Combining form that means stone:
   a. azot/o
   b. cyst/o
   c. lith/o
   d. olig/o

8. Term meaning painful urination:
   a. pyuria
   b. dysuria
   c. diuresis
   d. hyperemia

9. Combining form meaning scant:
   a. glyc/o
   b. hydr/o
   c. meat/o
   d. olig/o

10. Term that describes renal failure that is acute:
    a. ARF
    b. ESRD
    c. HD
    d. BPH

URINARY SYSTEM—PATHOPHYSIOLOGY

Renal Failure

Acute Renal Failure
Sudden onset of renal failure

Cause
Trauma

Infection

Inflammation

Toxicity

Symptoms
Uremia

Oliguria (decreased output) or anuria (no output)

Hyperkalemia (high potassium in blood)

Pulmonary edema

Types
Prerenal

- Associated with poor systemic perfusion
- Decreased renal blood flow
  - Such as with congestive heart failure

Intrarenal

- Associated with renal parenchyma disease (functional tissue of kidney)
  - Such as acute interstitial nephritis

Postrenal

- Resulting from urine flow obstruction out of kidney

Treatment
Underlying condition

Dialysis

Monitoring of fluid and electrolyte balance

Chronic Renal Failure
Gradual loss of function

- Progressively more severe renal insufficiency until end stage of
  - End-stage renal disease
  - Irreversible kidney failure

Stages
Stage I: Blood flow through kidney increases, kidney enlarges

Stage II: (mild) Small amounts of blood protein (albumin) leak into urine (microalbuminuria)

Stage III: (moderate) Albumin and other protein losses increase; patient may develop high blood pressure and kidney loses ability to filter waste

Stage IV: (severe) Large amounts of urine pass through kidney; blood pressure increases

Stage V: Ability to filter waste nearly stops; dialysis or transplant only option

Cause

Long-term exposure to nephrotoxins

Diabetes

Hypertension

Symptoms

No symptoms until well advanced

Polyuria

Nausea or anorexia

Dehydration

Neurologic manifestations

Stages of nephron loss

Decreased reserve

- 60% loss

Renal insufficiency

- 75% loss

End-stage renal failure

- 90% loss

Treatment

No cure

Dialysis

Kidney transplant

Urinary Tract Infections (UTI)

Cystitis—Bacterial

Cause

Bacteria, usually *E. coli*

Symptoms

Lower abdominal pain

Dysuria

Lower back pain

Urinary frequency and urgency

Cloudy, foul-smelling urine

Systemic signs

Fever

Malaise

Nausea

Treatment
Antibiotics

Increased fluid intake

Cystitis—Nonbacterial
Cause
Unknown

May later produce bacterial infection

Treatment
No known treatment

Acute Pyelonephritis (Figure 1-34)
Infection of the renal pelvis and medullary tissue

• May involve one or both kidneys

Cause
E. coli

Proteus

Pseudomonas

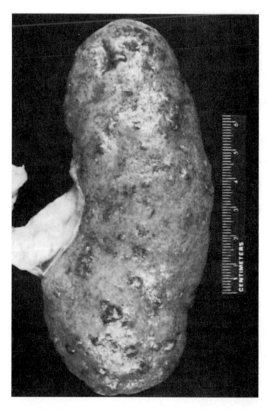

Figure **1-34** Acute pyelonephritis. Cortical surface is dotted with abscesses. (From Cotran R, Kumar V, Robbins S: *Robbins pathologic basis of disease,* Philadelphia, 1994, WB Saunders, p 969.)

Symptoms

Fever

Chills

Groin or flank pain

Dysuria

Pyuria

Nocturia

Treatment

Antibiotics

Chronic Pyelonephritis

Recurrent infection that causes scarring of kidney

Cause is difficult to determine

- Repeated infections
- Obstructive conditions

Symptoms

Hypertension

Dysuria

Flank pain

Increased frequency of urination

Glomerular Disorders

Function of the glomerulus is blood filtration

Nephrotic Syndrome

Disease of the kidneys that includes damage to the membrane of the glomerulus

Accompanied by

- Hypoalbuminemia
- Hypercholesterolemia
- Edema

Damage to the glomerulus results from

- Infection
- Immune response
  - Most predominant cause of dysfunction is exposure to toxins

May be a manifestation of an underlying condition, such as diabetes

Symptoms

Edema

Weight gain

Pallor

Treatment

Glucocorticoids, such as prednisone

- Reduces inflammation

Sodium reduction

Careful monitoring for continued inflammation

Acute Poststreptococcal Glomerulonephritis (APSGN)

Cause

Streptococcus infection

- With certain types of group A beta-hemolytic *Streptococcus*

Creates an antigen-antibody complex

- Infiltrates the glomerular capillaries

- Results in inflammation in kidneys

- Inflammation interferes with normal kidney function

- Fluid and waste build-up

- Can lead to acute renal failure and scarring

Usually occurs in children 3 to 7 years of age

- Most often in boys

Symptoms

Back and flank pain

Cloudy, dark urine

Oliguria (decreased output)

Edema

Elevated blood pressure

Fatigue

Malaise

Headache

Nausea

Elevated blood pressure

Treatment

Sodium reduction

Antibiotics

Careful monitoring for continued inflammation

Urinary Tract Obstructions

Interference with urine flow

Causes dilation of urinary system

Increased urinary tract infection

Obstruction can be

- Functional

- Anatomic

  - Also known as obstructive uropathy

Kidney Stones

Formed of mineral salts

Develop anywhere in urinary tract

Tend to form in presence of excess salt and decreased fluid intake

- Most stones are formed of calcium salts

- Staghorn calculus form in the renal pelvis

Symptoms

Asymptomatic until obstruction occurs

Obstruction results in renal colic

- Extremely intense pain in flank

- Nausea

- Vomiting

- Cold, clammy skin

- Increased pulse rate

Treatment

Stone usually passes spontaneously

May use extracorporeal shock wave lithotripsy (ESWL) to break up stone

- Laser lithotripsy may also be used

Drugs may be used to dissolve the stone

Preventative treatment to adjust pH level

- Increased fluid intake

Bladder Carcinoma

Tumors originate in the transitional epithelial lining

Tends to recur

Often metastatic to the liver and bone

Symptoms

Often asymptomatic in early stage

Hematuria

Dysuria

Frequent urination

Infections common

Increased Risks
Cigarette smoking

Working with industrial chemicals

Analgesics used in large amounts

Recurrent bladder infections

Treatment
Immunotherapy (bacillus Calmette-Guérin vaccine, BCG)

Excision

Chemotherapy

Radiation therapy

Hydronephrosis
Distention of kidney with urine

- Due to an obstruction

- Usually as a result of a kidney stone

- May also be due to scarring, tumor, edema from infection, or other obstruction

Symptoms
Usually asymptomatic

Mild flank pain

Infection may develop

May lead to chronic renal failure

Treatment
Treat the underlying condition, such as removal of the stone or antibiotics for infection

Dilation of the stricture

Vascular Disorders

Nephrosclerosis
Excessive hardening and thickening of vascular structure of kidney
- Reduces blood supply
  - Increases blood pressure
  - Results in atrophy and ischemia of structures
  - May lead to chronic renal failure

Symptoms
Asymptomatic in early stages

Treatment
Diuretics

ACE inhibitors (angiotensin-converting enzyme)

Beta blockers that block the release of resin

Antihypertensive drugs

Sodium intake reduction

Congenital Disorders

Polycystic Kidney
Numerous kidney cysts

Genetic disease

Symptoms
Asymptomatic until 40s

Develops chronic renal failure

Cysts may spread to other organs, such as liver

Treatment
As for chronic renal failure

Wilms' Tumor
Usually unilateral kidney tumors

Most common tumor in children

Usually advanced at time of diagnosis

• Metastasis to lungs at time of diagnosis is common

Symptoms
Asymptomatic until abdominal mass becomes apparent at age 1 to 5

Treatment
Excision

Radiation therapy

Chemotherapy

Usually a combination of above

URINARY SYSTEM PATHOPHYSIOLOGY QUIZ

1. Which of the following is NOT a type of acute renal failure?
   a. prerenal
   b. intrarenal
   c. interrenal
   d. postrenal

2. The loss of nephron function in end-stage renal disease is:
   a. 60%
   b. 70%
   c. 80%
   d. 90%

3. The cause of bacterial cystitis is usually:
   a. proteus
   b. *Pseudomonas*
   c. *Staphylococci*
   d. *E. coli*

4. The primary treatment for acute pyelonephritis would be:
   a. prednisone
   b. sodium reduction
   c. antibiotics
   d. BCG

5. APSGN stands for:
   a. advanced poststaphylococcal glomerulonephritis
   b. acute poststreptococcal glomerulonephritis
   c. acute poststaphylococcal glomerulonephritis
   d. advanced poststreptococcal glomerulonephritis

6. Obstructive uropathy is also known as:
   a. pyelonephritis
   b. renal failure
   c. urinary tract obstruction
   d. nephrotic syndrome

7. A treatment for kidney stone may be:
   a. ESWL
   b. prednisone
   c. open surgical procedure
   d. diuretics

8. The treatment for hydronephrosis involves:
   a. an open surgical procedure
   b. use of diuretics
   c. treatment of the underlying condition
   d. BCG

9. This is a congential condition in which numerous cysts form in the kidney:
   a. Wilms'
   b. polycystic kidney
   c. nephrosclerosis
   d. nephrotic syndrome

10. The treatment of Wilms' would NOT include which of the following?
    a. excision
    b. chemotherapy
    c. diuretic
    d. radiation therapy

■ DIGESTIVE SYSTEM

DIGESTIVE SYSTEM—ANATOMY AND TERMINOLOGY

Function: digestion, absorption, and elimination

Includes gastrointestinal tract (alimentary canal) and accessory organs

Mouth (Figure 1-35)

Roof: hard palate, soft palate, uvula (projection at back of mouth)

Floor: contains tongue (Figure 1-36), muscles, taste buds, and lingual frenulum, which anchors tongue to floor of mouth

Teeth

Thirty-two teeth (permanent)

Names of teeth: incisor, cuspid, bicuspid, and tricuspid

Tooth has crown (outer portion), neck (narrow part below gum line), root (end section), and pulp cavity (core)

Salivary Glands (Figure 1-37)

Surround the mouth and produce saliva

Parotid

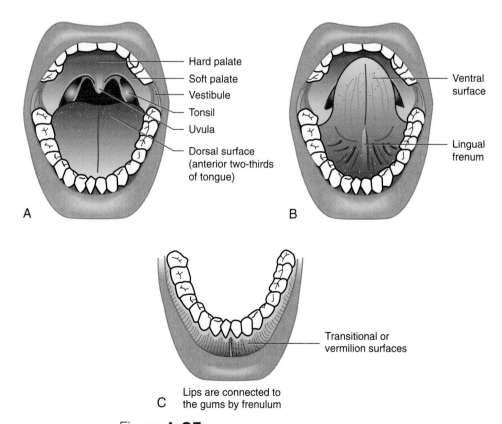

Figure **1-35** Anatomic structure of the mouth.

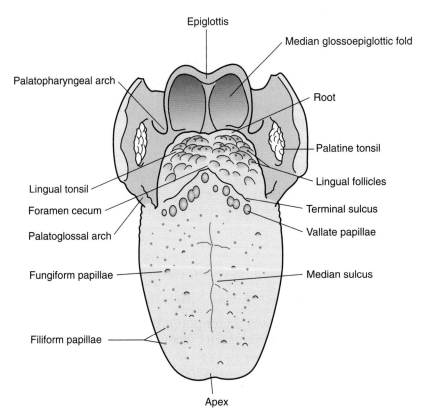

Figure **1-36** Dorsum of the tongue.

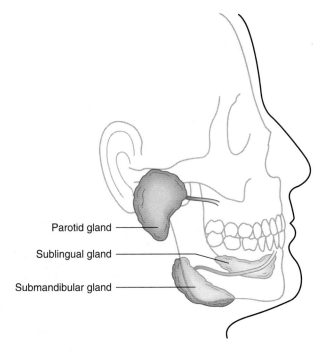

Figure **1-37** Major salivary glands.

Submandibular

Sublingual

Pharynx or Throat (Figure 1-38)

Muscular tube through which air and food/water travel

Epiglottis covers larynx when swallowing

Esophagus

Muscular tube that carries food to stomach by means of peristalsis (rhythmic contractions)

Stomach

Sphincter (ring of muscles) at entry into stomach (gastroesophageal or cardiac)

Three parts of stomach: fundus (upper part), body (middle part), antrum/pylorus (lower part)

Lined with rugae (folds of mucosal membrane)

Pyloric sphincter opens to allow food to leave stomach and enter small intestine

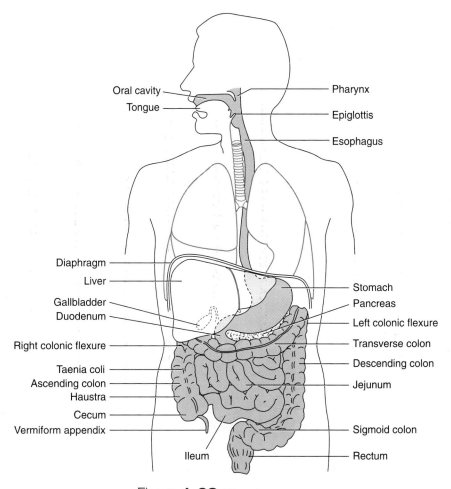

Figure **1-38** Digestive system.

Small Intestine

Duodenum

Jejunum

Ileum

Large Intestine

Extends from ileum to anus

Cecum, from which appendix extends, connects ileum and colon

Colon, divided into ascending, transverse, descending, and sigmoid

Sigmoid colon, connected to rectum that terminates at anus

Accessory Organs

Liver produces bile, sent to gallbladder via hepatic duct and cystic duct

Gallbladder stores bile, sent to duodenum via common bile duct

Pancreas produces enzymes sent through pancreatic duct to common bile duct then to duodenum

Islets of Langerhans produce insulin and glucagon

Peritoneum

Serous membrane lines abdominal cavity and maintains organs in correct anatomic place

COMBINING FORMS

1.	abdomin/o	abdomen
2.	an/o	anus
3.	appendic/o	appendix
4.	bil/i	bile
5.	bilirubin/o	bile pigment
6.	cec/o	cecum
7.	celi/o	abdomen
8.	chol/e	gall/bile
9.	cholangio/o	bile duct
10.	cholecyst/o	gallbladder
11.	choledoch/o	common bile duct
12.	col/o	colon
13.	dent/i	tooth
14.	diverticul/o	diverticulum
15.	duoden/o	duodenum
16.	enter/o	small intestine

17. esophag/o	esophagus
18. gastr/o	stomach
19. gingiv/o	gum
20. gloss/o	tongue
21. hepat/o	liver
22. herni/o	hernia
23. ile/o	ileum
24. jejun/o	jejunum
25. lapar/o	abdomen
26. lingu/o	tongue
27. lip/o	fat
28. lith/o	stone
29. or/o	mouth
30. palat/o	palate
31. pancreat/o	pancreas
32. peritone/o	peritoneum
33. polyp/o	polyp
34. proct/o	rectum
35. pylor/o	pylorus
36. rect/o	rectum
37. sial/o	saliva
38. sigmoid/o	sigmoid colon
39. steat/o	fat
40. stomat/o	mouth
41. uvul/o	uvula

SUFFIXES

1. -cele	hernia
2. -chezia	defecation
3. -phagia	eating

MEDICAL ABBREVIATIONS

1. EGD	esophagogastroduodenoscopy
2. EGJ	esophagogastric junction
3. ERCP	endoscopic retrograde cholangiopancreatography
4. GERD	gastroesophageal reflux disease
5. GI	gastrointestinal

6. HJR	hepatojugular reflux
7. LLQ	left lower quadrant
8. LUQ	left upper quadrant
9. PEG	percutaneous endoscopic gastrostomy
10. RLQ	right lower quadrant
11. RUQ	right upper quadrant

MEDICAL TERMS

Anastomosis	Surgical connection of two tubular structures, such as two pieces of the intestine
Biliary	Refers to gallbladder, bile, or bile duct
Cholangiography	Radiographic recording of the bile ducts
Cholecystectomy	Surgical removal of the gallbladder
Cholecystoenterostomy	Creation of a connection between the gallbladder and intestine
Colonoscopy	Fiberscopic examination of the entire colon that may include part of the terminal ileum
Colostomy	Artificial opening between the colon and the abdominal wall
Diverticulum	Protrusion in the wall of an organ
Dysphagia	Difficulty swallowing
Enterolysis	Releasing of adhesions of intestine
Eventration	Protrusion of the bowel through an opening in the abdomen
Evisceration	Pulling the viscera outside of the body through an incision
Exstrophy	Condition in which an organ is turned inside out
Fulguration	Use of electric current to destroy tissue
Gastrointestinal	Pertaining to the stomach and intestine
Gastroplasty	Operation on the stomach for repair or reconfiguration
Gastrostomy	Artificial opening between the stomach and the abdominal wall
Hernia	Organ or tissue protruding through the wall or cavity that usually contains it
Ileostomy	Artificial opening between the ileum and the abdominal wall
Imbrication	Overlapping
Incarcerated	Regarding hernias, a constricted, irreducible hernia that may cause obstruction of an intestine
Intussusception	Slipping of one part of the intestine into another part
Jejunostomy	Artificial opening between the jejunum and the abdominal wall
Laparoscopy	Exploration of the abdomen and pelvic cavities using a scope placed through a small incision in the abdominal wall
Lithotomy	Incision into an organ or a duct for the purpose of removing a stone

Lithotripsy	Crushing of a stone by sound wave or force
Paraesophageal hiatus hernia	Hernia that is near the esophagus
Proctosigmoidoscopy	Fiberscopic examination of the sigmoid colon and rectum
Sialolithotomy	Surgical removal of a stone of the salivary gland or duct
Varices	Varicose veins
Volvulus	Twisted section of the intestine

DIGESTIVE SYSTEM ANATOMY AND TERMINOLOGY QUIZ

1. This is NOT a part of the small intestine:
   a. ileum
   b. cecum
   c. duodenum
   d. jejunum

2. Term meaning a ring of muscles:
   a. pyloric
   b. parotid
   c. epiglottis
   d. sphincter

3. The throat is also known as the:
   a. larynx
   b. epiglottis
   c. esophagus
   d. pharynx

4. The three parts of the stomach:
   a. pyloric, rugae, fundus
   b. fundus, body, antrum
   c. antrum, pyloric, rugae
   d. ilium, fundus, pyloric

5. The projection at the back of the mouth:
   a. palate
   b. sublingual
   c. uvula
   d. parotid

6. Mucosal membrane that lines the stomach:
   a. cecum
   b. rugae
   c. frenulum
   d. fundus

7. The parts of the colon are:
   a. ascending, transverse, descending, sigmoid
   b. ascending, descending, sigmoid
   c. transverse, descending, sigmoid
   d. descending, sigmoid

8. Combining form meaning abdomen:
   a. an/o
   b. cec/o
   c. celi/o
   d. col/o

9. Term that means tying together of two ends of a tube:
   a. anastomosis
   b. amylase
   c. aphthous stomatitis
   d. atresia

10. Abbreviation that means a scope placed through the esophagus, into the stomach, and to the duodenum:
    a. ERCP
    b. EGD
    c. GERD
    d. PEG

DIGESTIVE SYSTEM—PATHOPHYSIOLOGY

Disorders of the Oral Cavity

Cleft Lip and Cleft Palate (Figure 1-39)
Congenital defect

Cleft lip and palate is a condition in which the lip and palate do not properly join together

Causes feeding problems

• Infants cannot create sufficient suction for feeding

• Danger of aspirating food

• Results in speech defects

Treatment
Surgical repair of defects

Ulceration
Canker sore

• Ulceration of the oral mucosa

Also known as

• Aphthous ulcer (aphtha: small ulcer)

• Aphthous stomatitis

Heals spontaneously

Infections
Candidiasis
Candida albicans is naturally found in mouth

Thrush (oral candidiasis) is overarching infection

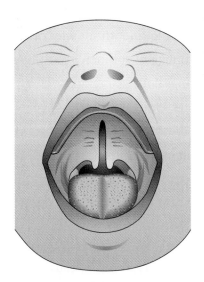

Figure **1-39** Cleft palate.

Causes

Antibiotic regimen

Chemotherapy

Glucocorticoids

Common in diabetics and AIDS patients

Treatment

Nystatin (topical fungal agent)

Herpes simplex type 1

Herpetic stomatitis

- Viral cold sores and blisters

- Associated with herpes simplex virus type 1 (HSV-1)

Treatment

No cure

May be alleviated somewhat by antiviral medications

Cancer of the Oral Cavity

Most common type is squamous cell carcinoma

- Kaposi's sarcoma is type seen in AIDS patients

Increased in smokers

Lip cancer also increased in smokers

Poor prognosis

Usually asymptomatic until later stages

Metastasis through lymph nodes

Esophageal Disorders

Scleroderma

Also known as progressive systemic sclerosis

Atrophy of the smooth muscles of the lower esophagus

Lower esophageal sphincter (LES) does not close properly

- Leads to esophageal reflux

- Strictures form

Symptom

Predominantly dysphagia

Esophagitis

Inflammation of esophagus

Types

Acute

Most common type is that caused by hiatal hernia

Infectious esophagitis is common in patients with AIDS

Ingestion of strong alkaline or acid substances

• Such as those in household cleaners

Inflammation leads to scarring

Chronic
Most common type is that caused by LES reflux

Cancer of the Esophagus
Most common type is leiomyoma (smooth muscle tumor)

Usually caused by continued irritation

• Smoking

• Alcohol

• Hiatal hernia

• Chronic esophagitis

Poor prognosis

Hiatal Hernia
Diaphragm goes over the stomach

• Esophagus passes through the diaphragm at natural opening (hiatus)

• Part of the stomach protrudes (herniates) through the opening in the diaphragm into the thorax

Types (Figure 1-40)
Sliding

• Stomach and gastroesophageal junction protrude through the hiatus

Paraesophageal

• Part of fundus protrudes

Symptoms
Heartburn

Reflux

Belching

Lying down causes discomfort

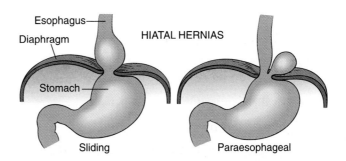

Figure **1-40** Sliding and paraesophageal hernias (hiatal hernias).

Dysphagia

Substernal pain after eating

Gastroesophageal Reflux Disease (GERD)
Associated with hiatal hernias

- Reflux of gastric contents

Lower esophageal sphincter does not constrict properly

Treatment
Reduce irritants, such as

- Smoking

- Spicy foods

- Alcohol

Antacids

Elevate the head of the bed

Avoid tight clothing

Stomach and Duodenum Disorders

Gastritis
Inflammation of the stomach

Acute superficial gastritis
Mild, transient irritation

Causes
Excessive alcohol

Infection

Food allergies

Spicy foods

Aspirin

Symptoms
Nausea

Vomiting

Anorexia

Bleeding in more severe cases

Epigastric pain

Treatment
Usually spontaneous remission in 2 to 3 days

Removal of underlying irritation

Antibiotics for infection

Chronic atrophic gastritis
Progressive atrophy of epithelium

Types

Type A, atrophic or fundal

- Involves the fundus of the stomach

- Autoimmune disease

  · Decreases acid secretion

  · Results in high gastrin levels

Type B, antral

- Involves the antrum region of the stomach

- Often associated with the elderly

  · May be associated with pernicious anemia

- Low gastrin levels

- Usually caused by infection

- Irritated by alcohol, drugs, and tobacco

Peptic Ulcers

Erosive area on the mucosa

- Extends below epithelium

- Chronic ulcers have scar tissue at the base of the erosive area

Ulcers can occur anyplace on the gastrointestinal tract but typically are found on the

- Lower esophagus

- Stomach

- Proximal duodenum

Some causes

Alcohol

Aspirin

Severe stress

Bacterial infection caused by *Helicobacter pylori (H. pylori)*, 90% of the time

Genetic factor

Symptoms

Epigastric pain when stomach is empty

- Relieved by food or antacid

Burning

May include

- Vomiting red blood

- Nausea

- Weight loss

- Anorexia

Severe cases may include

- Obstruction

- Hemorrhage

- Perforation

Treatment
Surgical intervention

Antacids

Dietary restrictions

Rest

Antibiotics

Gastric Cancer
Most often occurs in men over 40

Cause is unknown

Predisposing Factors
Atrophic gastritis

Pernicious anemia

History of nonhealing gastric ulcer

Blood type A

Geographic factors

Environmental factors

Carcinogenic foods

- Smoked meats

- Nitrates

- Pickled foods

Symptoms
Usually asymptomatic in early stages

Treatment
Excision

Chemotherapy

Radiation

Prognosis is poor

Pyloric Stenosis
Narrowing of the pyloric sphincter

Signs appear soon after birth

- Failure to thrive

- Projectile vomiting

Treatment
Surgery to relieve the stenosis (pyloromyotomy)

Intestinal Disorders

■ Small Intestine

Malabsorption Conditions

Celiac disease

Most important malabsorption condition

Villi atrophy in response to food containing gluten and lose ability to absorb

• Gluten is a protein found in wheat, rye, oats, and barley

Symptoms

Malnutrition

Muscle wasting

Distended abdomen

Diarrhea

Fatigue

Weakness

Steatorrhea (excess fat in feces)

Treatment

Gluten-free diet

Steroids when necessary

Lactase deficiency

Enzyme deficiency

• Secondary to gastrointestinal damage, such as

  • Regional enteritis

  • Infection

• Genetic defect

Symptoms

Intolerance to milk

Treatment

Elimination of milk

Crohn's disease (regional enteritis)
Cause
Unknown

Symptoms
Vary greatly

Diarrhea

Gas

Fever

Abdominal pain

Malaise

Anorexia

Weight loss

Treatment
No specific treatment

Antidiarrheal drugs

Palliative medications based on symptoms

Resection of the affected section of intestine

Appendicitis
Inflammation of vermiform appendix that projects from the cecum

Obstruction of lumen leads to infection

- Appendix becomes hypoxic (decreased oxygen levels)
- May cause gangrene
- May rupture, causing peritonitis

Symptoms
Periumbilical (around umbilicus) pain, initially

Right lower quadrant (RLQ) pain as inflammation progresses

Nausea

Vomiting

Possible diarrhea

Treatment
Management of any perforation or abscess

Peritonitis
Inflammation of the peritoneum (membrane that lines the abdominal cavity)

Usually a result of

- Spread of infection from abdominal organ
- Puncture wound to abdomen
- Rupture of gastrointestinal tract

Abscesses form, resulting in adhesions

- May result in obstruction

Types
Acute

Chronic

Symptoms
Abdominal pain

Vomiting

Rigid abdomen

Fever

Leukocytosis (increased white cells in blood)

Treatment
Antibiotics

Suction of stomach and intestines

If possible, surgical removal of origin of infection, such as appendix

Fluid replacement

Bed rest

Obstruction
Any interference with passage of intestinal contents

May be

- Acute

- Chronic

- Partial

- Total

Types
Nonmechanical

- Paralytic ileus

- Result of trauma or toxin

Mechanical

- Result of tumors, adhesions, hernias

- Simple mechanical obstruction

  - One point of obstruction

- Closed-loop obstruction

  - At least two points of obstruction

Symptoms
Abdominal distention

Pain

Vomiting

Total constipation

Treatment
Surgical intervention

Symptomatic treatment

■ Large Intestine

Diverticulosis

Herniation of intestinal mucosa

- Forms sacs in the lining, called diverticula

Diverticulitis

Sacs fill and become inflamed

- Common in aged

Symptoms

Diarrhea or constipation

Gas

Abdominal discomfort

Complications

Perforation

Bleeding

Peritonitis

Abscess

Obstruction

Treatment

Antimicrobials as necessary

Stool softeners

Dietary restrictions of solid foods

Surgical intervention if necessary

Ulcerative Colitis (Figure 1-41)

Inflammation of rectum that progresses to colon

May develop into toxic megacolon

- Leads to obstruction and dilation of colon

Increased risk of colorectal cancer

Symptoms

Diarrhea

- Blood and mucus may be present

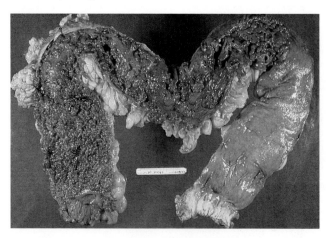

Figure **1-41** Ulcerative colitis. (From Damjanov I: *Pathology for the health-related professions,* ed 2, Philadelphia, 2000, WB Saunders.)

Cramping

Fever

Weight loss

Treatment
Remove physical or emotional stressors

Antiinflammatory medications

Antimotility agents

Nutritional supplementation

Surgical intervention, if necessary

Colorectal Cancer
Usually develop from polyp

- In those 55 and older

Increased risks
Genetic factors

40 years of age and older

Diets high in

- Fat
- Sugar
- Red meat

Low-fiber diets

Symptoms
Asymptomatic until advanced

Some may experience

- Cramping
- Ribbon stools
- Feeling of incomplete evacuation
- Fatigue
- Weight loss
- Change in bowel habits
- Blood in the stool

Treatment
Surgical excision

Radiation

Chemotherapy

Combination of above

Disorders of Liver, Gallbladder, and Pancreas

■ Disorders of the Liver

Jaundice (Hyperbilirubinemia)

A symptom of biliary disease, not a disease itself

- Results in yellow eyes and skin

Types

Prehepatic

- Excess destruction of red blood cells
- Result of hemolytic anemia or reaction to transfusion

Intrahepatic

- Impaired uptake of bilirubin and decreased blending of bilirubin by hepatic cells
- Result of liver disease, such as cirrhosis or hepatitis

Posthepatic

- Excess bile flows into blood
- Result of obstruction
  - Due to conditions such as inflammation of liver, tumors, cholelithiasis

Treatment

Removal of the cause

Viral Hepatitis

Liver cells are damaged

Results in inflammation and necrosis

Damage can be mild or severe

Scar tissue forms in liver

- Leads to ischemia

Hepatitis A (HAV)

Infectious hepatitis

Transmission

- Most commonly the oral-fecal route
- Homosexual sexual transmission has occurred

Does not have a chronic state

Vaccine available for those who are traveling

Gamma globulin may be administered to those just exposed

Hepatitis B (HBV)

Serum hepatitis

Carrier state is common

- Asymptomatic but contagious

Long incubation period

Transmission

- Intravenous drug users

- Transfusion

- Exposure to blood and bodily fluids

- Sexual transmission

- Mother-to-fetus transmission

- Immune globulin is temporary prophylactic

- Vaccine is now routine for children

Hepatitis C (HCV)
Transmission

- Most commonly by transfusion

Half of the cases develop into chronic hepatitis

Increases the risk of hepatocellular cancer

Carrier state may develop

Hepatitis D (HDV)
Transmission

- Blood

- Intravenous drug users

Hepatitis B is present for this type to develop

Hepatitis E (HEV)
Transmission

- Oral-fecal

Does not develop into chronic or carrier

Symptoms of hepatitis
Stages
Preicteric

- Anorexia

- Nausea

- Fatigue

- Malaise

Icteric

- Jaundice

- Hepatomegaly (enlarged liver)

- Biliary obstruction

- Light-colored stools

- Pruritus

Posticteric (recovery)

- Reduction of symptoms

Treatment
None

In early stages gamma globulins may be used

Interferon may be used for cases of chronic hepatitis B and C

Nonviral hepatitis
Hepatitis that results from hepatotoxins

Symptoms

- Similar to viral hepatitis

Treatment

- Removal of hepatotoxin

Cirrhosis
Profuse liver damage

- Extensive fibrosis
  - Results in inflammation

Progressive disorder

Leads to liver failure

Types
Alcoholic liver

- Known as Laënnec's cirrhosis or portal
- Largest group

Biliary

- Associated with immune disorders
- Obstructions occur and disrupt normal function

Postnecrotic

- Associated with chronic hepatitis and exposure to toxins

Symptoms
Asymptomatic in early stages

Nausea

Vomiting

Fatigue

Weight loss

Pruritus

Jaundice

Edema

Treatment
Symptomatic

Dietary restrictions

• Reduced protein and sodium

• Increased vitamins and carbohydrates

Diuretics

Antibiotics

Liver transplant

■ Disorders of the Gallbladder

Cholecystitis
Inflammation of gallbladder and cystic duct

Cholangitis
Inflammation of bile duct

Cholelithiasis
Formation of gallstones (Figure 1-42)

• Consists of cholesterol or bilirubin

• Occurs most often in those with high levels of cholesterol or bile salts

Stones cause irritation and inflammation

• May lead to infection

• Obstruction

  • May result in pancreatitis

  • Rupture is possible

Symptoms
Often asymptomatic

Upper right quadrant (URQ) pain

Pain in back and/or shoulder

Epigastric discomfort

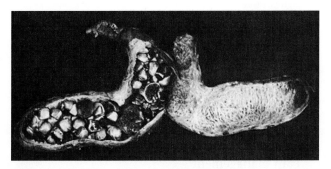

Figure **1-42** Resected gallbladder containing mixed gallstones. (From Kissane JM, editor: *Anderson's pathology,* ed 9, St Louis, 1990, Mosby.)

Bloating

Belching

Treatment
Surgical intervention (cholecystectomy)

Lithotripsy

Medical management by use of drugs that break down stone

■ Disorders of the Pancreas

Pancreatitis
Inflammation of pancreas

Acute and chronic forms

Symptoms
Severe pain

Fever

Acute form is a medical emergency

Neurogenic shock

Septicemia

General sepsis

Complications
Adult respiratory distress syndrome (ARDS)

Renal failure

Treatment
No oral intake

• IV fluids given and carefully monitored

Analgesics

Pancreatic Cancer
Increased risk
Cigarette smoking

Diet high in fat and protein

Symptoms
Weight loss

Jaundice

Anorexia

Most types of pancreatic cancer are asymptomatic until well advanced

Treatment
Palliative

Pain management

DIGESTIVE SYSTEM PATHOPHYSIOLOGY QUIZ

1. This type of hyperbilirubinemia is hallmarked by excess bile flow into the blood:
   a. intrahepatic
   b. prehepatic
   c. posthepatic
   d. jaundice

2. This type of hepatitis is transmitted by the oral-fecal route:
   a. A
   b. B
   c. C
   d. D

3. Which of the following is the recovery stage of hepatitis?
   a. prehepatic
   b. posthepatic
   c. preicteric
   d. posticteric

4. This type of cirrhosis is also known as portal cirrhosis:
   a. biliary
   b. alcoholic liver
   c. postnecrotic
   d. traumatic

5. This condition is the inflammation of the bile ducts:
   a. cholangitis
   b. cholecystitis
   c. cholelithiasis
   d. cholangioma

6. Formation of gallstones most often occurs with high levels of the following:
   a. bile salts and toxins
   b. cholesterol and toxins
   c. cholesterol and bile salts
   d. toxins

7. The primary factor that increases the risk of pancreatic cancer is:
   a. smoking
   b. alcohol
   c. intravenous drug use
   d. hepatitis

8. A potential complication of this condition is ARDS:
   a. hyperbilirubinemia
   b. hepatitis
   c. pancreatitis
   d. pancreatic cancer

9. The primary treatment for jaundice is:
   a. removal of cause
   b. antibiotics
   c. dialysis
   d. vaccine

10. This condition has as the largest group those that abuse alcohol:
    a. cirrhosis
    b. hepatitis
    c. pancreatitis
    d. pancreatic cancer

■ MEDIASTINUM AND DIAPHRAGM

MEDIASTINUM AND DIAPHRAGM—ANATOMY AND TERMINOLOGY

Not an organ system

Mediastinum

That area between lungs that a median (partition) divides (Figure 1-43) into

- superior
- anterior
- posterior
- middle

Diaphragm

A dome-shaped muscular partition that separates abdominal cavity from thoracic cavity

- Assists in breathing
  - Expands to assist lungs in exhalation/relaxation of the diaphragm
  - Flattens out during inspiration/contraction of diaphragm
- Diaphragmatic hernia: esophageal hernia

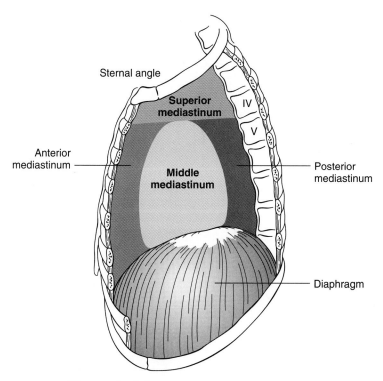

Figure **1-43** Mediastinum and diaphragm.

MEDIASTINUM AND DIAPHRAGM ANATOMY AND TERMINOLOGY QUIZ

1. The mediastinum is not an organ system:
   a. true
   b. false

2. The mediastinum is divided into:
   a. superior, anterior, posterior
   b. superior, anterior, posterior, middle
   c. anterior, posterior, middle
   d. middle, anterior, superior

3. During inspiration, the diaphragm:
   a. expands
   b. moves upward
   c. collapses
   d. flattens out

4. The term means partition:
   a. middle
   b. aspect
   c. median
   d. diaphragm

5. The diaphragm is said to be this shape:
   a. square
   b. flat
   c. dome
   d. round

6. This separates the abdominal cavity from the thoracic cavity:
   a. mediastinum
   b. diaphragm
   c. superior
   d. inferior

7. This is the area between the lungs:
   a. mediastinum
   b. diaphragm
   c. superior
   d. inferior

8. This is an esophageal hernia:
   a. mediastinal
   b. diaphragmatic
   c. paraesophageal
   d. hiatal

9. A diaphragmatic hernia is also known as:
   a. esophageal
   b. epiglottis
   c. partitional
   d. medial

10. The diaphragm assists in:
    a. percussion
    b. auscultation
    c. contraction
    d. breathing

■ HEMIC AND LYMPHATIC SYSTEM

HEMIC AND LYMPHATIC SYSTEM—ANATOMY AND TERMINOLOGY

Hemic refers to blood

Lymphatic system removes excess tissue fluid

- Located throughout body
- Composed of lymph, vessels, and organs

Lymph

Colorless fluid containing lymphocytes and monocytes

Originates in blood and after filtering, returns to blood

Transports fluids and proteins that have leaked from blood system back to veins

Absorbs and transports fats from villi of small intestine to blood system

Assists in immune function

Lymph Vessels

Similar to veins

Scattered throughout body

Lymph Organs

Lymph nodes, spleen, bone marrow, thymus, and tonsils

Lymph nodes, areas of concentrated tissue (Figure 1-44)

Spleen, located in upper left quadrant (ULQ) of abdomen

- Composed of lymph tissue
  - Function is to filter blood; activates lymphocytes and B-cells to filter antigens
  - Stores blood

Thymus secretes thymosin causing T-cells to mature

- Larger in infants and shrinks with age

Tonsils

- Palatine tonsils
- Pharyngeal tonsils/adenoids

Hematopoietic Organ

Bone marrow, contains tissue that produces RBCs, WBCs, and platelets

- Produces stem cells

COMBINING FORMS

1.	aden/o	gland
2.	adenoid/o	adenoids
3.	axill/o	armpit

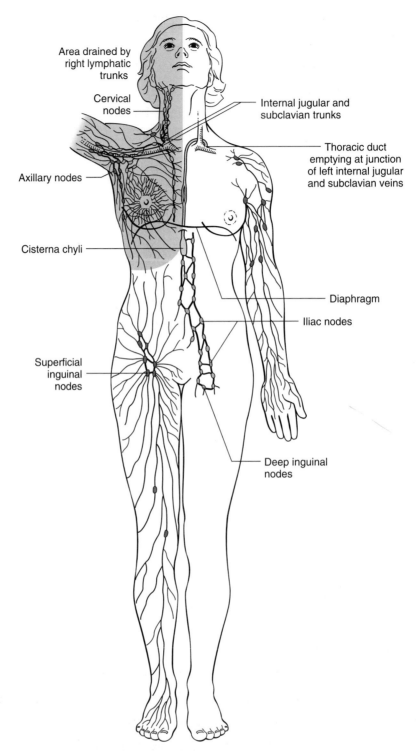

Area drained by
right lymphatic
trunks

Cervical
nodes

Internal jugular and
subclavian trunks

Thoracic duct
emptying at junction
of left internal jugular
and subclavian veins

Axillary nodes

Cisterna chyli

Diaphragm

Iliac nodes

Superficial
inguinal
nodes

Deep inguinal
nodes

Figure **1-44** Lymphatic system.

4. cervic/o   neck/cervix
5. immun/o   immune
6. inguin/o   groin
7. lymph/o   lymph
8. lymphaden/o   lymph gland
9. splen/o   spleen
10. thym/o   thymus gland
11. tonsill/o   tonsil
12. tox/o   poison

PREFIXES

1. hyper-   excess
2. inter-   between
3. retro-   behind

SUFFIXES

1. -ectomy   removal
2. -edema   swelling
3. -itis   inflammation
4. -megaly   enlargement
5. -oid   resembling
6. -oma   tumor
7. -penia   deficient
8. -pexy   fixation
9. -phylaxis   protection
10. -poiesis   production

MEDICAL TERMS

Axillary nodes	Lymph nodes located in the armpit
Cloquet's node	Also called a gland; it is the highest of the deep groin lymph nodes
Inguinofemoral	Referring to the groin and thigh
Jugular nodes	Lymph nodes located next to the large vein in the neck
Lymph node	Station along the lymphatic system
Lymphadenectomy	Excision of a lymph node or nodes
Lymphadenitis	Inflammation of a lymph node
Lymphangiography	Radiographic recording of the lymphatic vessels and nodes
Lymphangiotomy	Incision into a lymphatic vessel

Parathyroid	Produces a hormone to mobilize calcium from the bones to the blood
Splenectomy	Excision of the spleen
Splenography	Radiographic recording of the spleen
Splenoportography	Radiographic procedure to allow visualization of the splenic and portal veins of the spleen
Stem cell	Immature blood cell
Thoracic duct	Collection and distribution point for lymph, and the largest lymph vessel located in the chest
Transplantation	Grafting of tissue from one source to another

HEMIC AND LYMPHATIC SYSTEM ANATOMY AND TERMINOLOGY QUIZ

1. The spleen is located in this quadrant of the abdomen:
   a. URQ
   b. ULQ
   c. LLQ
   d. LRQ

2. Produces RBCs and platelets:
   a. thymus
   b. tonsils
   c. lymph node
   d. bone marrow

3. Which of the following is NOT a lymph organ?
   a. adrenal
   b. spleen
   c. thymus
   d. tonsil

4. Lymph transports fluids and _____ that have leaked from the blood system back to veins.
   a. stem cells
   b. lymphocytes
   c. B-cells
   d. proteins

5. This is largest in infants and shrinks with age:
   a. tonsils
   b. spleen
   c. thymus
   d. bone marrow

6. Combining form meaning gland:
   a. axill/o
   b. thym/o
   c. aden/o
   d. tox/o

7. Prefix meaning excess:
   a. hyper-
   b. hypo-
   c. inter-
   d. retro-

8. Suffix meaning enlargement:
   a. -edema
   b. -poiesis
   c. -penia
   d. -megaly

9. Lymph node located on neck:
   a. thoracic
   b. jugular
   c. Cloquet's
   d. axillary

10. These cells originate in the bone marrow:
    a. B-cells
    b. antigens
    c. lymphocytes
    d. stem cells

HEMIC AND LYMPHATIC SYSTEM—PATHOPHYSIOLOGY

Anemia

Reduction in number of erythrocytes or decrease in quality of hemoglobin

- Less oxygen is transported in the blood

Aplastic Anemia

Diverse group of anemias

Characterized by bone marrow failure with reduced number of hematopoietic cells

Causes
Genetic

Toxin

Radiation

Immunologic

Idiopathic (unknown)

Treatment
Blood transfusion

Bone marrow transplant

Iron Deficiency Anemia
Characterized by small erythrocytes and a reduced amount of hemoglobin

Caused by low or absent iron stores or serum iron concentrations

- Blood loss
- Decreased intake of iron
- Malabsorption of iron

Symptoms
Pallor

Headache

Stomatitis

Oral lesions

Gastrointestinal complaints

Retinal hemorrhages

Thinning, brittle nails and hair

Treatment
Iron supplement

Pernicious Anemia
Megaloblastic anemia (large stem cells)

Usually in older adults

Caused by impaired intestinal absorption of vitamin B_{12}

Symptoms
Pallor

Weakness

Neurologic manifestations

Gastric discomfort

Treatment
Injections of vitamin B_{12}

Hemolytic Anemia
May be acute or chronic

Shortened survival of mature erythrocytes

- Inability of bone marrow to compensate for decreased survival of erythrocytes

Treatment
Treat the cause

Sickle Cell Anemia
Occurs primarily in those of West African descent

Abnormal sickle-shaped erythrocytes (sickle cell)

Symptoms
Abdominal pain

Ulceration of lower extremities

Fatigue

Dyspnea

Increased heart rate

Treatment
Symptomatic

Granulocytosis

Increase in granulocytes

- Neutrophils

- Eosinophils

- Basophils

Eosinophilia

Increase in number of eosinophils

Cause
Allergic disorders

Dermatologic disorders

Parasitic invasion

Drugs

Malignancies

Monocytosis

Increased number of monocytes

Cause

Infection

Hematologic factors

Leukocytosis

Increased number of leukocytes

Cause

Acute viral infections, such as hepatitis

Chronic infections, such as syphilis

Leukocytopenia

Decreased number of leukocytes

Cause

Neoplasias

Immune deficiencies

Drugs

Virus

Radiation

Infectious Mononucleosis

Acute Infection of B Cells

Epstein-Barr virus the most common cause

Symptoms

Fatigue

Lymph node enlargement

Splenomegaly

Hepatomegaly

Transmission

Saliva

• Known as kissing disease

Treatment

Rest

Treatment of symptoms

Leukemia

Malignant disorder of the blood and blood-forming organs

Leads to dysfunction of cells

• Primarily leads to proliferation of abnormal leukocytes

Acute Leukemia

Rapid onset

Short survival time

Most cases occur in children

Types

Lymphocytic

Myelogenous

Monocytic

Symptoms

Anemia

Bleeding

Fever

Infection

Anorexia

Treatment

Chemotherapy

Bone marrow transplant

Chronic Leukemia

Types

Myelogenous

Lymphocytic

Cells are more differentiated

Gradual onset with milder symptoms

Survival time is longer than with acute leukemia

• Majority of cases are in adults

Symptoms

Extreme fatigue

Weight loss

Splenomegaly

Night sweats

Fever

Infections

Treatment

Chemotherapy

Bone marrow transplant

Lymphadenopathy

Lymphadenopathy
Any abnormality of lymph node

Enlargement of lymph node

Lymphangitis
Inflammation of lymphatic vessel

Lymphadenitis
Inflammation of lymph node

Localized inflammation associated with inflamed lesion

Generalized inflammation associated with disease

Inflammation can occur as result of

- Trauma
- Infection
- Drug reaction
- Autoimmune disease
- Immunologic disease

Malignant Lymphoma

Hodgkin Disease
Initial sign is a painless mass commonly located on the neck

Giant Reed-Sternberg cells are present in the lymphatic tissue

Presentation
Enlarged spleen (splenomegaly)

Abdominal mass

Mediastinal mass

Localized node involvement

- Orderly spreading of node involvement

Symptoms
Night sweats

Fever

Weight loss

Itching (pruritus)

Anorexia

Treatment
Radiation therapy

Chemotherapy

Prognosis depends of the stage of the disease when diagnosed

Non-Hodgkin Lymphoma

No giant Reed-Sternberg cells present

Involves multiple nodes scattered throughout the body

• Noncontiguous spread of node involvement

Usually begins as a painless enlargement of node

Symptoms
Presents similar to Hodgkin disease

Treatment
Chemotherapy

Radiation

Prognosis depends on stage

Burkitt Lymphoma

Type of non-Hodgkin lymphoma

Usually found in Africa

Characterized by lesions in the jaw

Epstein-Barr (herpes virus) has been found in Burkitt's lymphoma

Myeloma

Multiple Myeloma

B cell cancer

• Also known as plasma cell myeloma

Increased plasma cells replace bone marrow

Multiple tumor sites cause bone destruction

Result in weakened bone

Cause is unknown

Treatment
Chemotherapy

Poor prognosis, with average life expectancy of 3 years

HEMIC AND LYMPHATIC SYSTEM PATHOPHYSIOLOGY QUIZ

1. This condition involves a reduced number of erythrocytes and decreased quality of hemoglobin:
   a. monocytosis
   b. eosinophilia
   c. anemia
   d. leukocytosis

2. This condition is hallmarked by a shortened survival of mature erythrocytes and inability of bone marrow to compensate for decreased survival:
   a. hemolytic anemia
   b. granulocytosis
   c. eosinophilia
   d. monocytosis

3. The most common cause of this disease is Epstein-Barr virus:
   a. leukocytopenia
   b. infectious mononucleosis
   c. leukocytosis
   d. hemolytic anemia

4. Inflammation of the lymphatic vessels is:
   a. lymphadenitis
   b. lymphoma
   c. lymphadenopathy
   d. lymphangitis

5. What giant cell is present in Hodgkin disease?
   a. B cell
   b. Reed-Sternberg
   c. T cell
   d. C cell

6. The average number of years of survival for multiple myeloma is:
   a. 5
   b. 10
   c. 3
   d. 20

7. Injection of vitamin B may be prescribed for this type of anemia:
   a. pernicious
   b. aplastic
   c. sideroblastic
   d. sickle cell

8. These are large stem cells:
   a. megaloblasts
   b. leukocytes
   c. erythrocytes
   d. granulocytes

9. This is known as the kissing disease:
   a. monocytosis
   b. leukocytopenia
   c. infectious mononucleosis
   d. granulocytosis

10. This lymphoma is usually found in Africa:
    a. multiple
    b. Burkitt
    c. B cell
    d. T cell

■ ENDOCRINE SYSTEM

ENDOCRINE SYSTEM—ANATOMY AND TERMINOLOGY

Regulates body through hormones

Affects growth, development, and metabolism

Endocrine Glands (Figure 1-45)

Pituitary (Hypophysis): Master Gland
Located at base of brain in a depression in skull (sella turcica)

Anterior pituitary (adenohypophysis)

- Adrenocorticotropic hormone (ACTH)—stimulates adrenal cortex

- Follicle-stimulating hormone (FSH)—males, stimulates sperm production; females, stimulates secretion of estrogen and stimulates follicle development

- Growth hormone (GH or somatotropin)—stimulates growth and fat metabolism, and maintains blood glucose levels

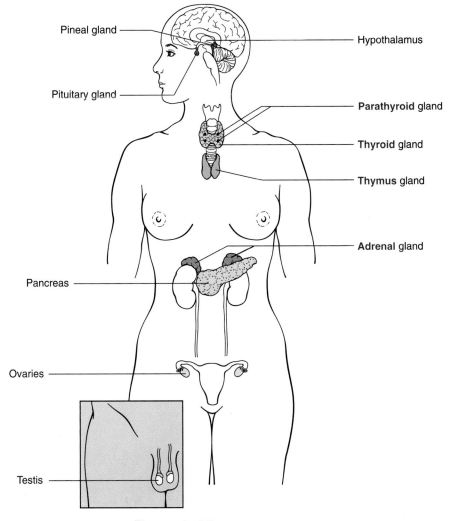

Figure **1-45** Endocrine system.

- Luteinizing hormone (LH)—male, stimulates testosterone; females, stimulates secretion of progesterone and estrogen

- Melanocyte-stimulating hormone (MSH)—increases pigmentation

- Prolactin (PRL)—stimulates milk production and breast development

- Thyroid-stimulating hormone (TSH or thyrotropin)—stimulates thyroid gland

Posterior pituitary (neurohypophysis)—stores hormones

- Antidiuretic hormone (ADH)—stimulates reabsorption of water by kidney tubules

- Oxytocin—stimulates contractions during childbirth and release of milk

Thyroid
Two lobes overlying trachea

Secretes two hormones that increase metabolism—thyroxine (T_4) and triiodothyronine (T_3)

Secretes one hormone that decreases blood calcium—thyrocalcitonin

Parathyroid (4)
Located on posterior side of thyroid

Secretes PTH (parathyroid hormone)

Mobilizes calcium from bones

Adrenal (Pair)
Located on top of each kidney

Adrenal cortex—outer region that secretes corticosteroids

- Cortisol—increases blood glucose

- Aldosterone—increases reabsorption of sodium (salt)

- Androgen, estrogen, progestin—sexual characteristics

Adrenal medulla—inner region that secretes catecholamines (epinephrine and norepinephrine)

Pancreas
Located behind stomach

Contains specialized cells (islets of Langerhans) that produce hormones

Produces insulin (decreases blood glucose), glucagon (converts glycogen to glucose), and somatostatin (regulates other cells of pancreas)

Thymus
Located behind sternum

Atrophies during adolescence

Produces thymosin—stimulates T-lymphocytes

Hypothalamus (Part of Brain)
Located below thalamus

Stimulates pituitary to release hormones

Pineal
Located behind hypothalamus

Secretes melatonin—affects brain and releases of hormones

Ovaries (Pair, Females)
Estrogen—female sex characteristics

Progesterone—maintains pregnancy

Placenta
Produces HCG (human chorionic gonadotropin) during pregnancy

Testes (Pair, Males)
Testosterone—male sex characteristics

COMBINING FORMS

1.	aden/o	in relationship to a gland
2.	adren/o	adrenal gland
3.	adrenal/o	adrenal gland
4.	andr/o	male
5.	calc/o, calc/i	calcium
6.	cortic/o	cortex
7.	crin/o	secrete
8.	dips/o	thirst
9.	estr/o	female
10.	gluc/o	sugar
11.	glyc/o	sugar
12.	gonad/o	ovaries and testes
13.	home/o	same
14.	hormon/o	hormone
15.	kal/i	potassium
16.	lact/o	milk
17.	myx/o	mucus
18.	natr/o	sodium
19.	pancreat/o	pancreas
20.	phys/o	growing
21.	pituitar/o	pituitary gland
22.	somat/o	body
23.	ster/o, stere/o	solid, having three dimensions
24.	thyroid/o	thyroid gland
25.	toxic/o	poison

PREFIXES

1.	eu-	good/normal
2.	oxy-	sharp, oxygen
3.	pan-	all
4.	tetra-	four
5.	tri-	three
6.	tropin-	act upon

SUFFIXES

1.	-agon	assemble
2.	-drome	run
3.	-in	a substance
4.	-ine	a substance
5.	-tropin	act upon
6.	-uria	urine

MEDICAL TERMS

Adrenals	Glands, located at the top of the kidneys, that produce steroid hormones
Contralateral	Opposite side
Hormone	Chemical substance produced by the body's endocrine glands
Isthmus	Connection of two regions or structures
Isthmus, thyroid	Tissue connection between right and left thyroid lobes
Isthmusectomy	Surgical removal of the isthmus
Lobectomy	Removal of a lobe
Thymectomy	Surgical removal of the thymus
Thymus	Gland that produces hormones important to the immune response
Thyroglossal duct	Connection between the thyroid and the tongue
Thyroid	Part of the endocrine system that produces hormones that regulate metabolism
Thyroidectomy	Surgical removal of the thyroid

ENDOCRINE SYSTEM ANATOMY AND TERMINOLOGY QUIZ

1. Which of the following is NOT affected by the endocrine system?
   a. digestion
   b. development
   c. progesterone
   d. metabolism

2. Gland that overlies the trachea:
   a. parathyroid
   b. adrenal
   c. pancreas
   d. thyroid

3. Gland that is located on the top of each kidney:
   a. parathyroid
   b. adrenal
   c. pancreas
   d. thyroid

4. The outer region of the adrenal gland that secretes corticosteroids:
   a. cortex
   b. medulla
   c. sternum
   d. medullary

5. Located on the thyroid:
   a. hypophysis
   b. thymus
   c. pineal
   d. parathyroid

6. Located at the base of the brain in a depression in the skull:
   a. pituitary
   b. thymus
   c. adrenal
   d. pineal

7. Stimulates contractions during childbirth:
   a. cortisol
   b. PTH
   c. ADH
   d. oxytocin

8. Produced only during pregnancy by the placenta:
   a. human chorionic gonadotropin
   b. melatonin
   c. thymosin
   d. adrenocorticotropic hormone

9. Combining form meaning secrete:
   a. dips/o
   b. crin/o
   c. gluc/o
   d. kal/i

10. Prefix meaning good:
    a. tri-
    b. tropin-
    c. pan-
    d. eu-

ENDOCRINE SYSTEM—PATHOPHYSIOLOGY

Diabetes Mellitus

Caused by a deficiency in insulin production or poor use of insulin by body cells

Types of Diabetes Mellitus

Type 1, IDDM (insulin-dependent diabetes mellitus), immune mediated
Onset before age 30

Acute onset

Positive family history

Requires insulin

Type 2, NIDDM (non–insulin dependent diabetes mellitus)
Adult onset, after age 30, but it is now occurring earlier

Insidious onset

Positive in immediate family

Dietary management and/or oral hypoglycemics and/or insulin

Most common type

Symptoms
Polyuria

Polydipsia

Glycosuria

Hyperglycemia

Acute complications
Hypoglycemia

Diabetic ketoacidosis

Chronic complications
Diabetic neuropathy (Figure 1-46)

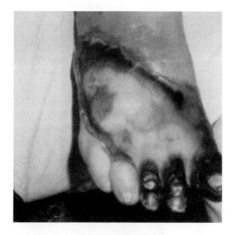

Figure **1-46** Diabetic patient with neuropathy. (From Levin ME: Pathogenesis and general management of foot lesions in the diabetic patient. In Bowker JH, Pfeifer MA, editors: *Levin and O'Neal's the diabetic foot,* ed 6, St Louis, 2001, Mosby.)

Retinopathy

Coronary artery disease

Stroke

Peripheral vascular disease

Infection

Pituitary Disorders

Tumors are the most common cause of pituitary disorders

Tumors may secrete hormones, such as prolactin and ACTH

Anterior Pituitary

Dwarfism
Can be caused by deficiency of somatotrophin (GH) hormone

Gigantism (Figure 1-47)
Can be caused by excess of somatotrophin (GH) hormone in childhood

Acromegaly
Increased GH in adulthood

Enlargement of facial bones, feet, and hands

Diabetes insipidus
Insufficient ADH

Causes polyuria, polydipsia, and dehydration

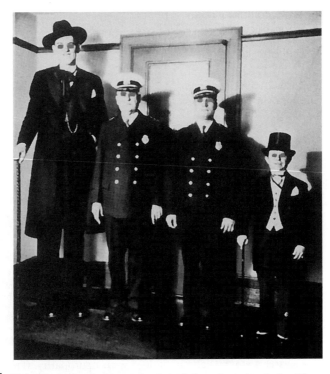

Figure **1-47** Gigantism. A pituitary giant and dwarf contrasted with normal-size men. (From Thibodeau GA, Patton KT: *Anatomy & physiology,* ed 5, St Louis, 2003, Mosby.)

Thyroid Disorders

Goiter (Figure 1-48)
Enlargement of thyroid gland

Cause
Hypothyroid disorders

Hyperthyroid disorders

Hyperthyroidism
Excessive thyroid hormone production

Characterized by
Goiter

Tachycardia

Atrial fibrillation

Pulse pressure

Palpitations

Fatigue

Tremor

Nervousness

Weight loss

Exophthalmos (protruding eyes)

• Decreased blinking

Treatment
Medication (antithyroid drugs)

Radioactive iodine

Surgical excision

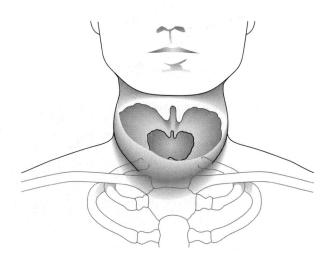

Figure **1-48** Goiter is an enlargement of the thyroid gland.

Hypothyroidism
Decreased levels of thyroid hormone production

Types
Cretinism

- Congenital

- Occurs in children

- If not treated, it will cause a severe delay in physical/mental development

Myxedema

- Severe form

- Occurs in adults

- Symptoms

  - Cold intolerance

  - Weight gain

  - Mental sluggishness

  - Fatigue

Hashimoto's thyroiditis

- Autoimmune disorder

Treatment
Medication (hormone replacement)

Parathyroid Disorders

Hyperparathyroidism
Leads to hypercalcemia

- Affects heart and bones

Symptoms
Brittle bones

Kidney stones

Cardiac disturbances

Treatment
Surgical excision

Hypoparathyroidism
Leads to hypocalcemia

Symptoms
Nerve irritability

Muscle cramps

Tetany

Treatment
Calcium and vitamin D

Adrenal Gland Disorders

Cushing Syndrome
Excess levels of circulating cortisol (glucocorticoid)

Cause

Hyperfunction of the adrenal cortex

Excess levels of ACTH from the pituitary

Long-term use of steroid medications

Symptoms

Weight gain

- Fat deposits on face and trunk

Glucose intolerance

- Diabetes may develop (20%)

Muscle wasting

Osteoporosis

Change in mental status

Delayed healing

Treatment

Medication

Radiation therapy

Surgical intervention

Hyperaldosteronism
Excess aldosterone secreted by the adrenal cortex

Types

Primary hyperaldosteronism (Conn's syndrome)

- Caused by an abnormality of the adrenal cortex
  - Usually an adrenal adenoma

Secondary hyperaldosteronism

- Caused by other than adrenal stimuli

Symptoms

Hypertension

Hypokalemia

Neurologic disorders

Treatment

Treat the underlying condition that caused hyperaldosteronism

- Such as adrenal adenoma

Androgen and Estrogen Hypersecretion
Androgen, male characteristic hormone

- Virilization, development of male characteristics

Estrogen, female characteristic hormone

Cause
Underlying condition

- Adrenal tumor

- Cushing syndrome

Treatment
Surgical intervention for tumor

Underlying condition

Addison's Disease
Deficiency of adrenocortical hormones
- Glucocorticoids

- Mineralocorticoids

Cause
Tumors

Autoimmune disorders

Viral

Tuberculosis

Infection

Symptoms
Decreased blood glucose levels

Fatigue

Lack of ability to handle stress

Weight loss

Infections

Hypotension

Decreased body hair

Hyperpigmentation

Treatment
Hormone replacement

ENDOCRINE SYSTEM PATHOPHYSIOLOGY QUIZ

1. This type of diabetes typically occurs before age 30:
   a. type 1
   b. type 2

2. The acronym that indicates that insulin is not required is:
   a. IDDM
   b. NIDDM
   c. PIDDM
   d. NDDMI

3. The most common cause of pituitary disorders is:
   a. hypersecretion
   b. hyposecretion
   c. tumor
   d. infection

4. In excess, this hormone can cause gigantism:
   a. somatotrophin
   b. thyroid
   c. mineralocorticoids
   d. adrenocortical

5. Goiter can be caused by which of the following:
   a. hypothyroidism
   b. parathyroidism
   c. hyperthyroidism
   d. both a and c

6. This type of hypothyroidism is an autoimmune disorder:
   a. myxedema
   b. Hashimoto's
   c. cretinism
   d. hypokalemia

7. Tetany can be caused by:
   a. hypoparathyroidism
   b. hyperthyroidism
   c. hyperparathyroidism
   d. hyperaldosteronism

8. Conn's syndrome is also known as:
   a. primary hypoparathyroidism
   b. primary hyperthyroidism
   c. primary hyperparathyroidism
   d. primary hyperaldosteronism

9. Development of male characteristics is known as:
   a. virilization
   b. feminization
   c. hypertrophy
   d. hyperaldosteronism

10. The treatment for Addison disease is often:
    a. chemotherapy
    b. radiation
    c. hormone replacement
    d. all of the above

■ NERVOUS SYSTEM

NERVOUS SYSTEM—ANATOMY AND TERMINOLOGY

Controlling, regulating, and communicating system

Organization

• Central nervous system (CNS), brain and spinal cord

• Peripheral nervous system (PNS), cranial and spinal nerves

Cells of the Nervous System (Figure 1-49)

Neurons

Classified according to function (afferent [sensory], efferent [motor])

• Dendrites (receive signals)

• Cell body (nucleus, within cell body)

• Axon (carries signals from cell body)

• Myelin sheath (insulation around axon)

Glia

Astrocytes

Microglia

Oligodendrocytes

Divisions (Figure 1-50)

Brain

Brainstem
Medulla oblongata

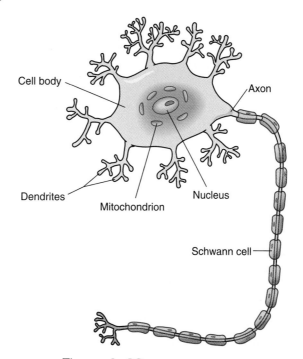

Figure **1-49** Myelinated axon.

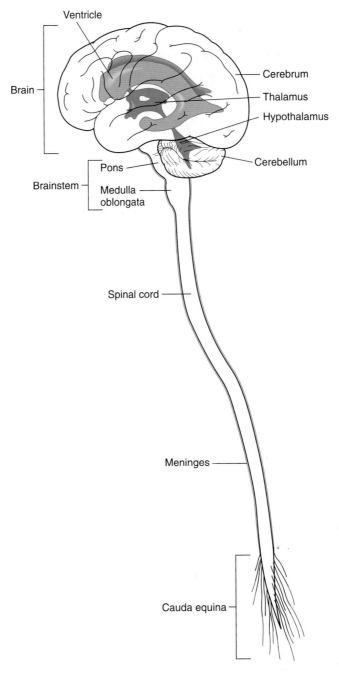

Figure **1-50** Brain and spinal cord.

Pons

Midbrain

Diencephalon

Hypothalamus controls autonomic nervous system

Thalamus relays impulses to cerebral cortex

Cerebellum

Controls muscle contractions

Balance

Cerebrum

Largest part of brain

Mental processes, sensory interpretation, etc.

Two hemispheres

Right controls left side of body

Left controls right side of body

Divided into five lobes

- Frontal
- Parietal
- Temporal
- Occipital
- Insula

Spinal Cord and Cranium

Spinal and cerebral meninges (coverings)

Spine and brain spaces containing cerebrospinal fluid (subarachnoid space)

Cavities within the brain containing cerebrospinal fluid (ventricles)

Peripheral Nervous System (PNS)

Cranial nerves, 12 pair

Spinal nerves, 31 pair

Autonomic Nervous System (ANS)

Two divisions

- Sympathetic system
- Parasympathetic system

COMBINING FORMS

1. cephal/o — head
2. cerebell/o — cerebellum
3. cerebr/o — cerebrum
4. crani/o — cranium
5. dur/o — dura mater
6. encephal/o — brain
7. gangli/o — ganglion
8. ganglion/o — ganglion
9. mening/o — meninges
10. meningi/o — meninges
11. ment/o — mind

12. mon/o   one
13. myel/o   bone marrow, spinal cord
14. neur/o   nerve
15. phas/o   speech
16. phren/o   mind
17. poli/o   gray matter
18. pont/o   pons
19. psych/o   mind
20. quadr/i   four
21. radic/o   nerve root
22. radicul/o   nerve root
23. rhiz/o   nerve root

PREFIXES

1. hemi-   half
2. per-   through
3. quadri-   four
4. tetra-   four

SUFFIXES

1. -algesia   pain sensation
2. -algia   pain
3. -cele   hernia
4. -esthesia   feeling
5. -iatry   medical treatment
6. -ictal   pertaining to
7. -paresis   incomplete paralysis
8. -plegia   paralysis

MEDICAL ABBREVIATIONS

1. ANS   autonomic nervous system
2. CNS   central nervous system
3. CSF   cerebrospinal fluid
4. CVA   stroke/cerebrovascular accident
5. EEG   electroencephalogram
6. LP   lumbar puncture
7. PNS   peripheral nervous system

8. TENS   transcutaneous electrical nerve stimulation

9. TIA   transient ischemic attack

MEDICAL TERMS

Burr	Drill used to create an entry into the cranium
Central nervous system	Brain and spinal cord
Craniectomy	Permanent, partial removal of skull
Craniotomy	Opening of the skull
Cranium	That part of the skeleton that encloses the brain
Diskectomy	Removal of a vertebral disk
Electroencephalography	Recording of the electric currents of the brain by means of electrodes attached to the scalp
Laminectomy	Surgical excision of the lamina
Peripheral nerves	12 pairs of cranial nerves, 31 pairs of spinal nerves, and autonomic nervous system; connects peripheral receptors to the brain and spinal cord
Shunt	An artificial passage
Skull	Entire skeletal framework of the head
Somatic nerve	Sensory or motor nerve
Stereotaxis	Method of identifying a specific area or point in the brain
Sympathetic nerve	Part of the peripheral nervous system that controls automatic body function and sympathetic nerves activated under stress
Trephination	Surgical removal of a disk of bone
Vertebrectomy	Removal of vertebra

NERVOUS SYSTEM ANATOMY AND TERMINOLOGY QUIZ

1. Portion of the nervous system that contains the cranial and spinal nerves:
   a. central
   b. peripheral
   c. autonomic
   d. parasympathetic

2. The part of the neuron that receives signals:
   a. dendrites
   b. cell body
   c. axon
   d. myelin sheath

3. NOT associated with glia:
   a. monocytes
   b. astrocytes
   c. microglia
   d. oligodendrocytes

4. Largest part of the brain:
   a. cerebellum
   b. cerebrum
   c. cortex
   d. pons

5. Divided into two hemispheres:
   a. cerebellum
   b. cerebrum
   c. cortex
   d. pons

6. The number of pairs of cranial nerves:
   a. 10
   b. 11
   c. 12
   d. 13

7. Controls the right side of the body:
   a. left cerebrum
   b. right cerebrum
   c. right cortex
   d. left cortex

8. Combining form that means brain:
   a. mening/o
   b. mon/o
   c. esthesi/o
   d. encephal/o

9. Prefix that means four:
   a. per-
   b. tetra-
   c. para-
   d. bi-

10. Combining form that means speech:
    a. phas/o
    b. rhiz/o
    c. poli/o
    d. myel/o

NERVOUS SYSTEM—PATHOPHYSIOLOGY

Dementias

Cognitive deficiencies

Causes

Alzheimer's disease

Vascular disease

Head trauma

Tumors

Infection

Toxins

Substance abuse

AIDS

Alzheimer's Disease

Most common type of dementia

Progressive intellectual impairment

- Results in damage to neurons (neurofibrillary tangles)

- Fatal within 3 to 20 years

Causes

Mostly unknown

Perhaps genetic defect, autoimmune reaction, or virus

Symptoms

Behavior change

Memory loss

Personality change

Irritability

Inability to complete activities of daily living

Treatment

- No cure

- Symptomatic treatment

- Support for the family

Vascular Dementia

Result of brain infarctions

Nutritional Degenerative Disease

Deficiency

- B vitamins

- Niacin

- Pantothenic acid

Associated with alcoholism

Amyotrophic Lateral Sclerosis (ALS)
Motor neuron disease (MND)

Also known as Lou Gehrig's disease

- Baseball player who died of ALS

Deterioration of neurons of the spinal cord and brain

Results in atrophy of muscles and loss of fine motor skills

Mental functioning remains normal

Survival is 2 to 10 years after diagnosis

- Death usually results from respiratory failure

Treatment
Symptomatic only

Emotional support

No cure

Huntington's Disease
Inherited progressive atrophy of brain

Symptoms
Restlessness

Rapid, jerky movements in the arms and face

Rigidity

Intellectual impairment

Treatment
No cure

Symptomatic

Parkinson's Disease
Decreased secretion of dopamine

Typically occurs after age 60

Symptoms
Muscle rigidity and weakness

Tremors

Masklike facial appearance

Treatment
Medications to reduce symptoms

Dopamine replacement

Multiple Sclerosis
Common neurologic condition

- Demyelination of the central nervous system

Affects young adults

Results in myelin destruction and gliosis of the white matter of the central nervous system

Speculation that it is an autoimmune condition or the result of a virus

Symptoms
Loss of feeling (paresthesias)

Vision problems

Bladder disorder

Mood disorders

Weakness of limbs

Treatment
Symptomatic

Myasthenia Gravis
Means grave muscle weakness

Speculation that it is an autoimmune condition

Symptoms
Muscle weakness and fatigability

May be localized or generalized

Often affects

- Swallowing

- Breathing

- Compromised swallowing and breathing may lead to crisis

Treatment
Anticholinesterase drugs

- Restores normal muscle strength and recoverability after fatigue

Poliomyelitis
Contagious viral disease

Affects motor neurons

Causes paralysis and respiratory failure

Prevent with vaccination

Postpolio Syndrome (PPS)
Also known as postpoliomyelitis neuromuscular atrophy

Progressive muscle weakness

- Past history of paralytic polio

Symptoms
Muscle weakness and fatigability

- May include atrophy and muscle twitching

Treatment
Symptomatic

Maintenance of respiratory function

Guillain-Barré Syndrome
Also known as

- Idiopathic polyneuritis

- Acute inflammatory polyneuropathy

- Landry's ascending paralysis

Demyelination of peripheral nerves

Symptoms
Primary ascending motor paralysis

Variable sensory disturbances

Treatment
Supportive

Congenital Neurologic Disorders

Hydrocephalus
Excessive amounts of cerebrospinal fluid in the head

Compresses brain

Treatment is placement of a shunt

Spina Bifida (Figure 1-51)
Defect in the vertebral column

- Myelomeningocele

  - Meninges and spinal cord protrude through the defect

- Meningocele

  - Meninges herniated through the defect

Results in neurologic deficiencies

Treatment
Surgical repair

Mental Disorders

Schizophrenia
Variety of syndromes

Results in changes in the brain

Hereditary factors are considered a cause

- Also, fetal brain damage is suspected

Stress usually precipitates onset

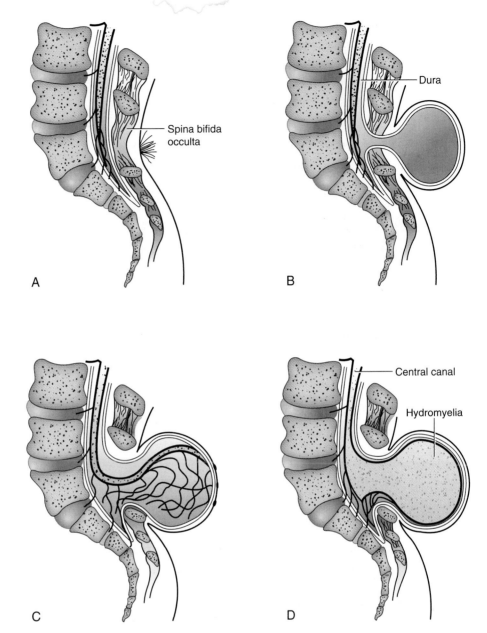

Figure **1-51** **A,** Spina bifida occulta. **B,** Meningocele. **C,** Myelomeningocele. **D,** Myelocystocele or hydromyelia.

Symptoms

Delusions of persecution and/or grandeur

Disorganized thought

Repetitive behaviors

Behavior issues

Decreased speech

Decreased ability to solve problems

Loss of emotions

Hallucinations

Types are based on characteristics

Treatment
Antipsychotic drugs

Drugs have very unpleasant side effects such as

- Excessive movement
- Grimacing
- Jerking
- Tremors
- Shuffling gait
- Dry mouth
- Blurred vision

Depression
Common mood disorder

Exact cause is unknown

Symptoms
Sadness

Hopelessness

Lethargy

Insomnia

Anorexia

Treatment
Antidepressant drugs

Electroconvulsive therapy

Central Nervous System (CNS) Disorders
■ Vascular Disorder
Transient Ischemic Attack (TIA)
Temporary reduction of blood flow to brain

Often a warning sign of cerebrovascular accident

Symptoms
Depend on location of ischemia

- Usual recovery in 24 hours

No loss of consciousness

May display muscle weakness in legs/arms

Paresthesia (numbness) of face

Mental confusion may be present

Repeated attacks common in the presence of atherosclerotic disease

Cerebrovascular Accident (CVA) or Stroke
Infarction of brain due to lack of blood flow

Necrosis of tissue with total occlusion of vessel

Causes
Atherosclerotic disease

Embolus

Hemorrhage

Symptoms
Depend on location of obstruction

- Thrombus
  - Gradual onset
  - Often occurs at rest
  - Intracranial pressure (ICP) minimal
  - Localized damage
- Embolus
  - Sudden onset
  - Occurs anytime
  - ICP minimal
  - Localized damage unless multiple emboli
- Hemorrhage
  - Sudden onset
  - Occurs most often with activity
  - ICP high
  - Widespread damage
  - May be fatal

Treatment
Anticoagulant drugs if caused by thrombus or embolus

Oxygen treatment

Underlying condition treated, such as

- Hypertension
- Atherosclerosis
- Thrombus

Aneurysm
Dilation of artery

- May be localized or multiple

Rupture possible, often on exertion

- Fatal if rupture is massive

Symptoms

May display visual effects, such as

- Loss of visual fields

- Photophobia

- Diplopia

Headache

Confusion

Slurred speech

Weakness

Stiff neck (nuchal rigidity)

Treatment

Dependent on diagnosis prior to rupture

Surgical intervention

Encephalitis

Infection of parenchymal tissue of brain or spinal cord

- Often viral

Accompanying inflammation

Usually results in some permanent damage

Symptoms

Stiff neck

Headaches

Vomiting

Fever

May have seizure

Lethargy

Some of the types of encephalitis

Herpes simplex

Lyme disease

West Nile fever

Western equine

Treatment

Symptomatic

Supportive

Reye's Syndrome

Associated with viral infection

- Especially when aspirin has been administered

Changes occur in brain and liver

- Leads to increased intracranial pressure

Symptoms
Headaches

Vomiting

Lethargy

Seizures

Treatment
Symptomatic treatment

Brain Abscess
Localized infection

Necrosis of tissue

Usually spread from infection elsewhere, such as ears or sinus

Symptoms
Neurologic deficiencies

Increased intracranial pressure

Treatment
Antibiotics for bacterial infections

Surgical drainage

■ Epilepsies
Chronic seizure disorder

Types
Partial
State of altered focus but conscious

Aura

- Auditory or visual sign that precedes a seizure

Generalized
Absence seizures

- Brief loss of awareness

- Most common in children

Tonic-clonic

- Loss of consciousness

- Alternate contraction and relaxation

- Incontinence

- No memory of seizure

Causes
Tumor

Hemorrhage

Trauma

Edema

Infection

Excessive cerebrospinal fluid

High fever

Treatment

Correct the cause

Anticonvulsant drugs

Neurosurgery

■ Trauma

Head Injury

Concussion

Mild blow to head

Results in reversible interference with brain function

- Recover in 24 hours with no residual damage

Contusion

Bruising of the brain

Force of the blow determines outcome

Hematomas

Compresses surrounding structures

Classified based on location

- Epidural

  - Develops between dura and skull

- Subdural

  - Develops between dura and arachnoid

    · Development within 24 hours is acute

    · Development within a week is subacute

  - ICP increases with enlargement of hematoma

- Subarachnoid

  - Develops between the pia and arachnoid

  - Blood mixes with cerebrospinal fluid

    · No localized hematoma forms

- Intracerebral

  - As a result of a contusion

Symptoms

Increased ICP

Others dependent on location and severity of injury

Treatment

Identification of the location of hematoma

Medications to decrease edema

Antibiotics

Surgical intervention if necessary to decrease the ICP

Spinal Cord Injury

Result of trauma to vertebra, cord, ligaments, intervertebral disc

Vertebra injuries classified as

Simple

Compression

Wedge (displaced angular section of bone)

- Flexion injury in which hyperflexion compresses vertebra

Dislocation

Rotation

Symptoms

Depend on location and severity

Paralysis

Loss of sensation

Drop in blood pressure

Loss of bladder and rectal control

Decreased venous circulation

Treatment

Identification of area of injury

Immobilization

Corticosteroids to decrease edema

Bladder and bowel management

Rehabilitation

■ Tumors of Brain and Spinal Cord

Increases the ICP

Life threatening

Rarely metastasize outside of central nervous system

Secondary brain tumors are common

Metastasize from lung or breast

Gliomas Common Type

Primary malignant tumor

Types based on cell from which tumor arises and location of tumor

Glioblastoma
Located in cerebral hemispheres

Highly aggressive

Oligodendrocytoma
Usually located in frontal lobes

Oligodendroblastoma, more aggressive form

Ependymoma
Located in ventricles

Most often occurs in children

Ependymoblastoma, more aggressive form

Astrocytoma
Located anywhere in brain and spinal cord

Invasive but slow growing

Pineal Region
Germ cell tumors
Usually in children

Rare

Variable growth rate

Several other pineal tumors
Pineocytoma

Teratoma

Germinoma

Blood Vessel
Angioma
Usually located in posterior cerebral hemispheres

Slow growing

Hemangioblastoma
Located in cerebellum

Slow growing

Medulloblastoma
Aggressive tumor

Located in posterior cerebellar vermis (fourth ventricle roof)

Meningioma
Originates in arachnoid

Slow growing

Pituitary Tumor
Related to aging

Slow growing

• Such as macroadenomas

Cranial Nerve Tumors

Neurilemmomas

Slow growing

Metastatic

Spinal Cord Tumors

Manifestations include
- Seizure

- Visual disturbance

- Loss of balance

Intramedullary

- Originates in neural tissue

Extramedullary

- Originates outside the spinal cord

Metastatic tumors of spinal cord are usually

- Myeloma

- Lymphoma

- Carcinomas

Most common type of primary extramedullary tumor

- Meningiomas

- Neurofibromas

NERVOUS SYSTEM PATHOPHYSIOLOGY QUIZ

1. The most common dementia is:
   a. Alzheimer's disease
   b. secondary
   c. nutritional degenerative disease
   d. Lou Gehrig's

2. MND stands for:
   a. maximal neuron disorder
   b. migrating niacin disorder
   c. motor neuron disease
   d. motor neuropathic disorder

3. Dopamine replacement is useful in treating:
   a. multiple sclerosis
   b. Parkinson's disease
   c. Huntington's disease
   d. CVA

4. The condition in which the primary symptoms are muscle weakness and fatigability:
   a. amyotrophic lateral sclerosis
   b. multiple sclerosis
   c. dyskinesis
   d. myasthenia gravis

5. Another name for idiopathic polyneuritis is:
   a. Guillain-Barré syndrome
   b. multiple sclerosis
   c. amyotrophic lateral sclerosis
   d. postpolio syndrome

6. This condition is thought to be caused by genetic factors and possibly fetal brain damage:
   a. Parkinson's
   b. schizophrenia
   c. spina bifida
   d. Guillain-Barré syndrome

7. This condition is associated with viral infection, especially when aspirin has been administered:
   a. Reye's syndrome
   b. Guillain-Barré syndrome
   c. Lou Gehrig's
   d. Conn's syndrome

8. Concussion is a mild blow to the head in which recovery is expected within _____ hours:
   a. 12
   b. 24
   c. 48
   d. 1 week

9. ICP means:
   a. intercranial pressure
   b. intracranial pressure
   c. interior cranial pressure
   d. intensive cranial pressure

10. In this type of hematoma, blood mixes with cerebrospinal fluid:
    a. epidural
    b. subdural
    c. subarachnoid
    d. intracerebral

■ SENSES

SENSES—ANATOMY AND TERMINOLOGY

Sight	Eyes
Hearing	Ears
Smell	Nose
Taste	Tongue
Touch	Skin

Sight: Three Layers of the Eye (Figure 1-52)

Sclera (Outer Layer)
White of eye

Cornea, front transparent portion of sclera

• Lies over iris

Choroid (Middle Layer)
Pigment layer

Ciliary muscle and iris on front portion of layer

• Contracts

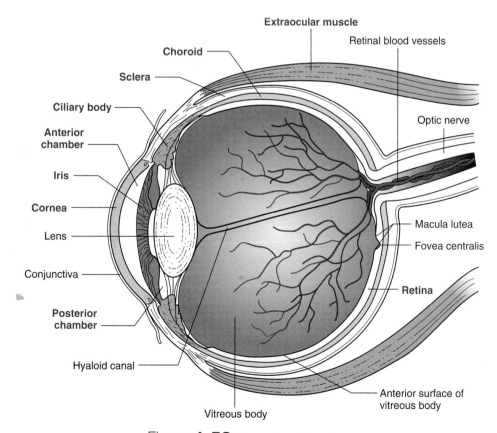

Figure **1-52** Eye and ocular adnexa.

Retina (Inner Layer)
Contains rods and cones

- Rods provide night vision

- Cones provide day and color vision

Conjunctiva
Covers front of sclera and lines eyelid

Lens
Behind pupil

Focuses light

Fluids
Aqueous humor (front of lens)

Vitreous humor (behind lens)

Hearing, Three Divisions of the Ear

External Ear
Auricle (pinna)

External auditory canal

Middle Ear
Begins with tympanic membrane

Ossicles

- Malleus

- Incus

- Stapes

Eustachian tube—leads to pharynx

Inner Ear
Vestibule

Semicircular canals/vestibular apparatus

Cochlea

Smell

Olfactory Sense Receptors
Located in nasal cavity

Closely related to sense of taste

Cranial nerve I

Taste

Gustatory sense

Taste buds located on tongue

Cranial nerves VII and IX

Touch

Mechanoreceptors

Widely distributed throughout body

Reacts to touch and pressure

- Meissner corpuscles (touch)

- Pacinian corpuscles (pressure)

Proprioceptors

Position and orientation

Thermoreceptors

Under skin

Sense temperature changes

Nociceptors

Pain sensors

In skin and internal organs

COMBINING FORMS

1.	ambly/o	dim
2.	aque/o	water
3.	audi/o	hearing
4.	blephar/o	eyelid
5.	conjunctiv/o	conjunctiva
6.	cor/o, core/o	pupil
7.	corne/o	cornea
8.	cycl/o	ciliary body
9.	dacry/o	tear
10.	essi/o, esthesi/o	sensation
11.	ir/o	iris
12.	irid/o	iris
13.	kerat/o	cornea
14.	lacrim/o	tear
15.	myring/o	ear drum
16.	ocul/o	eye
17.	ophthalm/o	eye
18.	opt/o	eye, vision
19.	optic/o	eye
20.	ot/o	ear
21.	palpebr/o	eyelid

22. papill/o	optic nerve
23. phac/o	eye lens
24. phak/o	eye lens
25. pupill/o	pupil
26. retin/o	retina
27. scler/o	sclera
28. staped/o	stapes
29. tympan/o	ear drum
30. uve/o	uvea
31. vitre/o	glassy

PREFIXES

1. audi-	hearing
2. eso-	inward
3. exo-	outward

SUFFIXES

| 1. -opia | vision |
| 2. -tropia | to turn |

MEDICAL ABBREVIATIONS

1. AD	right ear
2. AS	left ear
3. AU	both ears
4. H or E	hemorrhage or exudate
5. IO	intraocular
6. IOL	intraocular lens
7. OD	right eye
8. OS	left eye
9. OU	each eye
10. PERL	pupils equal and reactive to light
11. PERRL	pupils equal, round, and reactive to light
12. PERRLA	pupils equal, round, and reactive to light and accommodation
13. REM	rapid eye movement
14. TM	tympanic membrane

MEDICAL TERMS

Anterior segment	Those parts of the eye in the front of and including the lens, orbit, extraocular muscles, and eyelid
Apicectomy	Excision of a portion of the temporal bone
Astigmatism	Condition in which the refractive surfaces of the eye are unequal
Aural atresia	Congenital absence of the external auditory canal
Cataract	Opaque covering on or in the lens
Cholesteatoma	Tumor that forms in middle ear
Conjunctiva	The lining of the eyelids and the covering of the sclera
Dacryostenosis	Narrowing of the lacrimal duct
Enucleation	Removal of an organ or organs from a body cavity
Episclera	Connective covering of sclera
Exenteration	Removal of an organ all in one piece
Exophthalmos	Protrusion of the eyeball
Exostosis	Bony growth
Fenestration	Creation of a new opening in the inner wall of the middle ear
Glaucoma	Eye diseases that are characterized by an increase of intraocular pressure
Hyperopia	Farsightedness, eyeball is too short from front to back
Keratomalacia	Softening of the cornea associated with a deficiency of vitamin A
Keratoplasty	Surgical repair of the cornea
Labyrinth	Inner connecting cavities, such as the internal ear
Labyrinthitis	Inner ear inflammation
Lacrimal	Related to tears
Mastoidectomy	Removal of the mastoid bone
Ménière's disease	Condition that causes dizziness, ringing in the ears, and deafness
Myopia	Nearsightedness, eyeball too long from front to back
Myringotomy	Incision into tympanic membrane
Ocular adnexa	Orbit, extraocular muscles, and eyelid
Ophthalmoscopy	Examination of the interior of the eye by means of a scope, also known as funduscopy
Otitis media	Noninfectious inflammation of the middle ear; serous otitis media produces liquid drainage (not purulent) and suppurative otitis media produces purulent (pus) matter
Otoscope	Instrument used to examine the ear
Papilledema	Swelling of the optic disk (papilla)
Posterior segment	Those parts of the eye behind the lens
Sclera	Outer covering of the eye
Strabismus	Extraocular muscle deviation resulting in unequal visual axes

Tarsorrhaphy	Suturing together of eyelids
Tinnitus	Ringing in the ears
Transmastoid	Creates an opening in mastoid for drainage antrostomy
Tympanolysis	Freeing of adhesions of the tympanic membrane
Tympanometry	Test of the inner ear using air pressure
Tympanostomy	Insertion of ventilation tube into tympanum
Uveal	Vascular tissue of the choroid, ciliary body, and iris
Vertigo	Dizziness

SENSES ANATOMY AND TERMINOLOGY QUIZ

1. The middle layer of the eye:
   a. sclera
   b. retina
   c. episclera
   d. choroid

2. The covering of the front of sclera and lining of eyelid:
   a. aqueous humor
   b. ossicles
   c. vitreous
   d. conjunctiva

3. Which of the following is NOT a bone of the middle ear?
   a. cochlea
   b. stapes
   c. malleus
   d. incus

4. This cranial nerve controls the sense of smell:
   a. I
   b. II
   c. III
   d. IV

5. Which of the following is NOT part of the inner ear?
   a. pinna
   b. vestibule
   c. semicircular canals
   d. cochlea

6. These receptors react to touch:
   a. nociceptors
   b. mechanoreceptors
   c. proprioceptors
   d. thermoreceptors

7. These react to position and orientation:
   a. nociceptors
   b. mechanoreceptors
   c. proprioceptors
   d. thermoreceptors

8. Combining form meaning eyelid:
   a. aque/o
   b. blephar/o
   c. optic/o
   d. uve/o

9. Combining form meaning eye lens:
   a. cor/o
   b. irid/o
   c. ocul/o
   d. phak/o

10. Abbreviation meaning the pupils are round, reactive to light, equal, and reactive to accommodation:
    a. PERRLA
    b. PERRL
    c. PERL
    d. PURL

SENSES—PATHOPHYSIOLOGY

Eye

Visual Disturbances

Astigmatism

Irregular curvature of the refractive surfaces of the eye

Can be congenital or acquired (as a result of disease or trauma)

Diplopia

Double vision

Amblyopia

Dimness of vision

Hyperopia

Farsightedness

Shortened eyeball

• Can see objects in the distance, not close up

Presbyopia

Age-related farsightedness

Myopia

Nearsightedness

Elongated eyeball

• Can see objects up close, not in the distance

Nystagmus

Rapid, involuntary eye movements

Movements can be

• Vertical

• Horizontal

• Rotational

• Combination of above

Due to underlying condition or adverse effect of drug

Various types, such as

• Vestibular nystagmus

• Rhythmic eye movements

Strabismus

Cross-eyed

Due to muscle weakness or neurologic defect

Treatment

• Eye exercises

• Corrective lenses

• Corrective surgery

Infections

Conjunctivitis (pink eye)

Inflammation of the conjunctival lining of the eyelid or covering of the sclera

Due to

- Infection

- Allergy

- Irritation

Treatment

- Varies with the cause

- Antibiotic eye drops

Hordeolum (stye)

Bacterial infection of eyelid hair follicle

- Usually *Staphylococci*

Results in mass on eyelid

Treatment

- Antibiotics

- Incision and drainage may be necessary

Keratitis

Corneal inflammation

Caused by herpes simplex virus

Causes tearing and photophobia

Macular Degeneration

Destruction of the fovea centralis

- Fovea centralis is the small pit in the center of the retina (fovea centralis retinae)

Usually age related

Results from exposure to ultraviolet rays or drugs

- Also may have a genetic component

Central vision is lost

Treatment

Surgical intervention with laser

Medications

Detached Retina

Retinal tear

- Vitreous humor then leaks behind retina

- Retina then pulls away from choroid

Results in increasing blind spot in visual field

Condition is painless

Pressure continues to build if left unattended

Final result is blindness

Treatment
Surgical intervention with laser to repair tear

Cataracts
Lens becomes opaque

Classified by morphology
Size

Shape

Location

Also may be classified by etiology (cause) or time cataract occurs

Examples of classification
Congenital cataract

- Bilateral opacity present at birth

- Also known as developmental cataract

Heat cataract

- Also known as glassblowers' cataract

- Caused by exposure to radiation

Traumatic cataract (Figure 1-53)

- Result of injury to eye

Senile cataract

- Age related

- Usually forms on corneal area of lens·

Symptoms
Blurring of vision

Halos around lights

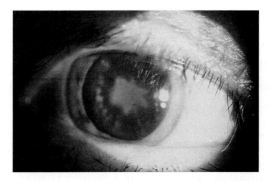

Figure **1-53** A concussion injury that resulted in a traumatic cataract. (From Yanoff M, Duker J: *Ophthalmology*, ed 2, St Louis, 2004, Mosby.)

Treatment
Removal of cataract with intraocular lens implantation

Glaucoma
Excess accumulation of intraocular aqueous humor

- Results in decreased blood flow and edema

- Damages the retinal cells and optic nerve

Narrow angle glaucoma
Acute type of glaucoma

Chronic glaucoma
Also known as

- Wide angle glaucoma

- Open angle glaucoma

Asymptomatic

Treatment
Medications that decrease output of aqueous humor and decreased intraocular pressure (IOP)

Laser treatment to provide drainage

Ear

■ Infections

Otitis Media
Infection or inflammation of middle ear cavity

Chronic infection produces adhesions

Results in loss of hearing

Often occurs in children in combination with URI (upper respiratory infection)

Causes severe ear pain (otalgia)

Treatment
Antibiotics

Surgical intervention with placement of tubes to allow for drainage

- Useful in patients with recurrent infection

Otitis Externa
Also known as swimmer's ear

Infection of external auditory canal and pinna (exterior ear)

Caused by bacteria or fungus

Results in pain and discharge

Treatment
Antibiotic

Encouraged to keep ear dry

■ Hearing Loss

Conductive Hearing Loss

Due to a defect of the sound-conducting apparatus

- Accumulation of wax

- Scar tissue on the tympanic membrane

Also known as:

- Transmission hearing loss

- Conduction deafness

Sensorineural

Due to a lesion of the cochlea or central neural pathways

Also known as

- Perceptive deafness

May be divided into

- Cochlear hearing loss
  - Due to a defect in the receptor or transducing mechanisms of cochlea
- Retrocochlear hearing loss
  - Due to defect located proximal to the cochlea (vestibulocochlear nerve or auditory area of brain)

Presbycusis is age-related sensorineural hearing loss

Ototoxic Hearing Loss

Due to ingestion of toxic substance

Also known as toxic deafness

Mèniére's Disease

Inner ear disturbance

Also known as idiopathic endolymphatic hydrops

Cause unknown

Most common cause of vertigo (dizziness) of the inner ear

Other symptoms include vertigo, hearing loss, and tinnitus

SENSES PATHOPHYSIOLOGY QUIZ

1. This condition can be acquired or congenital and results in an irregular curvature of the refractive surfaces of the eye:
   a. diplopia
   b. hyperopia
   c. nystagmus
   d. astigmatism

2. In this condition the eyeball is shorter than normal and results in being able to see objects in the distance but not close up:
   a. diplopia
   b. hyperopia
   c. nystagmus
   d. astigmatism

3. Rapid, involuntary eye movement is the predominant symptom of this condition:
   a. diplopia
   b. hyperopia
   c. nystagmus
   d. astigmatism

4. Age-related farsightedness is:
   a. presbyopia
   b. hyperopia
   c. diplopia
   d. myopia

5. Another name for a stye is:
   a. keratitis
   b. hordeolum
   c. hyperopia
   d. strabismus

6. An inflammation of the cornea that is caused by herpes simplex virus is:
   a. keratitis
   b. hordeolum
   c. hyperopia
   d. strabismus

7. In this condition there is destruction of the fovea centralis:
   a. macular degeneration
   b. detached retina
   c. glaucoma
   d. cataract

8. This is an infection that occurs in the middle ear cavity:
   a. otitis media
   b. otitis externa
   c. ototoxic
   d. retrocochlear

9. The hearing loss that can be due to a lesion on the cochlea is:
   a. conductive
   b. sensorineural
   c. ototoxic
   d. transmission

10. This condition is also known as perceptive deafness:
    a. conductive
    b. sensorineural
    c. otitis media
    d. transmission

ANATOMY AND TERMINOLOGY QUIZ ANSWERS

Integumentary System Anatomy and Terminology Quiz

1. c	6. c
2. d	7. d
3. a	8. b
4. b	9. c
5. d	10. c

Musculoskeletal System Anatomy and Terminology Quiz

1. b	6. d
2. c	7. b
3. a	8. d
4. c	9. a
5. a	10. c

Respiratory System Anatomy and Terminology Quiz

1. b	6. c
2. d	7. c
3. c	8. b
4. a	9. d
5. a	10. d

Cardiovascular System Anatomy and Terminology Quiz

1. d	6. b
2. a	7. d
3. c	8. a
4. a	9. d
5. d	10. d

Female Genital System and Pregnancy Anatomy and Terminology Quiz

1. d	6. a
2. a	7. b
3. a	8. b
4. b	9. c
5. c	10. d

Male Genital System Anatomy and Terminology Quiz

1. c   6. a
2. a   7. a
3. d   8. d
4. b   9. d
5. a   10. b

Urinary System Anatomy and Terminology Quiz

1. c   6. d
2. d   7. c
3. a   8. b
4. c   9. d
5. b   10. a

Digestive System Anatomy and Terminology Quiz

1. b   6. b
2. d   7. a
3. d   8. c
4. b   9. a
5. c   10. b

Mediastinum and Diaphragm Anatomy and Terminology Quiz

1. a   6. b
2. b   7. a
3. d   8. b
4. c   9. a
5. c   10. d

Hemic and Lymphatic System Anatomy and Terminology Quiz

1. b   6. c
2. d   7. a
3. a   8. d
4. d   9. b
5. c   10. d

Endocrine System Anatomy and Terminology Quiz

1. c
2. d
3. b
4. a
5. d

6. a
7. d
8. a
9. b
10. d

Nervous System Anatomy and Terminology Quiz

1. b
2. a
3. a
4. b
5. b

6. c
7. a
8. d
9. b
10. a

Senses Anatomy and Terminology Quiz

1. d
2. d
3. a
4. a
5. a

6. b
7. c
8. b
9. d
10. a

PATHOPHYSIOLOGY QUIZ ANSWERS

Integumentary System Pathophysiology Quiz

1. c	6. c
2. c	7. d
3. a	8. b
4. d	9. d
5. b	10. a

Musculoskeletal System Pathophysiology Quiz

1. d	6. d
2. c	7. a
3. b	8. c
4. a	9. b
5. d	10. d

Respiratory System Pathophysiology Quiz

1. b	6. a
2. a	7. c
3. d	8. b
4. d	9. a
5. d	10. c

Cardiovascular Pathophysiology Quiz

1. b	6. a
2. a	7. c
3. d	8. c
4. c	9. a
5. d	10. d

Female Genital System and Pregnancy Pathophysiology Quiz

1. b	6. a
2. d	7. a
3. a	8. c
4. c	9. b
5. b	10. c

Male Genital System Pathophysiology Quiz

1. a	6. b
2. b	7. d
3. d	8. b
4. a	9. a
5. c	10. b

Urinary System Pathophysiology Quiz

1. c	6. c
2. d	7. a or c
3. d	8. c
4. c	9. b
5. b	10. c

Digestive System Pathophysiology Quiz

1. c	6. c
2. a	7. a
3. d	8. c
4. b	9. a
5. a	10. a

Hemic and Lymphatic System Pathophysiology Quiz

1. c	6. c
2. a	7. a
3. b	8. a
4. d	9. c
5. b	10. b

Endocrine System Pathophysiology Quiz

1. a	6. b
2. b	7. a
3. c	8. d
4. a	9. a
5. d	10. c

Nervous System Pathophysiology Quiz

1. a   6. b
2. c   7. a
3. b   8. b
4. d   9. b
5. a   10. c

Senses Pathophysiology Quiz

1. d   6. a
2. b   7. a
3. c   8. a
4. a   9. b
5. b   10. b

Reimbursement Issues

REIMBURSEMENT ISSUES

Your Responsibility

Ensure accurate coding based upon services provided and documented

Obtain correct reimbursement for services rendered

Upcoding (maximizing) or downcoding is never appropriate

Stay abreast of current and changing

- Reimbursement policies
- Coding guidelines
- HIPAA changes utilizing various resources such as
  - Centers for Medicare and Medicaid Policy Manuals
  - National Correct Coding Guidelines

Population Changing = Reimbursement Change

Elderly fastest growing patient segment, due to "Baby Boomers"

By 2030, one elderly person for each person younger than 19 years

Medicare primarily for elderly

Medicare

Getting Bigger All the Time!
By 2008, Medicare spending will exceed $364 billion

Health care will continue to expand to meet enormous future demands

- Job security for coders!

Those Covered
Originally established for those 65 and older

Later disabled and ESRD added

Persons covered are called "beneficiaries"

Basic Structure
Medicare program established in 1965

Part A: Hospital and Institutional Care Coverage

Part B: Supplemental—nonhospital

   Example: Physician services and medical equipment

Part C: Medicare + Choice—health care options (added later)

Part D: Prescription Drug Coverage (added January 1, 2006)

Officiating Office
Department of Health and Human Services (DHHS)

Delegated to Centers for Medicare and Medicaid Services (CMS) (formerly HCFA)

- CMS runs Medicare and Medicaid
- CMS delegates daily operation to fiscal intermediaries (FI) and Part B carriers
- FIs and carriers usually insurance companies

Funding for Medicare
Social security taxes

Equal match from government

CMS sends money to FI/carriers

FIs and carriers handle paperwork and pay claims

Medicare Covers
Medical necessity and frequency limitations
Defined in

- LMRPs (Local Medical Review Policies) and
- NCDs (National Coverage Decisions)

Beneficiary pays
20% of Medicare-approved amount after deductible is met for Part B

Plus annual deductible

For Part A, patient pays deductible for service rendered

Medicare pays
80% of Medicare-allowed amount of covered services

For Part A, all covered costs except deductible

Participating Providers
Signed agreement with FI and carrier

Provider agrees to accept what FI and carrier pays as payment in full

- Accepting assignment

Block 27 on CMS-1500 (Figure 2-1)

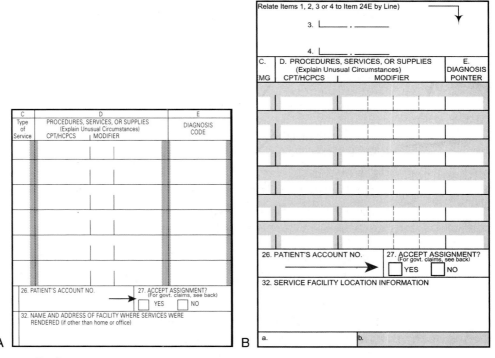

Figure **2-1 A,** Block 27, Accept Assignment on the CMS-1500 (12-90) Health Insurance Claim Form. **B,** Block 27, Accept Assignment on the CMS-1500 (08-05) Health Insurance Claim Form. (Courtesy U.S. Department of Health and Human Services, Centers for Medicare and Medicaid Services.)

National Provider Identification (NPI)
10-digit number assigned to all covered healthcare providers
- Required by 05/28/08

Good reasons to participate
FIs usually do not reimburse non-PAR providers
- Significant decrease in reimbursed amount
Participating providers (PARs) receive 5% more than non-PARs
Check sent directly from FIs/carriers to PAR
Faster claims processing
Provider names listed in PARs directory
- Sent to all beneficiaries

Part A, Hospital Inpatient
Hospitals submit charges on UB-92 form
ICD-9-CM codes primary basis for payment

Covered in-hospital expenses
Semiprivate room
Meals and special diets in hospital
All medically necessary services

Noncovered in-hospital expenses
Personal convenience items
   Example: Slippers, TV
Not medically necessary services or procedures

Types of covered expenses
Rehabilitation
Skilled nursing
Some personal convenience items for long-term illness or disabilities
Home health visits
Hospice care
Not automatically covered
- Must meet certain criteria

Part B, Supplemental
Part B pays services and supplies not covered under Part A
Not automatic
Beneficiaries purchase
- Pay monthly premiums

Types of items covered in part B
Physician services
Outpatient hospital services
Ambulatory surgical services
Home health care
Medically necessary supplies and equipment

Coding for Medicare Part B services
Three coding systems used to report Part B
- CPT
- HCPCS
- ICD-9-CM

NATIONAL CORRECT CODING INITIATIVE

Developed by the Centers for Medicare and Medicaid Services to

- Promote national correct coding methods
- Control improper coding that results in inappropriate payment of Part B claims (physician) and hospital outpatient claims

Unbundling

CMS defines unbundling as

- Billing multiple procedure codes for a group of procedures that are covered by a single comprehensive code

  Example: Dividing one service into parts and coding for each part separately, such as:

  Reporting bilateral procedures unilaterally

  > Reporting 31231, bilateral or unilateral diagnostic nasal endoscopy, with the -50 (bilateral procedure), rather than correctly as 31231

  Downcoding to use an additional code

  > Reporting one of two lacerations of the same complexity and site with a lesser code to enable reporting two separate repairs

  Separating the surgical approach from the major surgical service

  > Coding separately for a thoracic approach during an anterior spine procedure

FEDERAL REGISTER

Government publishes updates, revisions (changes), deletions in laws (Figure 2-2)

November and December issues contain outpatient facility updates

PEER REVIEW ORGANIZATION (PRO)

Social Security Act (SSA) was amended to establish PRO

Also known as Quality Improvement Organizations (QIO)

Purpose: Ensure hospitals adhere to payment system

PRO Reviews

Admission

Discharge

Quality of care

DRG validation

Coverage

Procedure

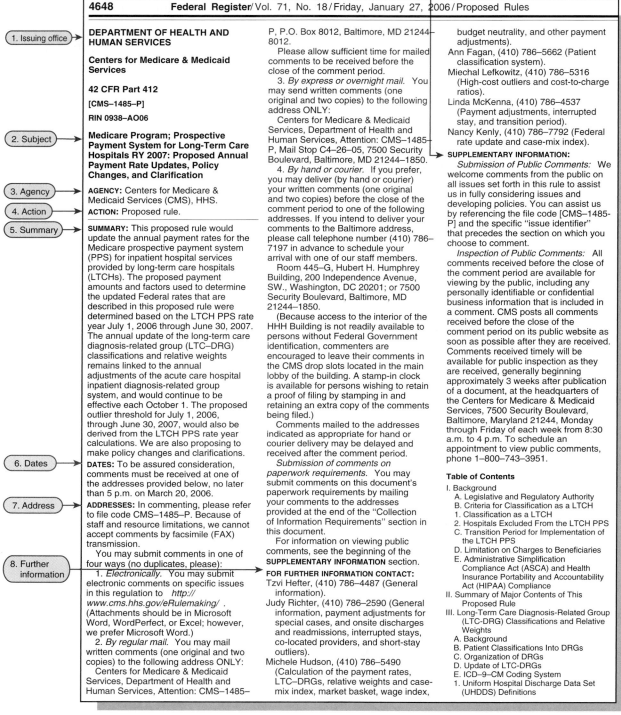

9. Supplementary information

4648 Federal Register/Vol. 71, No. 18/Friday, January 27, 2006/Proposed Rules

1. Issuing office

DEPARTMENT OF HEALTH AND HUMAN SERVICES

Centers for Medicare & Medicaid Services

42 CFR Part 412

[CMS–1485–P]

RIN 0938–AO06

2. Subject

Medicare Program; Prospective Payment System for Long-Term Care Hospitals RY 2007: Proposed Annual Payment Rate Updates, Policy Changes, and Clarification

3. Agency

AGENCY: Centers for Medicare & Medicaid Services (CMS), HHS.

4. Action

ACTION: Proposed rule.

5. Summary

SUMMARY: This proposed rule would update the annual payment rates for the Medicare prospective payment system (PPS) for inpatient hospital services provided by long-term care hospitals (LTCHs). The proposed payment amounts and factors used to determine the updated Federal rates that are described in this proposed rule were determined based on the LTCH PPS rate year July 1, 2006 through June 30, 2007. The annual update of the long-term care diagnosis-related group (LTC–DRG) classifications and relative weights remains linked to the annual adjustments of the acute care hospital inpatient diagnosis-related group system, and would continue to be effective each October 1. The proposed outlier threshold for July 1, 2006, through June 30, 2007, would also be derived from the LTCH PPS rate year calculations. We are also proposing to make policy changes and clarifications.

6. Dates

DATES: To be assured consideration, comments must be received at one of the addresses provided below, no later than 5 p.m. on March 20, 2006.

7. Address

ADDRESSES: In commenting, please refer to file code CMS–1485–P. Because of staff and resource limitations, we cannot accept comments by facsimile (FAX) transmission.

You may submit comments in one of four ways (no duplicates, please):

8. Further information

1. *Electronically.* You may submit electronic comments on specific issues in this regulation via *http:// www.cms.hhs.gov/eRulemaking/* . (Attachments should be in Microsoft Word, WordPerfect, or Excel; however, we prefer Microsoft Word.)

2. *By regular mail.* You may mail written comments (one original and two copies) to the following address ONLY:

Centers for Medicare & Medicaid Services, Department of Health and Human Services, Attention: CMS–1485–P, P.O. Box 8012, Baltimore, MD 21244–8012.

Please allow sufficient time for mailed comments to be received before the close of the comment period.

3. *By express or overnight mail.* You may send written comments (one original and two copies) to the following address ONLY:

Centers for Medicare & Medicaid Services, Department of Health and Human Services, Attention: CMS–1485–P, Mail Stop C4–26–05, 7500 Security Boulevard, Baltimore, MD 21244–1850.

4. *By hand or courier.* If you prefer, you may deliver (by hand or courier) your written comments (one original and two copies) before the close of the comment period to one of the following addresses. If you intend to deliver your comments to the Baltimore address, please call telephone number (410) 786–7197 in advance to schedule your arrival with one of our staff members.

Room 445–G, Hubert H. Humphrey Building, 200 Independence Avenue, SW., Washington, DC 20201; or 7500 Security Boulevard, Baltimore, MD 21244–1850.

(Because access to the interior of the HHH Building is not readily available to persons without Federal Government identification, commenters are encouraged to leave their comments in the CMS drop slots located in the main lobby of the building. A stamp-in clock is available for persons wishing to retain a proof of filing by stamping in and retaining an extra copy of the comments being filed.)

Comments mailed to the addresses indicated as appropriate for hand or courier delivery may be delayed and received after the comment period.

Submission of comments on paperwork requirements. You may submit comments on this document's paperwork requirements by mailing your comments to the addresses provided at the end of the "Collection of Information Requirements" section in this document.

For information on viewing public comments, see the beginning of the **SUPPLEMENTARY INFORMATION** section.

FOR FURTHER INFORMATION CONTACT:
Tzvi Hefter, (410) 786–4487 (General information).
Judy Richter, (410) 786–2590 (General information, payment adjustments for special cases, and onsite discharges and readmissions, interrupted stays, co-located providers, and short-stay outliers).
Michele Hudson, (410) 786–5490 (Calculation of the payment rates, LTC–DRGs, relative weights and case-mix index, market basket, wage index,

budget neutrality, and other payment adjustments).
Ann Fagan, (410) 786–5662 (Patient classification system).
Miechal Lefkowitz, (410) 786–5316 (High-cost outliers and cost-to-charge ratios).
Linda McKenna, (410) 786–4537 (Payment adjustments, interrupted stay, and transition period).
Nancy Kenly, (410) 786–7792 (Federal rate update and case-mix index).

SUPPLEMENTARY INFORMATION:

Submission of Public Comments: We welcome comments from the public on all issues set forth in this rule to assist us in fully considering issues and developing policies. You can assist us by referencing the file code [CMS–1485-P] and the specific "issue identifier" that precedes the section on which you choose to comment.

Inspection of Public Comments: All comments received before the close of the comment period are available for viewing by the public, including any personally identifiable or confidential business information that is included in a comment. CMS posts all comments received before the close of the comment period on its public website as soon as possible after they are received. Comments received timely will be available for public inspection as they are received, generally beginning approximately 3 weeks after publication of a document, at the headquarters of the Centers for Medicare & Medicaid Services, 7500 Security Boulevard, Baltimore, Maryland 21244, Monday through Friday of each week from 8:30 a.m. to 4 p.m. To schedule an appointment to view public comments, phone 1–800–743–3951.

Table of Contents

I. Background
  A. Legislative and Regulatory Authority
  B. Criteria for Classification as a LTCH
    1. Classification as a LTCH
    2. Hospitals Excluded From the LTCH PPS
  C. Transition Period for Implementation of the LTCH PPS
  D. Limitation on Charges to Beneficiaries
  E. Administrative Simplification Compliance Act (ASCA) and Health Insurance Portability and Accountability Act (HIPAA) Compliance
II. Summary of Major Contents of This Proposed Rule
III. Long-Term Care Diagnosis-Related Group (LTC-DRG) Classifications and Relative Weights
  A. Background
  B. Patient Classifications Into DRGs
  C. Organization of DRGs
  D. Update of LTC-DRGs
  E. ICD–9–CM Coding System
    1. Uniform Hospital Discharge Data Set (UHDDS) Definitions

Figure **2-2** Example of page from the *Federal Register*. (From *Federal Register,* Proposed Rules, January 27, 2006, vol. 71, no. 18.)

The Review

Begins with nurse who screens records based on PRO guidelines

Out-of-compliance cases forwarded to physician reviewer

Violations can result in severe sanctions

RESOURCE-BASED RELATIVE VALUE SCALE (RBRVS)

Physician payment reform implemented in 1992

Prior to reform, physicians were paid lowest of

- Physician's charge for service
- Physician's customary charge
- Prevailing charge in locality

National Fee Schedule (NFS)

Replaced RBRVS

Termed Medicare Fee Schedule (MFS)

Payment 80% of MFS, after patient deductible

Used for physicians and suppliers

Relative Value Units (RVUs)

Assigns national unit values to each CPT code

Local adjustments made

- Work and skill required
- Overhead costs
- Malpractice costs

Often referred to as fee schedule

Annually, CMS updates RVU based on national and local factors

MEDICARE FRAUD AND ABUSE

Program established by Medicare

- To decrease and eliminate fraud and abuse

Beneficiary signatures on file

- Service, charges submitted without need for patient signature

Presents opportunity for fraud

Fraud

Intentional deception to benefit

   Example: Submitting for services not provided

Anyone who submits for Medicare services can be violator

- Physicians
- Hospitals

- Laboratories
- Billing services
- YOU

Fraud Can Be

Billing for services not provided

Misrepresenting diagnosis or CPT/HCPCS codes

Kickbacks

Unbundling services

Falsifying medical necessity

Systematic waiver of copayment

Office of the Inspector General (OIG)

Develops and publishes work plan annually

Outlines Medicare monitoring program

FI/carrier monitors those areas identified in plan

Complaints of Fraud or Abuse

Submitted orally or in writing to FI or carrier

Allegations made by anyone against anyone

Allegations followed up by FI or carrier

Abuse

Generally involves

- Impropriety
- Lack of medical necessity for services reported

Review takes place after claim submitted

- FI/carrier goes back and does historical review of claims

Kickbacks

Bribe or rebate for referring patient for any service covered by Medicare

Any personal gain kickback

A felony

- $25,000 fine or
- 5 years in jail or
- Both

Protect Yourself

Use your common sense

Submit only truthful and accurate claims

If you are unsure about charges, services, or procedures

- Check with physician or supervisor

MANAGED HEALTH CARE

Network health care providers that offer health care services under one organization

Group hospitals, physicians, or other providers

90% of people with health care coverage are covered by an organization (e.g., HMO, PPO, POS)

Managed Care Organizations

Responsible for health care services to an enrolled group or person

Coordinate various health care services

Negotiate with providers and groups

Preferred Provider Organization (PPO)

Providers form network to offer health care services as group

Enrollees who seek health care outside PPO pay more

Point of Service (POS)

In-network or out-of-network providers may be used

Benefits are paid at a higher rate to in-network providers

Subscribers are not limited to providers, but to amount covered by plan

Health Maintenance Organization (HMO)

Total package health care

Out-of-pocket expenses minimal

Assigned physician that acts as gatekeeper to refer patient outside organization

REIMBURSEMENT TERMINOLOGY

Advance Beneficiary Notice	ABN, notification in advance of services that Medicare probably will not pay for and the estimated cost to patient (Figure 2-3) (formerly WOL, waiver of liability)
Ancillary Service	A service that is supportive of care of a patient, such as laboratory services
Assignment	A legal agreement that allows the provider to receive direct payment from a payer and the provider to accept payment as payment in full for covered services
Attending Physician	The physician legally responsible for oversight of an inpatient's care (in residency programs, the teaching physician that monitors the resident's work)
Beneficiary	The person who benefits from insurance coverage; also known as subscriber, dependent, enrollee, member, or participant
Birthday Rule	When both parents have insurance coverage, the parent with the birthday earlier in the year carries the primary coverage for a dependent

Patient's Name: _____   Medicare # (HICN): _____

ADVANCE BENEFICIARY NOTICE (ABN)

NOTE: You need to make a choice about receiving these health care items or services.

We expect that Medicare will not pay for the item(s) or service(s) that are described below. Medicare does not pay for all of your health care costs. Medicare only pays for covered items and services when Medicare rules are met. The fact that Medicare may not pay for a particular item or service does not mean that you should not receive it. There may be a good reason your doctor recommended it. Right now, in your case, **Medicare probably will not pay for –**

Items or Services:

Because:

The purpose of this form is to help you make an informed choice about whether or not you want to receive these items or services, knowing that you might have to pay for them yourself. Before you make a decision about your options, you should **read this entire notice carefully.**
- Ask us to explain, if you don't understand why Medicare probably won't pay.
- Ask us how much these items or services will cost you (**Estimated Cost: $_____**), in case you have to pay for them yourself or through other insurance.

PLEASE CHOOSE **ONE** OPTION. CHECK **ONE** BOX. **SIGN & DATE** YOUR CHOICE.

☐ **Option 1. YES. I want to receive these items or services.**
I understand that Medicare will not decide whether to pay unless I receive these items or services. Please submit my claim to Medicare. I understand that you may bill me for items or services and that I may have to pay the bill while Medicare is making its decision. If Medicare does pay, you will refund to me any payments I made to you that are due to me. If Medicare denies payment, I agree to be personally and fully responsible for payment. That is, I will pay personally, either out of pocket or through any other insurance that I have. I understand I can appeal Medicare's decision.

☐ **Option 2. NO. I have decided not to receive these items or services.**
I will not receive these items or services. I understand that you will not be able to submit a claim to Medicare and that I will not be able to appeal your opinion that Medicare won't pay.

_____   _____
Date   **Signature of patient or person acting on patient's behalf**

NOTE: **Your health information will be kept confidential.** Any information that we collect about you on this form will be kept confidential in our offices. If a claim is submitted to Medicare, your health information on this form may be shared with Medicare. Your health information which Medicare sees will be kept confidential by Medicare.

OMB Approval No. 0938-0566   Form No. CMS-R-131-G   (June 2002)

Figure **2-3** Centers for Medicare and Medicaid Services Advance Beneficiary Notice (ABN).

Certified Registered Nurse Anesthetist	CRNA, an individual with specialized training and certification in nursing and anesthesia
"Clean Claim"	A properly completed CMS-1500 form submitted to a payer with all data boxes containing current and accurate information and submitted within the timely filing period required by the insurer
Coinsurance	Cost-sharing of covered services
Compliance Plan	Written strategy developed by medical facilities to ensure appropriate, consistent documentation within the medical record and ensure compliance with third-party

	payer guidelines and the Office of the Inspector General (OIG) Workplan guidelines
Concurrent Care	More than one physician providing care to a patient at the same time
Coordination of Benefits	COB, management of multiple third-party payments to ensure overpayment does not occur
Co-payment	Cost-sharing between beneficiary and payer
Deductible	That portion of covered services paid by the beneficiary before third-party payment begins
Denial	Statement from a payer that coverage is denied
Documentation	Detailed chronology of facts and observations, procedures, services, and diagnoses relative to the patient's health
Durable Medical Equipment	DME, medically related equipment that is not disposable, such as wheelchairs, crutches, and vaporizers
Electronic Data Interchange	EDI, computerized submission of health care insurance information exchange
Employer Identification Number	EIN, an Internal Revenue Services (IRS)–issued identification number used on tax documents
Encounter Form	Medical document that contains information regarding a patient visit for health care services, can serve as a billing and/or coding document
Explanation of Benefits	EOB or EOMB, written, detailed listing of medical service payments by third-party payer to inform beneficiary and provider of payment
Fee Schedule	List of established payment for medical services arranged by CPT and HCPCS codes
Follow-up Days	FUD, established by third-party payers and listing the number of days after a procedure for which a provider must provide services to a patient for no fee. Also known as *global days*, *global package,* and *global period*
Group Provider Number	GPN, a numeric designation for a group of providers that is used instead of the individual provider number
HMO	Health Maintenance Organization
Invalid Claim	Claim that is missing necessary information and cannot be processed or paid
Medical Record	Documentation about the health care of a patient to include diagnoses, services, and procedures rendered
Noncovered Services	Any service not included by a third-party payer in the list of services for which payment is made
National Provider Identifier	NPI, 10-digit number assigned to provider and used for identification purposes when submitting services to third-party payers
Point of Service	POS, a plan in which either an in-network or out-of-network provider may be used with a higher rate paid to in-network providers

Preferred Provider Organization	PPO, providers form a network to offer health care services to a group
Prior Authorization	Also known as preauthorization, which is a requirement by the payer to receive written permission prior to patient services in order to be considered for payment by the payer
Provider Identification Number	PIN, or UPIN, is a number assigned by a third-party payer to providers to be used for identification purposes when submitting claims
Reimbursement	Payment from a third-party payer for services rendered to a patient covered by the payer's health care plan
Rejection/Denial	A claim that did not pass the edits and is returned to the provider as rejected
Resource-based Relative Value Scale	RBRVS, a list of physician services with assigned units of monetary value
State License Number	Identification number issued by a state to a physician who has been granted the right to practice in that state
Usual, Customary, and Reasonable	UCR, used by some third-party payers to establish a payment rate for a service in an area with the usual (standard fee in area), customary (standard fee by the physician), and reasonable (as determined by payer) fee amounts

REIMBURSEMENT QUIZ

1. Any person who is identified as receiving life or medical benefits:
   a. primary
   b. beneficiary
   c. participant
   d. recipient

2. According to the Birthday Rule, if both parents are covered by an employer-provided health policy, the insurance policy that would be primary for reporting their child's health services is:
   a. parent with the birthday earlier in the year
   b. parent with the birthday later in the year
   c. either parent
   d. parent whose birthday is closer to the child's

3. Abbreviation for reusable medical equipment is:
   a. DRG
   b. CRN
   c. DME
   d. DIM

4. Management of multiple third-party payments to ensure that overpayment does not occur:
   a. PRO
   b. COB
   c. DME
   d. FUD

5. CMS delegates the daily operation of the Medicare program to:
   a. DHHS
   b. PRO
   c. RVU
   d. FI and carrier

6. A PAR physician is one who:
   a. signs an agreement with the FI
   b. submits charges directly to CMS
   c. receives 5% less than some other physicians
   d. can bill the patient the total remaining balance after payment from Medicare

7. This part of Medicare covers the inpatient portion of covered costs after the deductible has been paid:
   a. Part A
   b. Part B
   c. Part C
   d. Part D

8. This issue of the *Federal Register* contains outpatient facility changes for CMS programs for the coming year:
   a. October/November
   b. November/December
   c. December/October
   d. November/August

9. This replaced the RBRVS:
   a. RAI
   b. OPPS
   c. APC
   d. MFS

10. Entity responsible for development of the plan that outlines monitoring of the Medicare program:
   a. FI
   b. OIG
   c. DHSS
   d. HEW

REIMBURSEMENT QUIZ ANSWERS

1. b	6. a
2. a	7. a
3. c	8. b
4. b	9. d
5. d	10. b

Overview of CPT, ICD-9-CM, and HCPCS Coding

■ INTRODUCTION TO MEDICAL CODING

Translates services/procedures/supplies/drugs into CPT/HCPCS codes

Translates diagnosis(es) into ICD-9-CM codes

Three Levels of Service Codes

1. Level I CPT

2. Level II HCPCS, National Codes

3. Level III Local Codes—phased out with implementation of HIPAA code sets

Diagnosis Codes, ICD-9-CM

ICD-9-CM, Volumes 1 and 2, *International Classification of Diseases,* 9th ed., Clinical Modification

Volume 1, Tabular List

Volume 2, Alphabetic List

Volume 3, Index and Tabular of Procedures (hospital version)

- Classification system
- Translates diagnosis (dx) into standardized codes that explain why service was provided
- Very specific in nature
- May be up to five numeric or alphanumeric places
- Diabetes becomes 250.XX

■ CPT

Developed by the AMA in 1966

Five-digit codes to report services provided to patients

Updated each November for use January 1

Types of CPT Codes

- Medical
- Surgical
- Diagnostic services
- Anesthesia

CPT Codes

Allow communication that is both effective and efficient

Inform third-party payers of services/procedures provided

Are used as a basis of payment

Incorrect Coding

Results in providers being paid inappropriately (either overpayment or underpayment)

Outpatient (Non-Hospital) Services

Reported on standardized insurance form

CMS-1500 = universal form (Figure 3-1)

CPT Format

Symbols. Used to convey information

- Bullet = New code symbol

▲ Triangle = Revised Code

►◄ Right and left triangles = Beginning and ending of text change

+ Plus = Add-on code

  - Can be used only with another specific code (primary code)
  - Never used alone
  - Full list in Appendix D of CPT

⊘ Circle with line = -51 cannot be used with these codes

  - Full list in Appendix E of CPT

⊙ Bullseye

  - Codes that include conscious sedation
    - Such as 45391, flexible colonoscopy
  - Full list in Appendix H of CPT

⚡ Lightning bolt symbol

  - Codes for which the FDA status pending

CPT Sections

1. Evaluation & Management (E/M)

2. Anesthesia

3. Surgery

4. Radiology

5. Pathology and Laboratory

6. Medicine

TIP: During your examination, the front section of the CPT (Introduction and Illustrations) is an excellent resource on the format, definitions of terms, medical terms, and instructions in the CPT. Review these well before the examination to familiarize yourself with where to find the information that is contained in the front section.

Also, flag the different sections of the CPT for easy access during the examination—for example, the illustrations section, E/M Guidelines, Appendices, and other major sections of the manual.

PLEASE
DO NOT
STAPLE
IN THIS
AREA

CARRIER →

HEALTH INSURANCE CLAIM FORM

| | PICA | | | | | | | PICA | | |

| PICA | | | | | | | | | PICA | |

1. MEDICARE ☐ (Medicare #)   MEDICAID ☐ (Medicaid #)   CHAMPUS ☐ (Sponsor's SSN)   CHAMPVA ☐ (VA File #)   GROUP HEALTH PLAN ☐ (SSN or ID)   FECA BLK LUNG ☐ (SSN)   OTHER ☐ (ID)   1a. INSURED'S I.D. NUMBER   (FOR PROGRAM IN ITEM 1)

2. PATIENT'S NAME (Last Name, First Name, Middle Initial)

3. PATIENT'S BIRTH DATE   MM ¦ DD ¦ YY   SEX   M ☐   F ☐

4. INSURED'S NAME (Last Name, First Name, Middle Initial)

5. PATIENT'S ADDRESS (No., Street)

6. PATIENT RELATIONSHIP TO INSURED
Self ☐   Spouse ☐   Child ☐   Other ☐

7. INSURED'S ADDRESS (No., Street)

CITY   STATE

8. PATIENT STATUS
Single ☐   Married ☐   Other ☐

CITY   STATE

ZIP CODE   TELEPHONE (Include Area Code)
(   )

Employed ☐   Full-Time Student ☐   Part-Time Student ☐

ZIP CODE   TELEPHONE (INCLUDE AREA CODE)
(   )

9. OTHER INSURED'S NAME (Last Name, First Name, Middle Initial)

10. IS PATIENT'S CONDITION RELATED TO:

11. INSURED'S POLICY GROUP OR FECA NUMBER

a. OTHER INSURED'S POLICY OR GROUP NUMBER

a. EMPLOYMENT? (CURRENT OR PREVIOUS)
YES ☐   NO ☐

a. INSURED'S DATE OF BIRTH   MM ¦ DD ¦ YY   SEX   M ☐   F ☐

b. OTHER INSURED'S DATE OF BIRTH   MM ¦ DD ¦ YY   SEX   M ☐   F ☐

b. AUTO ACCIDENT?   PLACE (State)
YES ☐   NO ☐

b. EMPLOYER'S NAME OR SCHOOL NAME

c. EMPLOYER'S NAME OR SCHOOL NAME

c. OTHER ACCIDENT?
YES ☐   NO ☐

c. INSURANCE PLAN NAME OR PROGRAM NAME

d. INSURANCE PLAN NAME OR PROGRAM NAME

10d. RESERVED FOR LOCAL USE

d. IS THERE ANOTHER HEALTH BENEFIT PLAN?
YES ☐   NO ☐   If yes, return to and complete item 9 a-d.

READ BACK OF FORM BEFORE COMPLETING & SIGNING THIS FORM.
12. PATIENT'S OR AUTHORIZED PERSON'S SIGNATURE I authorize the release of any medical or other information necessary to process this claim. I also request payment of government benefits either to myself or to the party who accepts assignment below.

SIGNED _____   DATE _____

13. INSURED'S OR AUTHORIZED PERSON'S SIGNATURE I authorize payment of medical benefits to the undersigned physician or supplier for services described below.

SIGNED _____

PATIENT AND INSURED INFORMATION →

14. DATE OF CURRENT: ◄ ILLNESS (First symptom) OR INJURY (Accident) OR PREGNANCY(LMP)   MM ¦ DD ¦ YY

15. IF PATIENT HAS HAD SAME OR SIMILAR ILLNESS. GIVE FIRST DATE   MM ¦ DD ¦ YY

16. DATES PATIENT UNABLE TO WORK IN CURRENT OCCUPATION
FROM MM ¦ DD ¦ YY   TO MM ¦ DD ¦ YY

17. NAME OF REFERRING PHYSICIAN OR OTHER SOURCE

17a. I.D. NUMBER OF REFERRING PHYSICIAN

18. HOSPITALIZATION DATES RELATED TO CURRENT SERVICES
FROM MM ¦ DD ¦ YY   TO MM ¦ DD ¦ YY

19. RESERVED FOR LOCAL USE

20. OUTSIDE LAB? $ CHARGES
YES ☐   NO ☐

21. DIAGNOSIS OR NATURE OF ILLNESS OR INJURY. (RELATE ITEMS 1,2,3 OR 4 TO ITEM 24E BY LINE)

1. L___ . ___   3. L___ . ___

2. L___ . ___   4. L___ . ___

22. MEDICAID RESUBMISSION CODE   ORIGINAL REF. NO.

23. PRIOR AUTHORIZATION NUMBER

24. A DATE(S) OF SERVICE			B Place of Service	C Type of Service	D PROCEDURES, SERVICES, OR SUPPLIES (Explain Unusual Circumstances)		E DIAGNOSIS CODE	F $ CHARGES	G DAYS OR UNITS	H EPSDT Family Plan	I EMG	J COB	K RESERVED FOR LOCAL USE
From MM DD YY	To MM DD YY				CPT/HCPCS	MODIFIER							
1													
2													
3													
4													
5													
6													

25. FEDERAL TAX I.D. NUMBER   SSN ☐ EIN ☐

26. PATIENT'S ACCOUNT NO.

27. ACCEPT ASSIGNMENT? (For govt. claims, see back)   YES ☐   NO ☐

28. TOTAL CHARGE $

29. AMOUNT PAID $

30. BALANCE DUE $

31. SIGNATURE OF PHYSICIAN OR SUPPLIER INCLUDING DEGREES OR CREDENTIALS (I certify that the statements on the reverse apply to this bill and are made a part thereof.)

SIGNED _____   DATE _____

32. NAME AND ADDRESS OF FACILITY WHERE SERVICES WERE RENDERED (If other than home or office)

33. PHYSICIAN'S, SUPPLIER'S BILLING NAME, ADDRESS, ZIP CODE & PHONE #

PIN# _____   GRP# _____

PHYSICIAN OR SUPPLIER INFORMATION →

(APPROVED BY AMA COUNCIL ON MEDICAL SERVICE 8/88)   **PLEASE PRINT OR TYPE**   APPROVED OMB-0938-0008 FORM CMS-1500 (12-90),   FORM RRB-1500,
APPROVED OMB-1215-0055 FORM OWCP-1500,   APPROVED OMB-0720-0001 (CHAMPUS)

Figure **3-1 A,** The CMS-1500 (12-90) Health Insurance Claim Form. (Courtesy U.S. Department of Health and Human Services, Centers for Medicare and Medicaid Services.)

1500

HEALTH INSURANCE CLAIM FORM

APPROVED BY NATIONAL UNIFORM CLAIM COMMITTEE 08/05

| | PICA | | | | | | | PICA | |

1. MEDICARE   MEDICAID   TRICARE   CHAMPVA   GROUP   FECA   OTHER   1a. INSURED'S I.D. NUMBER   (For Program in Item 1)
          CHAMPUS   HEALTH PLAN   BLK LUNG
   (Medicare #) (Medicaid #) (Sponsor's SSN) (Member ID#) (SSN or ID) (SSN) (ID)

2. PATIENT'S NAME (Last Name, First Name, Middle Initial)   3. PATIENT'S BIRTH DATE   SEX   4. INSURED'S NAME (Last Name, First Name, Middle Initial)
                                                          MM   DD   YY   M   F

5. PATIENT'S ADDRESS (No., Street)   6. PATIENT RELATIONSHIP TO INSURED   7. INSURED'S ADDRESS (No., Street)
                                      Self Spouse Child Other

CITY   STATE   8. PATIENT STATUS   CITY   STATE
                 Single Married Other

ZIP CODE   TELEPHONE (Include Area Code)   Employed Full-Time Student Part-Time Student   ZIP CODE   TELEPHONE (Include Area Code)
          (   )   (   )

9. OTHER INSURED'S NAME (Last Name, First Name, Middle Initial)   10. IS PATIENT'S CONDITION RELATED TO: 11. INSURED'S POLICY GROUP OR FECA NUMBER

a. OTHER INSURED'S POLICY OR GROUP NUMBER   a. EMPLOYMENT? (Current or Previous)   a. INSURED'S DATE OF BIRTH   SEX
                                            YES   NO   MM   DD   YY   M   F

b. OTHER INSURED'S DATE OF BIRTH   SEX   b. AUTO ACCIDENT?   PLACE (State)   b. EMPLOYER'S NAME OR SCHOOL NAME
   MM   DD   YY   M   F   YES   NO

c. EMPLOYER'S NAME OR SCHOOL NAME   c. OTHER ACCIDENT?   c. INSURANCE PLAN NAME OR PROGRAM NAME
                                      YES   NO

d. INSURANCE PLAN NAME OR PROGRAM NAME   10d. RESERVED FOR LOCAL USE   d. IS THERE ANOTHER HEALTH BENEFIT PLAN?
                                                                        YES   NO   If yes, return to and complete item 9 a-d.

READ BACK OF FORM BEFORE COMPLETING & SIGNING THIS FORM.
12. PATIENT'S OR AUTHORIZED PERSON'S SIGNATURE I authorize the release of any medical or other information necessary to process this claim. I also request payment of government benefits either to myself or to the party who accepts assignment below.

SIGNED _____   DATE _____

13. INSURED'S OR AUTHORIZED PERSON'S SIGNATURE I authorize payment of medical benefits to the undersigned physician or supplier for services described below.

SIGNED _____

14. DATE OF CURRENT: ILLNESS (First symptom) OR   15. IF PATIENT HAS HAD SAME OR SIMILAR ILLNESS.   16. DATES PATIENT UNABLE TO WORK IN CURRENT OCCUPATION
   MM   DD   YY   INJURY (Accident) OR   GIVE FIRST DATE MM   DD   YY   MM   DD   YY   MM   DD   YY
                   PREGNANCY(LMP)   FROM   TO

17. NAME OF REFERRING PROVIDER OR OTHER SOURCE   17a.   18. HOSPITALIZATION DATES RELATED TO CURRENT SERVICES
                                                  17b. NPI   MM   DD   YY   MM   DD   YY
                                                            FROM   TO

19. RESERVED FOR LOCAL USE   20. OUTSIDE LAB? $ CHARGES
                              YES   NO

21. DIAGNOSIS OR NATURE OF ILLNESS OR INJURY (Relate Items 1, 2, 3 or 4 to Item 24E by Line)   22. MEDICAID RESUBMISSION CODE   ORIGINAL REF. NO.

1. L___ . ___   3. L___ . ___

2. L___ . ___   4. L___ . ___   23. PRIOR AUTHORIZATION NUMBER

24. A. DATE(S) OF SERVICE						B. PLACE OF SERVICE	C. EMG	D. PROCEDURES, SERVICES, OR SUPPLIES (Explain Unusual Circumstances)		E. DIAGNOSIS POINTER	F. $ CHARGES	G. DAYS OR UNITS	H. EPSDT Family Plan	I. ID. QUAL.	J. RENDERING PROVIDER ID. #
From			To					CPT/HCPCS	MODIFIER						
MM	DD	YY	MM	DD	YY										
1														NPI	
2														NPI	
3														NPI	
4														NPI	
5														NPI	
6														NPI	

25. FEDERAL TAX I.D. NUMBER   SSN EIN   26. PATIENT'S ACCOUNT NO.   27. ACCEPT ASSIGNMENT? (For govt. claims, see back)   28. TOTAL CHARGE   29. AMOUNT PAID   30. BALANCE DUE
                                                                       YES   NO $ $ $

31. SIGNATURE OF PHYSICIAN OR SUPPLIER INCLUDING DEGREES OR CREDENTIALS (I certify that the statements on the reverse apply to this bill and are made a part thereof.)   32. SERVICE FACILITY LOCATION INFORMATION   33. BILLING PROVIDER INFO & PH # (   )

SIGNED _____   DATE _____   a.   b.   a.   b.

OMB APPROVAL PENDING

Figure **3-1**, cont'd **B,** The CMS-1500 (08-05) Health Insurance Claim Form. This has been revised from the CMS-1500 (12-90) form to accommodate reporting of the National Provider Identifier (NPI) number mandated for May 2007. The CMS-1500 (08-05) version will be effective October 1, 2006, but will not be mandated for use until February 1, 2007. For more information: http://www.cms.hhs.gov/transmittals/downloads/R899CP.pdf. (Courtesy U.S. Department of Health and Human Services, Centers for Medicare and Medicaid Services.)

(Side margin labels: CARRIER — PATIENT AND INSURED INFORMATION — PHYSICIAN OR SUPPLIER INFORMATION)

Categorized by

Sections

Subsections

Subheadings

Categories

   Anatomy

      Knee or Shoulder

   Procedure

      Incision or Excision

   Condition

      Fracture or Dislocation

   Description

      Cast or Strap

   Surgical approach

      Anterior Cranial Fossa or Middle Cranial Fossa

Guidelines

Section-specific information begins each section

Must read

Notes

Located throughout CPT

Two Types of Code Descriptions

1. **Stand-alone:** Full description

   Example: 10080 Incision and drainage of pilonidal cyst; simple

2. **Indented:** Dependent on preceding stand-alone for meaning

   Example: 10080 Incision and drainage of pilonidal cyst; simple

          10081   complicated

Semicolon

- The description preceding the semicolon is the common part of the description and applies to any indented codes under it

- You must return to stand-alone for full description

Modifiers Add Information

CPT Modifier

Added at the end of the CPT/HCPCS code

Some modifiers are informational; others affect reimbursement

   Example: 43820 gastrojejunostomy

   - -62 two surgeons

   - 43820-62 two surgeons performed a gastrojejunostomy

Level II HCPCS Modifiers

"-AS" physician's assistant

"-F1" Left hand, second digit

All modifiers used on CPT or HCPCS codes

All HCPCS modifiers begin with a letter

Modifiers are placed in 24D field on CMS-1500 (see Figure 3-1)

Unlisted Services

Codes end in "99" = "no specific code"

Equals = Miscellaneous

Used when a more specific code could not be assigned

Written report must accompany claim form indicating

- Nature
- Extent
- Need
- Time
- Effort
- Equipment used

Category II Codes—Supplemental Tracking Codes

Used for performance measurements

These codes collect data concerning the quality of care and test required

Alphanumeric and end in the letter "F" (0005F)

Located after the Medicine section in CPT

Category III Codes—New Technology

Temporary codes—may be used up to 3 years

Identify emerging technology, services, and procedures

Located after Category II codes

Alphanumeric (0003T)

- May or may not receive future Category I code status
- Category I codes (00100-99602)
- Approved by AMA and the Food and Drug Administration (FDA)
- Proven clinical effectiveness (efficacy)
- Category III has not been approved and has no proven clinical effectiveness (efficacy); not historically on certification examination
- Use Category III code instead of unlisted code
- Use unlisted code if no Category III code exists

The Index

Used to locate service/procedure terms and codes

Speeds up code location

Serves as a dictionary

- First entries and last entries on top of page
- Code display in index
  - Single code: 38115
  - Multiple codes: 26645, 26650
  - Range of codes: 22305-22325

Location Methods

Service/procedure: Repair, excision

Anatomic site: Medial nerve, elbow

Condition or disease: Cleft lip, clot

Synonym: Toe and interphalangeal joint

Eponym: Jones procedure, Heller operation

Abbreviation: ECG, PEEP (positive end-expiratory pressure)

"See" in index

Cross-reference terms: "Look here for code"

Index: Stem, Brain: *See* Brainstem

Appendices of CPT

Appendix A: Modifiers

Appendix B: Additions, Deletions, Revisions

Appendix C: Clinical Examples, E/M Codes

Appendix D: Add-On Codes

Appendix E: -51 Exempt Codes

Appendix F: -63 Exempt Codes

Appendix G: Conscious (Moderate) Sedation

Appendix H: Performance Measures, Category II Modifiers

Appendix I: Genetic Testing Modifiers

Appendix J: Electrodiagnostic Medicine Listing of Sensory, Motor, and Mixed Nerves

Appendix K: Products Pending FDA Approval

Appendix L: Vascular Families

Appendix M: Crosswalk to Deleted CPT Codes

Review information in the CPT appendices prior to examination

■ EVALUATION AND MANAGEMENT (E/M) SECTION (99201-99499)

> Your job is to code only from what is documented in medical record
> Optimize—never maximize
> Accurately report documented services
> Coding for services not provided is a punishable CRIME

Subsections by type of service

Types of service

- Consultation

- Office Services

- Hospital Services, etc.

Integral Factors When Selecting E/M Codes

1. Place of Service
Explains setting of service

- Office

- Emergency Department

- Nursing Home

2. Type of Service
Physicians provide many types of services

- Consultations

- Admissions

- Office visits

3. Patient Status
The four status types are

1. New patient

2. Established patient

3. Outpatient

4. Inpatient

New patient
Has not received any professional service in last 3 years from the same physician or another physician of the same specialty and in the same group

New patients are more labor-intensive for physician, medical staff, and clerical staff

Established patient
Has received professional services in last 3 years from the same physician or another physician of the same specialty in the same group

Medical record available with current, relevant information

Outpatient

One who has not been admitted to a health care facility

> ***Example:*** Patient receives services at clinic or same-day surgery center

Inpatient

One who has been formally admitted to a health care facility

Physician dictates:

- Admission orders

- H&P (history and physical)

- Requests for consultations

On certification examinations, the level of E/M service is indicated

- DO NOT challenge the indicated levels

Levels of E/M Service Based on

Skill required to provide service

Time spent

Level of knowledge necessary to treat the patient

Effort required

Responsibility required

E/M Levels Divided Based on

Key Components (KC)
- History (Hx)

- Physical examination (PE)

- Medical decision making (MDM)

Contributing Factors (CF)
- Counseling

- Coordination of care

- Nature of presenting problem

- Time

Every Encounter Contains Varying Amount of KC and CF
More extensive component/factor

- Higher level of service

Less extensive component/factor

- Lower level of service

KEY COMPONENTS

Four Elements of a History

1. Chief Complaint (CC)

2. History of Present Illness (HPI)

3. Review of Systems (ROS)

4. Past, Family, or Social History (PFSH)

Chief Complaint (CC)—Subjective

Reason for encounter or presenting problem: Patient's current complaint in patient's own words

Documented in medical record for each encounter

History of Present Illness (HPI)—Subjective

Description of development of current illness, e.g., date of onset

Patient describes HPI

PHYSICIAN AND PATIENT DIALOGUE

Development of a CC of Abdominal Pain (HPI):

"Started Thursday night and was mild. During the night, it got worse. Friday morning I went to work but had to leave because the pain got so bad."

Location. Specific source of pain

"Pain was in lower left-hand side, a little toward back."

Quality. Is pain sharp, intermittent, burning?

"Pain is really sharp and constant."

Severity. Is pain intense, moderate, mild?

"Pain is terrible, worst pain I have ever had." (intensity of pain/scale)

Duration. How long has pain been present?

"Pain has been going on now for 3 days."

Timing. Is pain present all of time or does it come and go?

"Pain just continues. It just doesn't go away."

Context. When does it hurt most?

"Pain is just there, it doesn't matter what I am doing."

Modifying factors. Does anything make it better or worse?

"Nothing I do makes it any better or any worse."

Associated signs and symptoms. Does anything else feel different when pain is present?

"Yes, I have nausea when pain is worst."

Review of Systems (ROS)—Subjective

Questions posed to the patient to identify signs and symptoms that have been or are being experienced relating to the HPI

Organ systems, e.g., respiratory system, cardiovascular system

Extent of ROS depends on CC

ROS Elements
Constitutional—General, Fever, Weight loss or gain

Eyes—Organ System (OS)

Ears, Nose, Mouth, Throat (OS)

Cardiovascular (OS)

Respiratory (OS)

Gastrointestinal (OS)

Genitourinary (OS)

Musculoskeletal (OS)

Integumentary (OS)

Neurologic (OS)

Psychiatric (OS)

Endocrine (OS)

Hematologic (OS)

Allergic/Immunologic (OS)

Past, Family, and Social History (PFSH)

Past. Contains relevant information about past illness, injury, or treatment, including

- Major illnesses/injuries
- Operations
- Hospitalizations
- Allergies
- Immunizations
- Dietary status
- Current medications

Family History
Health status or cause of death of family members

- Parents
- Siblings
- Children

Family history items related to CC

- Hereditary diseases

Social History
Review of past and current activities

- Marital status

- Employment

- Occupational history

- Use of drugs/alcohol

- Educational activities

- Sexual history

- Other relevant or contributory factors

Four History Levels

1. Problem Focused (PF)

2. Expanded Problem Focused (EPF)

3. Detailed (Det)

4. Comprehensive (Comp)

Problem Focused History
CC

Brief HPI

No ROS

No PFSH

Expanded Problem Focused History
CC

Brief HPI

Problem focused ROS

No PFSH

Detailed History
CC

Extended HPI

Problem pertinent ROS, extended to include a limited number of additional systems

Pertinent PFSH directly related to problem

Comprehensive History
CC

Extended HPI

Complete ROS directly related to CC, plus review of all additional systems

Complete PFSH

Summary of elements required for each level of history (Figure 3-2)

History Elements

Chief Complaint (CC)
Reason for the encounter in the patient's words

History of Present Illness (HPI)
Location
Quality
Severity
Duration
Timing
Context
Modifying factors
Associated signs and symptoms

Review of Systems (ROS)
Constitutional symptoms
Ophthalmologic (eyes)
Otolaryngologic (ears, nose, mouth, throat)
Cardiovascular
Respiratory
Gastrointestinal
Genitourinary
Musculoskeletal
Integumentary
Neurologic
Psychiatric
Endocrine
Hematologic/Lymphatic
Allergic/Immunologic

Past, Family, and/or Social History (PFSH)
Past illnesses, operations, injuries, and treatments
Family medical history for heredity and risk
Social activities, both past and current

Elements Required for Each Level of History

		Problem Focused	Expanded Problem Focused	Detailed	Comprehensive
History	CC	CC	CC	CC	CC
	HPI	Brief HPI	Brief HPI	Extended HPI	Extended HPI
	ROS	None	Problem pertinent ROS	Extended ROS	Complete ROS
	PFSH	None	None	Pertinent PFSH	Complete PFSH

Figure **3-2** History elements required for each level of history.

Four Examination Levels (Objective)

Problem Focused Examination
Limited examination of affected body area or organ system

Expanded Problem Focused Examination
Limited examination of affected body area or organ system

Other related body area(s) or organ system(s)

Detailed Examination
Extended examination of affected body area(s) and other symptomatic or related organ system(s)

Comprehensive Examination

Complete single specialty or complete multisystem examination

Summary of elements required for each level of examination (Figure 3-3)

Medical Decision Making Complexity (MDM)

Management Options

Based on number of possible diagnoses or various ways condition can be treated (e.g., aggressive intervention versus palliative care)

Levels: Minimal, limited, multiple, or extensive

Data Reviewed

Laboratory, radiology; any test/procedure results are documented along with the data reviewed and the identity of the reviewer in medical record

- "Hemoglobin within normal limits."

- "Chest x-ray, negative."

Old medical records (data) from others may be requested and reviewed

Levels: Minimal, limited, moderate, or extensive

Examination Elements

General
  Constitutional

Body Areas (BA)
  Head (including the face)
  Neck
  Chest (including breasts and axillae)
  Abdomen
  Genitalia, groin, buttocks
  Back
  Each extremity

Organ System (OS)
  Ophthalmologic (eyes)
  Otolaryngologic (ears, nose, mouth, throat)
  Cardiovascular
  Respiratory
  Gastrointestinal
  Genitourinary
  Musculoskeletal
  Integumentary
  Neurologic
  Psychiatric
  Hematologic/Lymphatic/Immunologic

Elements Required for Each Level of Examination

	Problem Focused	Expanded Problem Focused	Detailed	Comprehensive
Examination	Limited to affected BA or OS	Limited to affected BA or OS and other related OS(s)	Extended of affected BA(s) and other related OS(s)	General multi-system or complete single OS

Figure **3-3** Examination elements required for each level of examination.

Risks

Risks of morbidity (poor outcome), complications, or mortality (death) associated with problem, diagnostic procedure, and/or treatment

Other diseases or factors

- Diabetes

- Extreme age

Urgency relates to risks

- Myocardial infarction

- Ruptured appendix

Levels: Minimal, low, moderate, or high

See Figure 3-4, CMS Table of Risk

Four Levels of MDM Complexity

1. Straightforward MDM

Number of diagnoses or management options: Minimal

Amount or complexity of data: Minimal/None

Risk of complications or death: Minimal

2. Low-complexity MDM

Number of diagnoses or management options: Limited

Amount or complexity of data: Limited

Risk of complications or death: Low

3. Moderate-Complexity MDM

Number of diagnoses or management options: Multiple

Amount or complexity of data: Moderate

Risk of complications or death: Moderate

4. High-Complexity MDM

Number of diagnoses or management options: Extensive

Amount or complexity of data: Extensive

Risk of complications or death: High

Summary of elements required for each level of MDM (Figure 3-5)

The diagnosis or management options, amount or complexity of data, and risk are totaled to arrive at the level of MDM

Only two of three categories must meet or exceed each other in any level to assign the MDM

Example: Moderate complexity for diagnosis or management options and moderate complexity of amount or complexity of data, but only a low risk would be assigned a moderate level MDM

Example: Low risk of death, moderate diagnosis or management options, and high amount or complexity of data: Assign the moderate level of MDM

TABLE OF RISK
(Total = highest risk in any one category)

Level of risk	Presenting problem(s)	Diagnostic procedure(s) ordered	Management options selected
Minimal	• One self-limited or minor problem, e.g., cold, insect bite, tinea corpus	• Laboratory tests requiring venipuncture • Chest x-rays • EKG/EEG • Urinalysis • Ultrasound, e.g., echo-cardiography • KOH prep	• Rest • Gargles • Elastic bandages • Superficial dressings
Low	• Two or more self-limited or minor problems • One stable chronic illness, e.g., well controlled hypertension or non-insulin dependent diabetes, cataract, BPH • Acute uncomplicated illness or injury, e.g., cystitis, allergic rhinitis, simple sprain	• Physiologic tests not under stress, e.g., pulmonary function tests • Non-cardiovascular imaging studies with contrast, e.g., barium enema • Superficial needle biopsies • Clinical laboratory tests requiring arterial puncture • Skin biopsies	• Over-the-counter drugs • Minor surgery with no identified risk factors • Physical therapy • IV fluids without additives
Moderate	• One or more chronic illnesses with mild exacerbation, progression, or side effects of treatment • Two or more stable chronic illnesses • Undiagnosed new problem with uncertain prognosis, e.g., lump in breast • Acute illness with systemic symptoms, e.g., pyelonephritis, pneumonitis, colitis • Acute complicated injury, e.g., head injury with brief loss of consciousness	• Physiologic tests under stress, e.g., cardiac stress test, fetal contraction stress test • Diagnostic endoscopies with no identified risk factors • Deep needle or incisional biopsy • Cardiovascular imaging studies with contrast and no identified risk factors, e.g., arteriogram, cardiac catheterization • Obtain fluid from body cavity, e.g., lumbar puncture, thora-centesis, culdocentesis	• Minor surgery with identified risk factors • Elective major surgery (open, percutaneous, or endoscopic) with no identified risk factors • Prescription drug management • Therapeutic nuclear medicine • IV fluids with additives • Closed treatment of fracture or dislocation without manipulation
High	• One or more chronic illnesses with severe exacerbation, progression, or side effects of treatment • Acute or chronic illnesses or injuries that pose a threat to life or bodily function, e.g., multiple trauma, acute MI, pulmonary embolus, severe respiratory distress, progressive severe rheumatoid arthritis • Psychiatric illness with potential threat to self or others • Peritonitis • Acute renal failure • An abrupt change in neurologic status, e.g., seizure, TIA, weakness, or sensory loss	• Cardiovascular imaging studies with contrast with identified risk factors • Cardiac electrophysiological tests • Diagnostic endoscopies with identified risk factors • Discography	• Elective major surgery (open, percutaneous, or endoscopic) with identified risk factors • Emergency major surgery (open, percutaneous or endoscopic) • Parenteral controlled substances • Drug therapy requiring intensive monitoring for toxicity • Decision not to resuscitate or to de-escalate care because of poor prognosis

Figure **3-4** Centers for Medicare and Medicaid Services (CMS) Table of Risk. (Courtesy U.S. Department of Health and Human Services, Centers for Medicare and Medicaid Services.)

Medical Decision-Making Elements

Number of Diagnoses or Management Options
Minimal
Limited
Multiple
Extensive

Amount or Complexity of Data to Review
Minimal/None
Limited
Moderate
Extensive

Risk of Complications or Death If Condition Goes Untreated
Minimal
Low
Moderate
High

Elements Required for Each Level of Medical Decision Making

	Straightforward	Low	Moderate	High
Number of diagnoses or management options	Minimal	Limited	Multiple	Extensive
Amount or complexity of data to review	Minimal/None	Limited	Moderate	Extensive
Risk	Minimal	Low	Moderate	High

Figure **3-5** Elements required for each level of medical decision making.

Contributing Factors

Counseling

Provided to patient or family members (must be stated in medical record)

Discussion of diagnosis, test results, impressions, recommendations, prognosis, risks/benefits of treatment options or lack thereof, and risk factor reduction

Coordination of Care

Work done on behalf of patient by physician to provide care

Nature of Presenting Problem

Type of problem patient presents to physician with or reason for encounter

Levels of Presenting Problem

Minimal Presenting Problem

May not require a physician

> ***Example:*** A dressing change or removal of an uncomplicated suture

Self-limiting or Minor Presenting Problem

Self-limiting problems are minor and with a good outcome and no complications predicted

Example: Sore throat or a slightly irritated skin tag

Low-Severity Presenting Problem
Without treatment, low risk

Example: A middle-aged, healthy male with an upper respiratory infection

Moderate-Severity Presenting Problem
Without treatment, moderate risk

Example: An elderly male with bacterial pneumonia

High-Severity Presenting Problem
Without treatment, high risk

Example: An elderly male in very poor health with diabetic ketoacidosis

Time
Direct face-to-face: Physician and patient together

Example: Clinic visit or at bedside in hospital

Calculated for code assignment beginning and ending times documented in medical record

Unit/Floor: Time spent by physician on patient's floor or unit, also at patient's bedside

Example: Reviewing patient records or at chart desk and then with patient

---

Over 50 percent of the total time should include counseling and/or coordination of care, and the documentation must reflect the total time of the visit and the time spent counseling and/or in coordination of care to qualify to assign the code based on time.

Use of E/M Code

Codes are grouped by type of service and place of service

- Consultation
- Office visit
- Hospital admission

Different codes are required for various levels of service assignment

New patient (99201-99205) services to new patient in office or other outpatient setting

Selection of Level of E/M Services

For the following categories/subcategories, all three of the key components must meet or exceed the level stated in the code description:

- Office, new patient
- Hospital observation service
- Initial hospital care
- Office consultation

- Inpatient consultation
- Emergency department services
- Initial nursing facility care
- Domiciliary care, new patient
- Home, new patient

For the following categories/subcategories, two of the three key components must meet or exceed the level stated in the code description:

- Office, established patient
- Subsequent hospital care
- Subsequent nursing facility care
- Domiciliary care, established patient
- Home, established patient

Established Patient (99211-99215)
99211 may not require a physician

No such code in New Patient category; all new patients are seen by physician

Hospital Observation Status (99217-99220, 99234-99236)
Not officially admitted to a hospital

Patient not ill enough to admit but is too ill not to be monitored or discharged

Read notes at beginning of subsection

Observation services are not codes for "inpatient" services

Observation admission can be reported only for first day of service

When patient admitted on observation status and discharged on same day:

- Use code from 99234-99236 (Observation or Inpatient Care Services category)

Patient in hospital overnight for observation but less than 48 hours:

- **First day:** 99218-99220 (Initial Observation Care)
- **Second day:** 99217 (Observation Care Discharge Services)

If observation stay longer than 48 hours

- **First day:** 99218-99220 (Initial Observation Care)
- **Second day:** 99212-99215 (Established Patient, Office)
- **Third day:** 99217 (Observation Care Discharge Services)

Initial Observation Care

- Beginning of observation care service
- Does not require a specific hospital unit; can be a regular bed on a floor or in emergency department (ED)
- Status specified as "observation"

E/M services immediately prior to admission bundled into observation service

> ***Example:*** Office visit prior to observation, bundled into observation service

Hospital Inpatient Services (99221-99239)
Officially admitted to a hospital setting

Total (all day and night)

Partial (all day and no night, all night and no day, or a variation)

• Time in and out must be specified in medical record

Types of Physician Status
Attending: Primary or admitting physician

Consultant: Physician whose opinion and advice requested by attending physician

Referring: Physician requesting a consultation from another physician regarding a patient's health status

Types of Care
Concurrent care given to patient by more than one physician

> *Example:* Pulmonologist and cardiologist both treating patient for different conditions at same time

Three Types of Hospital Inpatient Services
Initial Hospital Care (99221-99223)
First service includes admission

Initial paperwork

Initial treatment plans and orders

Used only once for each admission

• Only one admission by the attending or admitting physician

Subsequent Hospital Care (99231-99233)
After initial service

Physician reviews patient's progress using documentation, information received from nursing staff, examination of patient

Hospital Discharge Services (99238, 99239)
Final day of hospital stay when patient in hospital more than 1 day

Documentation indicates final patient status

Final Status of Patient
Summary of stay
Condition (final examination)

Medications

Plan for return (follow-up care) to physician

How hospital stay progressed

Discharged destination (to home, nursing facility, etc.)

Only attending physician can use discharge code (only one discharge per admission)

Code based on time spent in service

Beginning and ending time must be documented to assign the extended discharge code or use lowest level code

Consultation Services (99241-99255)

One physician requests another physician's opinion or advice

Either inpatient or outpatient; outpatient consultations include those provided in ED

Outpatient consultations (99241-99245)

Inpatient consultations (99251-99255)

Third-Party-Payer Consultations

Request consult for

- Past medical treatment

- Current condition

- Payers may request prior to approving procedure

- Report services with -32, mandatory services

Emergency Department Services (99281-99285)

No distinction between new and established patients

Must be open 24 hours a day to qualify as ED (ER)

ED services often require additional codes from Critical Care Services

Critical Care Services (99291-99300)

Example: Multiple organ failure

Critical Care Services are provided to patients in life-threatening (critically ill/injured) situations

Critical Care Services (99291, 99292)

Time must be documented in medical record to select from this code range

99291 and 99292 used to report length of time a physician spends caring for critically ill patient

99291: 30-74 minutes

99292: Each additional 30 minutes

Pediatric Critical Care Patient Transport (99289, 99290)

Physician services to critically ill patients during transport to a facility

- Face-to-face or work directly related to patient care

Codes divided on first 30-74 minutes

- Then each additional 30 minutes

- Total time under 30 minutes should be reported with an E/M code

Inpatient Pediatric Critical Care (99293, 99294)

29 days through 24 months of age

Reported per day

Inpatient Neonatal Critical Care (99295, 99296)
1-28 days of age

99295: Reserved for date of admission

99296: Subsequent evaluations, per day

Continuing (Non-Critical) Intensive Care Service (99298-99300)
Intensive care of VLBW (very low birth weight) or LBW (low birth weight) (<2500 grams)

- 1000 grams = 2.2 pounds

Subsequent to admission based on VLBW (<1500 grams) or LBW (1500-2500 grams)

Reported per day

Nursing Facility Services (99304-99318)
Non-hospital settings with professional staff

- Provide continuous health care services to patients who are not acutely ill

Formerly known as Skilled Nursing Facility (SNF), Intermediate Care Facility (ICF), and Long-Term Care Facility (LTCF)

Various levels of nursing facility services

Initial Nursing Facility Assessment (99304-99306)
Provided at time of patient's initial admission

Provided periodically during stay as established by facility regulations

Subsequent Nursing Facility Care codes (99307-99310)
99307 stable, recovering, or improving

99308 not responding or minor complication

99309 significant complication or new problem

99310 significant new problem requiring immediate physician attention

Nursing Facility Discharge Services (99315, 99316)
For final discharge service

Time-based

Domiciliary, Rest Home, or Custodial Care Services (99324-99337)
Health care services are not available on site

Types of services provided are lodging, meals, supervision, personal care, leisure activities

Residents cannot live independently

Codes for either new or established patients

Home Services (99341-99350)
Care provided in patient's home

Services based on key components and contributing factors

Codes for new or established patients

Prolonged Services (99354-99359)
Time codes for direct face-to-face and without direct face-to-face contact

Report time beyond the usual service

• Must be documented in medical record

Codes for first 30-74 minutes and each additional 30 minutes

If less than 30 minutes, do not report service as prolonged

Standby Service (99360)
Physician not caring for other patient(s) to use these codes

Physician standing by only for that patient, if needed

• Must be documented in medical record

Report in 30-minute increments

Less than 30 minutes—do not report

Can report for subsequent 30 minutes only if a full 30 minutes

Carriers have strict policies regarding reimbursement for this service

Case Management Services (99361-99373)
Used to report coordination of care with other health professionals

Reported in increments of approximately 30 or 60 minutes

• Must be documented in medical record

Team conferences or telephone calls

Most third-party payers will not pay for telephone calls

Care Plan Oversight Services (99374-99380)
Used to report physician supervision of patient care in home health agency, domiciliary, or equivalent environment

Patient not present

Codes are time based

• 15-29 minutes

• 30 minutes or more

• Must be documented in medical record

Reported once for each 30-day period

Preventive Medicine (E/M) Services (99381-99429)
Used to report services when patient is not currently ill

Example: Annual checkup

Codes divided by new or established and age

If significant problem is encountered during preventive examination

• E/M code also reported

Counseling and/or Risk Factor Reduction Intervention (99401-99429)
Patient is seen specifically to promote health and/or wellness

Example: Diet, exercise program

Patient does not have symptoms or an established diagnosis to use these codes

Codes based on

- Document time
- Time
- Individual or group
- Physician review of assessment data

Newborn Care Services (99431-99440)

Services are for normal newborns

- Newborn H&P
- Physical exam of newborn
- Attendance at delivery to stabilize newborn requested by delivering physician
- Subsequent hospital care for normal newborn, per day charge subsequent to delivery day
- Newborn resuscitation

Special E/M Services (99450-99456)

99450 is reported for services provided for insurance or disability assessments

Involves no treatment; any treatment provided would be coded separately

Codes divided

- **99455:** Assessment by treating physician
- **99456:** Assessment by nontreating physician

For new/established patients in any setting

Unlisted E/M Service (99499)

Seldom used

Requires a written report with submission

■ ANESTHESIA SECTION (00100-01999)

Anesthesiologist

Doctor of medicine specializing in anesthesia

Usually outside practices, e.g., Anesthesia Associates, Inc., or Pain Clinic, Ltd.

Professional services reported separately

CRNA

Certified Registered Nurse Anesthetist

Uses of Anesthesia

Manage unconscious patients, life functions, and resuscitation

Analgesia

Relieve pain

Some Methods of Anesthesia

Endotracheal: Through mouth (general anesthesia)

Local: Application to area (injection or topical)

Epidural: Between vertebral spaces

Regional: Field or nerve

MAC: monitored anesthesia care

Patient-Controlled Analgesia (PCA)

Patient administers drug

Used to relieve chronic pain or temporarily for severe pain following surgery

Moderate (Conscious) Sedation

To be used when surgeon administers sedation

• No anesthesia personnel are present

Decreased level of consciousness

Report with 99143-99145 (Medicine)

Presence of trained observer, such as a nurse, is required

Second physician administered sedation, report 99148-99150

Anesthesia Formula

$(B + T + M) \times$ conversion factor = Anesthesia payment

B is for Basic Units

Published in *Relative Value Guide (RVG)* by American Society of Anesthesiologists

National unit values for anesthesia services based on complexity of service

T is for Time

Patient record indicates time, e.g., 60 minutes

Usually, 15 minutes = 1 unit

> **Example:** 60 minutes = 4 units

Begins: Anesthesiologist begins to prepare patient for induction—preoperative

Continues throughout procedure—intraoperative

Ends: Patient no longer under care of anesthesiologist—postoperative

M is for Modifying Unit

Additional units based on physical status of patient (see modifiers that follow)

Physical Status Modifiers, P1-P6
Located in Anesthesia Guidelines

Not reported to Medicare

Help to show complexity of service

- P1 Normal healthy
- P2 Mild systemic disease
- P3 Severe systemic disease
- P4 Severe systemic disease is constant threat to life
- P5 Not expected to survive without the operation
- P6 Clinically brain dead

Qualifying Circumstances Codes (99100-99140)
Anesthesia services provided under difficult circumstances

Located in both Anesthesia Guidelines and Medicine section

Listed in addition to primary anesthesia code

Summing Up Formula
Basic units (from *RVG*) based on CPT codes

Time units (usually 15 min is a unit)

- Total time ÷ 15 = time units

Modifiers [Qualifying Circumstances (99100-99140) and/or Physical Status (P1-P6)]

Conversion Factors
CMS anesthesia conversion factors

Sum of money allocated by payer, per unit for payment of anesthesia services

Anesthesia for Multiple Surgical Procedures
Once anesthetized, length of time, not number of procedures performed during session

Report highest service units only

> *Example:* Two procedures during same session

- One, 10 units; the other, 5 units
- Report only 10 units and combined time for all procedures

■ CPT/HCPCS LEVEL I MODIFIERS (-21 to -99)

Alters CPT or HCPCS code

Full list, CPT, Appendix A

- Two separate lists
  - One for physician use
  - One for hospital outpatient use

Modifier Functions

Altered (i.e., increased or reduced service)

Bilateral

Multiple

Only portions of service (i.e., professional service only)

More than one surgeon

-21 Prolonged E/M Service

Used only with highest-level E/M codes (99205-99397)

Indicates extended service above highest level in category

-22 Unusual Procedural Service

Indicates services significantly greater than usual

Accompanied by written report and supportive documentation

-23 Unusual Anesthesia

Use of general anesthesia where local or regional is norm

>   *Example:* Highly agitated senile patient

Used only with anesthesia codes

Written report with submission of modifier

-24 Unrelated E/M Services by Same Physician During a Postoperative Period

Service not related to surgery

If E/M provided during postoperative global period, no payment considered without -24

-25 Significant, Separately Identifiable E/M Service, Same Physician/and Day of Procedure/Service

Documentation must support service

>   *Example:* Patient seen for sinus congestion, physician performs H&P, prescribes decongestant, notes and removes lesion on back

>   Code: Procedure + E/M-25

-26 Professional Component

Professional component (physician, -26)

Technical component (technician + equipment, -TC)

-32 Mandated Service

Mandated by payer, worker's comp, or official body or court of law

Not requests of patient, patient's family, or another physician

> ***Example:*** Worker's Compensation requests examination of person currently receiving disability benefits

-47 Anesthesia by Surgeon

Physician administers regional or general anesthesia

Surgeon acts as both surgeon and anesthesiologist

Used only with Surgery codes

-50 Bilateral Procedure

Body is bilateral

> ***Example:*** Procedure on hands

Caution: Some codes describe bilateral procedures

Typically not used on Integumentary System codes

-51 Multiple Procedure—Three Types

Same procedure, different sites

Multiple operation(s), same operative session

Procedure performed multiple times

List most resource-intense procedure first, then descending order of importance

Next, other procedure(s) + -51 (unless code is -51 exempt)

Usual procedure payment: 1st 100%, 2nd 50%, 3rd 25%-50%, depending on payer

-52 Reduced Services

Service reduced or not performed to the extent described in code description

Physician directed reduction

Documentation substantiates reduction

Not to be used for patient unable to pay

-53 Discontinued Procedure

Surgical/diagnostic procedures

Started then stopped due to patient's condition

Does not apply to presurgical discontinuance

DO NOT USE -53

- When patient cancels scheduled procedure
- With E/M codes
- With time-based code

-54 Surgical Care Only

Physician provides only procedure (intraoperative); other physician does preoperative and postoperative service

Documented patient transfer must be in record

Some payers require copy of transfer order

-55 Postoperative Management Only

Physician provides only the care after hospital discharge

If transferred while patient hospitalized, report postoperative management with subsequent hospital codes 99231-99233

Documentation of transfer in medical record

-56 Preoperative Management Only

Physician provided only preoperative care

Not acceptable for Medicare

Requires E/M code

Usual reimbursement for portions, surgical package

- 10% preoperative
- 70% intraoperative
- 20% postoperative

Each payer determines reimbursement for portions

-57 Decision for Surgery Used With

E/M, 99201-99499

Medicine, 92012 and 92014 ophthalmologic services

Medicare: Only for preoperative period of major surgery (day before or day of)

-58 Staged/Related by Same Physician During Postoperative Period

Subsequent procedure planned at time of initial surgery

- During postoperative period of previous surgery in series

    Example: Multiple skin grafts completed in several sessions

- Do not use when code describes a session

    Example: 67208 destruction of lesion of retina, one or more sessions

- More extensive than original procedure or
- For therapy following diagnostic procedure (e.g., breast biopsy and subsequent mastectomy)

-59 Distinct Procedural Service

Used to report services not normally reported together

Different session or encounter

Different procedure

Different site

Separate incision, excision, lesion, injury

> *Example:* Physician removes several lesions from patient's leg; also notes a suspicious lesion on torso and biopsies it

- Excision code for lesion removal + biopsy code for torso lesion with -59
- Indicates biopsy as distinct procedure, not part of lesion removal

-62 Two Surgeons

Both function as cosurgeons (equals)

Usually of different specialties

Each reports same code + -62

-63 Procedure Performed on Infants Less Than 4 kg

Kilogram: 2.2 pounds (4 kg = 8.8 lb)

Small size increases complexity

Use with all Surgery section codes except Integumentary System

-66 Surgical Team

Team: Several physicians with various specialties plus technicians and other support personnel

Very complex procedures

Payers may increase payment up to 50%

- Each physician's service must be documented in the medical record

-76 Repeat Procedure/Service by Same Physician

Note: "Same Physician"

Used to indicate necessary service

> *Example:* X-rays before and after fracture repair

-77 Repeat Procedure/Service by Another Physician

Note: "Another Physician"

Performed by one physician, repeated by another physician

Submitted with written report to establish medical necessity and identity of performing physician

-78 Return to Operating Room for a Related Procedure During Postoperative Period

For complication of first procedure

> **Example:** Patient had outpatient procedure in morning; was returned to operating room in afternoon with severe hemorrhage

Indicates not typographical error

- Medical record must specifically document need for service provided

-79 Unrelated Procedure or Service by Same Physician During Postoperative Period

> **Example:** Several days after discharge for procedure, patient returns for unrelated problem

Diagnosis code would also be different

-80 Assistant Surgeon

Reimbursed at 15% to 30%

Payers identify procedures for which they reimburse assistant at surgery

-81 Minimum Assistant Surgeon

Services at a level less than that described in -80

Reimbursed at 10% if services reported with the modifier are recognized by payer

-82 Assistant Surgeon

Teaching hospitals

- Have residents who assist as part of education
- Must demonstrate no qualified resident available to use -82
  - Unavailability must be documented in written report

-90 Reference (Outside) Laboratory

Physician has business relationship with outside lab

Physician pays lab

Physician bills payer for lab services

-91 Repeat Clinical Diagnostic Laboratory Test

Repeat same laboratory tests on same day for multiple test results

- e.g., serial troponin levels for acute MI confirmation

Not tests rerun to confirm or negate original test results

Not assigned for malfunction of equipment, loss of specimen, or technician error

-99 Multiple Modifiers

Used when service needs more than one modifier but payer allows for only one modifier with each code

Placement of modifier -99 on CMS-1500 (Figure 3-6)

HCPCS Level II Modifiers

Examples of HCPCS Anatomical Modifiers

-LT   Left side

-RT   Right side

-E1   Upper left, eyelid

-E2   Lower left, eyelid

-E3   Upper right, eyelid

-E4   Lower right, eyelid

-FA   Left hand, thumb

-F1   Left hand, second digit

-F2   Left hand, third digit

-F3   Left hand, fourth digit

-F4   Left hand, fifth digit

-F5   Right hand, thumb

-F6   Right hand, second digit

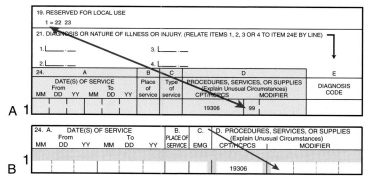

Figure **3-6** **A,** CMS-1500 (12-90) only allowed for one modifier. **B,** CMS-1500 (08-05) allows for multiple placement of modifiers. (Courtesy U.S. Department of Health and Human Services, Centers for Medicare and Medicaid Services.)

-F7   Right hand, third digit

-F8   Right hand, fourth digit

-F9   Right hand, fifth digit

-TA   Left foot, great toe

-T1   Left foot, second digit

-T2   Left foot, third digit

-T3   Left foot, fourth digit

-T4   Left foot, fifth digit

-T5   Right foot, great toe

-T6   Right foot, second digit

-T7   Right foot, third digit

-T8   Right foot, fourth digit

-T9   Right foot, fifth digit

-LC   Left circumflex, coronary artery

-LD   Left anterior descending coronary artery

-RC   Right coronary artery

Anatomical modifiers are not used with skin procedures

> ***Example:*** Removal of skin tags, any area

Exception is with codes that indicate feet, hands, fingers, legs, arms, and eyelids

■ SURGERY SECTION (10021-69990)

Largest CPT Section

Section Format

Divided by subspecialty, e.g., Integumentary, Cardiovascular

Notes and Guidelines

Throughout section

Information varied and extensive

"Must reading"

Subsection notes apply to entire subsection

Subheading notes apply to entire subheading

Category notes apply to entire category

Parenthetical information (Figure 3-7)

Unlisted Procedure Codes

Used only when more specific code not found

Written report accompanies submission

Each unlisted code service paid on case-by-case basis

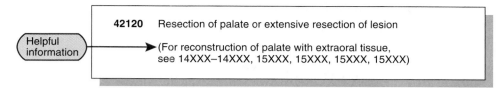

Figure **3-7** Parenthetical information in the CPT manual.

Separate Procedures

"(Separate procedure)" follows code description

Usually minor surgical procedure

Incidental to more major procedure

- Breast biopsy before radical mastectomy would not be coded
- Appendectomy performed routinely when other abdominal surgery is performed

Separate procedures reported when

- Only procedure performed
- With another procedure
  - On different site
  - Unrelated to major procedure

Major Guideline of Surgical Packages

Usually include

- Preoperative (before, preop)
- E/M service subsequent to decision for surgery but prior to surgery date
- Intraoperative (during, intraop)
- Postoperative (after—also known as global period, postop)
  - Post-anesthesia recovery (PAR)
  - Follow-up office visits
- Local/topical anesthesia and digital block

To report these bundled services separately is unbundling

Remember to use modifiers during global period for unrelated E/M, return to OR, etc.

Supplies

Supplies that are beyond those typically included in the procedure are reported separately

Example: Report surgical tray with

- 99070 CPT, Medicine section
- A4550 HCPCS

Special Report

Submitting an unlisted service or one that is unusual, variable, or new may require a special report

Demonstrates medical necessity/appropriateness of service

Contains pertinent information describing service in terms of

- Nature
- Extent
- Need for procedure
- Time
- Effort
- Equipment necessary

May also include complexity of symptoms, final diagnosis, physical findings, procedures, concurrent problems, and follow-up care

GENERAL SUBSECTION (10021, 10022)

Fine needle aspirations with or without (w/wo) imaging guidance

- Excludes bone marrow aspirations (38220)

Pathology 88172 and 88173 for evaluation of aspirate

INTEGUMENTARY SYSTEM SUBSECTION (10040-19499)

Often used in all specialties of medicine

Not just surgeons or dermatologists; wide range of physicians

Subheadings of Integumentary Subsection

- Skin, Subcutaneous, and Accessory Structures
- Nails
- Repair (Closure)
- Destruction
- Breast

Skin, Subcutaneous, and Accessory Structures (10040-11646)

Incision and Drainage (10040-10180)

I&D of abscess, carbuncle, boil, cyst, infection, hematoma, pilonidal cyst

- Lancing (cutting of skin)
- Aspiration (removal by puncturing lesion with a needle and withdrawing fluid)

Gauze or tube may be inserted for continued drainage

Pilonidal cyst

- Also known as a pilonidal abscess
- May be incised and drained (10080, 10081) or excised (11770-11772)

Excision—Debridement (11000-11044)
Dead tissue cut away and washed away with sterile saline

11000, 11001 Eczematous or infected skin

11004-11006 Debridement of infected area based on location and depth of necrotizing tissue (subcutaneous tissue, muscle, and fascia)

11008 Removal of prosthetic material or mesh from abdominal wall

11010-11012 Foreign material with fracture or dislocation

11040-11044 Skin, subcutaneous muscle, bone

Paring or Cutting (11055-11057)
Removal by scraping or peeling (e.g., removal of corn or callus)

Codes indicate number: 1, 2-4, 4+

Biopsy (11100, 11101)
Skin, subcutaneous tissue, or mucous membrane biopsy

Not all of lesion removed

- All lesion removed = excision

Do not use modifier -51

Codes indicate number: 1 or each additional

Tissue removed during excision, shaving, etc., and submitted to pathology is NOT reported separately as a biopsy

- Rather, it is included in the code for the excision

Skin Tag Removal (11200, 11201)
Benign lesions

Removed with scissors, blade, chemicals, electrosurgery, etc.

Do not use -51

- Codes indicate number: Up to 15 and each additional 10 lesions

Shaving of Lesions (11300-11313)
Removed by transverse incision or sliced horizontally

Based on

- Size (e.g., 1.1-2.0 cm)
- Location (e.g., arm, hand, nose)

Does not require suture closure

- Report most extensive lesion first with no modifier, then least extensive lesions with modifier -51

Benign/Malignant Lesions (11400-11646)
Codes divided: Benign or malignant

Physician assesses lesion as benign or malignant

Codes include local anesthesia and simple closure

Report each excised lesion separately

Lesion size

- Taken from physician's notes

- Includes greatest diameter plus margins (Figure 3-8)

  Example: A benign lesion measuring 0.5 cm at widest point is removed with 0.5-cm margin at narrowest point (each side, 0.5 + 0.5 = 1.0 cm). Reported as 1.5-cm lesion excision (11402)

  - Do not take size from pathology report—storage solution shrinks tissue

  - Margins (healthy tissue) are also taken for comparison with unhealthy tissue

  - Re-excisions following initial excision of malignant lesion

    Coded as excision of malignant lesion

All excised tissue pathologically examined

Codes 11400-11646 report excision of lesion

Codes 17260-17286 report destruction

Destroyed lesions have no pathology samples

  Example: Laser or chemical

Lesion closure

- Simple or subcutaneous closure included in removal

- Reported separately

  - Layered or intermediate, 12031-12057 (Repair—Intermediate)

  - Complex, 13100-13153 (Repair—Complex)

Nails (11719-11765)

Both toes and fingers

Types of services

- Trimming, debridement, removal, biopsy, repair

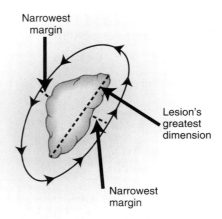

Figure **3-8** Calculating the size of a lesion.

Introduction (11900-11983)

Types of services

- Lesion injections (therapeutic or diagnostic), tattooing, tissue expansion, contraceptive insertion/removal, hormone implantation services, and insertion/removal of nonbiodegradable drug delivery implant

Repair (12001-13160)

Repair Factors in Wound Repair

As types of wounds vary, types of wound repair also vary

Length, complexity (simple, intermediate, complex), and site must be documented

- Length measured in centimeters

- Measured prior to closure

Types of Wound Repair

Simple. Superficial, epidermis, dermis, or subcutaneous tissue
- One-layer closure

- Dermabond closure

- Medicare report G0168

Intermediate. Layered closure of deeper layers of subcutaneous tissue and superficial fascia with skin closure

- Single-layer closure can be coded as intermediate if extensive debridement required

Complex. Greater than layered; may include multiple layers of tissue and fascia or extensive debridement

   Example: Scar revision, complicated debridement, extensive undermining, stents, extensive retention sutures

Included in Wound Repair Codes

Simple ligation of vessels in an open wound

Simple exploration of nerves, blood vessels, and exposed tendons

Normal debridement

- Additional codes for debridement can be used when

  - Gross contamination requires prolonged cleaning

  - Appreciable amounts of devitalized/contaminated tissue are removed to expose healthy tissue

  - Debridement is provided without immediate primary closure

Grouping of Wound Repair

Add together lengths by

- **Complexity** of Wound

  - Simple, intermediate, complex

- **Location** of Wound
  - e.g., face, ears, eyelids, nose, lips

1 inch = 2.54 cm

Example: **Same complexity, same codes description location:** Intermediate repairs of 2.9-cm laceration of leg and 1.1-cm laceration of buttocks. 2.9 + 1.1 = 4.0 cm (12032)

Example: **Different complexity:** Intermediate repair of 2.9-cm laceration of leg and simple repair of 1.1-cm laceration of buttocks. 2.9-cm intermediate repair (12032) and 1.1-cm simple repair (12001)

Example: **Same complexity, different code description locations:** Intermediate repair of 2.9-cm laceration of leg and intermediate repair of 1.1-cm laceration of nose. 2.9-cm intermediate repair of leg (12032) and 1.1-cm intermediate repair of nose (12051)

Do not Group Wound Repairs that are
Different complexities

Example: Simple repair and complex repair

Different locations as stated in the code description

Example: Simple repairs of scalp (12001) and nose (12011)

Adjacent Tissue Transfer, Flaps, and Grafts

Information Needed to Code Graft
Type of graft—adjacent, free, flap, etc.

Donor site (from)

Recipient site (to)

Any repair to donor site

Size of graft

Adjacent Tissue Transfer/Rearrangement (14000-14350)
Includes excision and/or repair (e.g., Z-plasty, W-plasty, V-plasty, Y-plasty, rotation flap, advancement flap)

Codes based on size and location of graft

Measure site of defect from excision plus size of defect from flap design

Skin Replacement Surgery and Skin Substitutes (15002-15431)
15002-15005 Site preparation based on size and site

15040 Harvest for tissue culture

15050-15261 Graft codes by type

Split-thickness: Epidermis and some dermis (Figure 3-9)

Full-thickness: Epidermis and all dermis

Grafts (15300-15431)
Bilaminate skin substitute

- Artificial skin, such as silicone covered nylon mesh

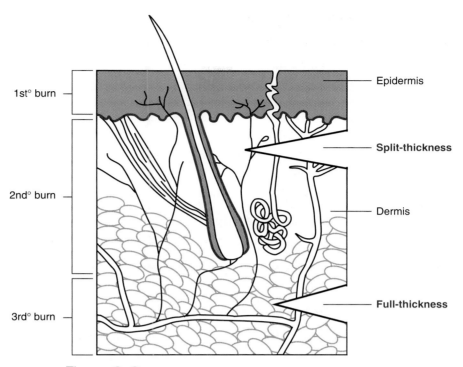

Figure **3-9** Split-thickness and full-thickness skin grafts.

Allograft: Donor graft

Xenograft: Nonhuman donor

Code is based on recipient site, not donor site

Flap (15570-15776)
Some skin left attached to blood supply

• Keeps flap viable

Donor site may be far from recipient site

Flaps may be in stages

Codes divided by location and size

Formation of flap (15570-15576)

• Based on location: Trunk, scalp, nose, etc.

Transfer of flap (15650): Previously placed flap released from donor site

• Also known as walking or walk up of flap

Muscle, Myocutaneous, or Fasciocutaneous Flaps (15732-15738)

• Repairs made with
  • Muscle
  • Muscle and skin
  • Fascia and skin

• Flaps rotated from donor to recipient site

• Includes closure donor site

Pressure (Decubitus) Ulcers (15920-15999)

Excision and various closures

- Primary, skin flap, muscle, etc.

Many codes "with ostectomy"

- Bone removal

Locations

- Coccygeal (end of spine)

- Sacral (between hips)

- Ischial (lower hip)

- Trochanteric (outer hip)

Site preparation only: 15936, 15946, or 15956

- Defect repair or donor site reported separately

Burns (16000-16036)

Codes for small, medium, and large

Most calculate percentage of body burn using Rule of Nines for adults (Figure 3-10)

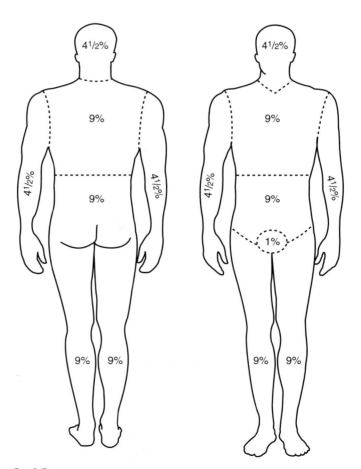

Figure **3-10** The Rule of Nines is used to calculate burn area on an adult.

- <5% small
- 5% to 10% medium
- >10% large

Lund-Browder for children (Figure 3-11)

- Proportions of children differ from adults
- Heads are larger

Often require multiple debridement and redressing

Based on

- Initial treatment of 1st-degree burn
- Size

The use of anesthesia not a factor in CPT burn codes as of 2006

Report percent of burn and depth

Destruction (17000-17286)
Ablation (destruction) of tissue

- Laser, electrosurgery, cryosurgery, chemosurgery, etc.

Benign/premalignant or malignant tissue

- Malignant tissue is based on location and size
- Benign/premalignant is based on the number of lesions removed

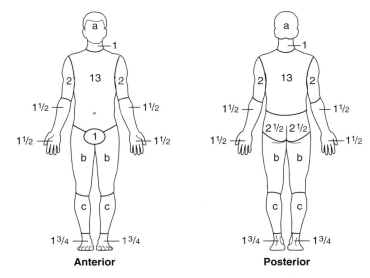

Relative percentage of body surface areas (% BSA) affected by growth

	0 yr	1 yr	5 yr	10 yr	15 yr
a – 1/2 of head	9 1/2	8 1/2	6 1/2	5 1/2	4 1/2
b – 1/2 of 1 thigh	2 3/4	3 1/4	4	4 1/4	4 1/2
c – 1/2 of lower leg	2 1/2	2 1/2	2 3/4	3	3 1/4

Figure **3-11** Lund-Browder chart for estimating the extent of burns on children.

Mohs' Micrographic Surgery (17311-17315)
Surgeon acts as pathologist and surgeon

Removes one layer of lesion at time

Continues until no malignant cells remain

Based on stages and number of specimens per stage indicated in medical record

Other Procedures (17340-17999)
Treatment of acne

- Cryotherapy

- Chemical exfoliation

Electrolysis

Unlisted procedures

Breast Procedures (19000-19499)
Divided based on procedure

- Incision

- Excision

- Introduction

- Repair/Reconstruction

Use excision of lesion codes if entire lesion is removed during incisional biopsy

Use additional code for placement of radiological marker

Mastectomies based on extent of procedure

- Wide excision

- Removal of neoplasm, capsule, and surrounding margins

- Radical

- Wide excision and anatomical structure surrounding neoplasm

    Example: Muscle or fascia

- Conservative mastectomy in which lesion is removed with adequate margins (19301)

- Axillary dissection and partial mastectomy, 19302

- Radical and modified radical 19305, 19306, and 19307 based on extent

Confirm whether pectoral muscles, axillary, or internal lymph nodes were removed

19307 most common and includes breast and axillary lymph node removal

Code removal of lymph node separately unless included in code description

Bilateral procedures, use -50

Biopsy/Removal of Lesion
Incisional biopsy: Incision made into lesion and small portion of lesion removed

Excisional biopsy: Entire lesion removed

Open incisional biopsy most complex (19101)

Percutaneous core needle biopsy without imaging guidance (19100)

- Same procedure without imaging guidance is 19102

Automated vacuum assisted or rotating biopsy device described in 19103 is the use of advanced breast biopsy instrumentation

- Image guidance performed by physician reported separately
- Complete, simple removal of a mass is reported with 19120

Lesion may be preoperatively marked by placing thin wire (radiologic marker) down to lesion

- Wire placement reported separately (19290)
- Additional wires reported with 19291
- Metallic localization clips may be placed during biopsy operative session so the site can be located later, if necessary
- Placement of clip reported with 19295, once for each clip placed
- Image guidance performed by physician reported separately

MUSCULOSKELETAL SYSTEM SUBSECTION (20000-29999)

Subsection divided: Anatomic site, then service (e.g., excision)

Used extensively by orthopedic surgeons

- Many codes commonly used by variety of physicians

Extensive notes

Most common

- Fracture and dislocation treatments
- "General" subheading
- Arthroscopic procedures
- Casting and strapping

Eponyms are "things" named after "people"

> **Example:** Barr procedure is a tendon transfer of the lower leg (27690-27692), and Mitchell Chevron procedure is a complex metatarsal osteotomy (bunion correction) (28296)

- Procedures are often referred to with eponyms
- Check the index of the CPT manual for directions to eponym codes

Fracture Treatment

Type of treatment depends on type and severity of fracture

Diagnosis codes must support the procedure codes and document the medical necessity

Open: Surgically opened to view or remotely opened to place nail across fracture site

- Open reduction with fixation is ORIF

Closed: Not surgically opened

Percutaneous: Insertion of devices through skin or a remote site

Treatment terms should not be confused with **types** of fractures:

- Open fracture: Fractured bone penetrates skin
- Closed fracture: Fractured bone does not penetrate skin

Traction

- Application of force to align bone
- Force applied by internal device (e.g., wire, pin) inserted into bone (skeletal fixation)
- Application of force by means of adhesion to skin (skin traction)

Manipulation

Use of force to return bone back to normal alignment by manual manipulation or temporary traction

Codes often divided based on whether manipulation was or was not used

Dislocation

Bone displaced from normal joint position

Treatment: Return bone to normal joint location

Subheading "General"

Begins "Incision" (20000, 20005)

Depth: Difference between Integumentary and Musculoskeletal incision codes

Musculoskeletal used when underlying bone or muscle is involved

Wound Exploration (20100-20103)

Traumatic penetrating wounds

Divided by wound location

Includes

- Enlargement
- Debridement
- Foreign body(ies) removal
- Ligation
- Repair of tissue and muscle

Use additional code for repair of major structures or blood vessels

Not used for integumentary repairs

- Unless the repair requires extension, enlargement, or exploration

Excision (20150-20251)

Biopsies for bone and muscle

Divided by

- Type of biopsy (bone/muscle)

- Depth
- Some by method

Can be percutaneous needle or excisional

Does not include tumor excision, which is coded separately

Biopsy with excision: Code only excision

Introduction or Removal (20500-20694)

Codes for

- Injections
- Aspirations
- Insertions
- Applications
- Removals
- Adjustments

Therapeutic sinus tract injection procedures

- Not nasal sinus
- Abscess or cyst with passage (sinus tract) to skin
- Antibiotic injected with use of radiographic guidance

Removal of foreign bodies lodged in muscle or tendon sheath

Integumentary removal codes for removal from skin

Injection into

- Tendon sheath
- Tendon origin
- Ligament
- Ganglion cyst
- Trigger points

Arthrocentesis injection "and/or" aspiration of a joint

- Both aspiration and injection reported with one code (20600-20610)
- Codes based on joint size: Small, intermediate, major
- Do not unbundle and report aspiration/injection with two codes

External Fixation (20690-20692)

Application of device that holds bone in place

Code fracture treatment and external fixation

- Unless treatment and fixation both included in fracture care code description

Replantation (20802-20838)

Used to report reattachment of amputated limb

Code by body area

Grafts (20900-20938)

Autogenous Grafts

Used to report harvesting through separate incision of

- Bone

- Cartilage

- Tendon

- Fascia lata

- Tissue

Fascia lata grafts: From lower thigh where fascia is thickest

Some codes include obtaining grafting material (not coded separately)

Other Procedures (20950-20999)

Monitoring muscle fluid pressure (interstitial for compartment syndrome, etc.)

- Pressure increases when blood supply decreases due to increased accumulation of fluids

Bone grafts identified by site taken from (donor site)

Free osseocutaneous flaps: Bone grafts

- Taken along with skin and tissue overlying bone

Electrical stimulation

- Used to speed bone healing

- Placement of stimulators externally or internally

- Ultrasound also used externally

Arthrodesis

Fixation of joint (arthro = joint, desis = fusion)

- Fixation with pins, wires, rods, etc. to immobilize the joint

Often performed with other procedure such as fracture repair

- Arthrodesis of the spine is also called spinal fusion

Subsequent Subheadings

After General subheading, divided by anatomic location

- Anatomic subheadings divided by type procedure

    Example: Subheading "Head" divided by procedure

- Incision

- Excision

- Introduction or Removal

- Repair, Revision, and/or Reconstruction

- Other Procedures

- Fracture and/or Dislocation

Spinal Instrumentation and Fixation

Insertion of spinal instrumentation reported in addition to arthrodesis (fusion)

Spine (Vertebral Column), 22100-22899, divided by repair location

- Cervical (C1-C7)

    C1 = Atlas

    C2 = Axis

- Thoracic (T1-T12)
- Lumbar (L1-L5)
- Sacral (S1)

Coccyx (tailbone)

Vertebral segment: Single complete vertebral bone with articular processes and laminae

Vertebral interspace: Non-bony compartment between two vertebral bodies which contains the disk

Single level = two vertebrae and the disk that separates them

Percutaneous vertebroplasty

- Use of polymethylmethacrylate injected into the vertebral space
    - Polymethylmethacrylate is a type of bone cement/glue like silicone but not silicone
    - Adheres bone fragments together
    - Fills vertebral body defects

Types of spinal instrumentation

Segmental: Devices at each end of repair area + at least one other attachment

Nonsegmental: Devices at each end of defect only

Approach: Pay special attention to the approach used to perform the surgery

- Several different approaches to spine: Most common anterior (front) and posterior (back)
- Most spinal instrumentation codes divided based on approach

Casting and Strapping (29000-29799)

Replacement procedure or initial placement to stabilize without additional restorative treatment

   Example: Application of wrist splint or cast for wrist sprain

Initial fracture treatment includes placement and removal of first cast

- Subsequent cast applications coded separately
- Payers have strict individual reimbursement policies for subsequent casting

Application not coded when part of surgical procedure

   Example: Application of wrist splint or cast for wrist sprain

Initial fracture treatment includes placement and removal of first cast

Ace bandage applications not billed separately

Removal bundled into surgical procedure

Supplies reported separately

Subheading Endoscopy/Arthroscopy (29800-29999)
Surgical arthroscopy always includes diagnostic arthroscopy

Codes divided by joint

• Subdivided by procedure

Be aware of subterms and bundled procedures within code descriptions

Note: Parenthetical information following codes indicates codes to use if procedure was an open procedure

RESPIRATORY SYSTEM SUBSECTION (30000-32999)

Anatomic site arrangement

• Nose

• Larynx

Further subdivided by procedure

• Incision

• Excision

Endoscopy

Endoscopy in all subheadings except Nose

Each preceded by "Notes"

Endoscopy Rule One
Code full extent of endoscopic procedure performed

> *Example:* Procedure begins at mouth and ends at bronchial tube

• Bronchial tube = full extent

Endoscopy Rule Two
Code correct approach

> *Example:* For removal:

  • Interior lung lesion via endoscopy inserted through mouth

  • Exterior lung lesion via laparoscope inserted through skin

Incorrect approach = incorrect code = incorrect or no reimbursement

Endoscopy Rule Three
Diagnostic always included in surgical

> *Examples:*

  • Diagnostic bronchial endoscopy begins

  • Identified foreign body

  • Removed foreign body (surgical endoscopy)

Multiple Procedures

Frequent in respiratory coding

- **Watch for bundled services**

Sequence primary procedure first, no modifier

Sequence secondary procedures next, with -51

Bilateral procedures often performed, use -50

Format for reporting chosen by payer

Example: Nasal lavage

- 31000 × 2
- 31000 and 31000-50
- 31000-50
- 31000-RT and 31000-LT

Nose (30000-30999)

Used extensively by otorhinolaryngologists (ear, nose, and throat [ENT] specialists)

Also used by wide variety of physicians in other specialties

When approach to nose

- External approach, use Integumentary System
- Internal approach, use Respiratory System

Incision (30000, 30020)

Bundled into Incision codes are drain or gauze insertion and removal

Supplies reported separately

Excision (30100-30160)

Contains intranasal biopsy codes

Polyp excision, by complexity

- Excision includes any method of destruction, even laser
- Use -50 (bilateral) for both sides

Turbinate excision and resection

- Three turbinates: Superior, middle, inferior
- Excision of inferior turbinate, 30130
- Excision of superior or middle turbinate, 30999
- Submucous resection of inferior turbinate, 30140

    Reduction of inferior turbinates, 30140-52

- Submucous resection of superior or middle turbinate, 30999

Introduction (30200-30220)

Common procedures

Example: Injections to shrink nasal tissue or displacement therapy (saline flushes) to remove mucus

- Displacement therapy performed through nose

Removal of Foreign Body (30300-30320)
Distinguished by the site of removal, whether at office or hospital (requires general anesthesia)

Repair (30400-30630)
Many plastic procedures

- Rhinoplasty (reshaping nose internal and/or external)

- Septoplasty (rearrangement or plastic repair of nasal septum)

Destruction (30801, 30802)
Use of cauterization or ablation (removing by cutting)

Used for removal of excess nasal mucosa or to reduce turbinate inflammation

Based on intramural or superficial extent of destruction

- **Intramural:** Deeper mucosa

- **Superficial:** Outer layer of mucosa

Other Procedures (30901-30999)
Control of nasal hemorrhage

- Packing

- Ligation

- Cauterization

Anterior packing for less severe bleeding

Posterior packing for more severe bleeding

Accessory Sinuses, Incision, Excision, Endoscopy (31000-31094)

Codes for lavage (washing) of sinuses

- Cannula (hollow tube) placed into sinus

- Sterile saline solution flushed through

Procedures may involve multiple codes when multiple locations are accessed

Example: 31020, Sinusotomy, maxillary, can be coded with 31050 sinusotomy, sphenoid, and 31070 sinusotomy, frontal

Use -50 (bilateral) for both sides

Maxillary sinusotomy may use an external and intranasal approach to creating passage between sinus and nose

- Used to clear blocked or infected sinus

- Intranasal sinusotomy, 31020

- External sinusotomy, radical (such as Caldwell-Luc)

Access through mouth

Incision above eyetooth

Sinus is cleaned

New opening created or old opening enlarged

Repair of fractures occurring during procedure may be coded separately if not included in code description

Larynx (31300-31599)

Excision (31300-31420)
Laryngotomy: Open surgical procedure to expose larynx

• For removal procedure (e.g., tumor)

May be confused with Trachea/Bronchi codes for tracheostomy used to establish airflow

Introduction (31500-31502)
Used to establish, maintain, and protect air flow

Endotracheal intubation, establishment of airway

Based on planned (ventilation support) or emergency procedure

Laryngoscopic Procedures (31505-31579)
Uses terms *indirect* and *direct*

• **Indirect:** Tongue depressor with mirror used to view larynx

• **Direct:** Endoscopy passed into larynx; physician directly views vocal cords

Repair (31580-31590)
Several plastic procedures and fracture repairs

Laryngoplasty procedures based on purpose

Fracture codes based on whether manipulation used

Trachea and Bronchi (31600-31899)

Incision (31600-31614)
Most codes: Tracheostomy divided by

• Planned (ventilation support)

• Emergency

Divided by type

• Transtracheal or cricothyroid (location of incision)

Endoscopy (31615-31656)
Bronchoscope may be inserted into nose or mouth

Rigid endoscopy performed under general anesthesia

Flexible endoscopy performed under local or conscious (moderate) sedation

Introduction (31715-31730)

Catheterization

Instillation

Injection

Aspiration

Tracheal tube placement

Some include inhaled gas as contrast material

Repair (31750-31830)

Plastic repairs of tracheoplasty and bronchoplasty

Lungs and Pleura (32000-32999)

Incision (32000-32225)

Thoracentesis. Needle inserted into pleural space for aspiration (withdrawal) of fluid or air

Thoracotomy. Surgical opening of chest to expose to view.

Used for

- Biopsy
- Cyst
- Foreign body removal
- Cardiac massage, etc.

Excision (32310-32540)

Biopsy codes in both Excision and Incision categories

- Excisional biopsy with percutaneous needle
- Incisional biopsy with chest open

Also services of pleurectomy, pneumocentesis, and lung removal

- **Segmentectomy:** 1 segment
- **Lobectomy:** 1 lobe
- **Bilobectomy:** 2 lobes
- **Total Pneumonectomy:** 1 lung

CARDIOVASCULAR (CV) SYSTEM SUBSECTION (33010-37799)

CV coding may require codes from

- **Radiology:** Diagnostic studies
- **Medicine:** Nonsurgical and percutaneous
- **Surgery:** Open and percutaneous

Cardiology Coding Terminology

Invasive: Enters body

- Incisional

Example: Opening chest for removal (i.e., tumor on heart)

- Percutaneously
  - Placement of catheter into artery or vein by means of wire threaded through needle and catheter slid over wire

  Example: PTCA (percutaneous transluminal coronary artery) procedure
- Cut down—small nick made and catheter inserted

  Example: Catheter inserted into femoral or brachial artery

Common catheters are:

- Broviac
- Hickman
- HydroCath
- Arrow multi-lumen
- Groshong
- Dual-lumen
- Triple-lumen

Both Medicine and Surgery sections contain invasive procedures

Noninvasive: Procedures that do not break skin

Example: Electrocardiogram

Electrophysiology (EPS): Study of electrical system of heart

Example: Study of irregular heartbeat (arrhythmia)

Nuclear Cardiology: Diagnostic and treatment specialty; uses radioactive substances to diagnose cardiac conditions

Example: MRI

■ Cardiovascular in Surgery Section

Codes for Procedures

Heart/Pericardium (33010-33999)

- Pacemakers, valve disorders

Arteries/Veins (34001-37799)

- Many of same types of procedures but noncoronary procedures

Heart/Pericardium (33010-33999)
Both percutaneous and open surgical

- Cardiologists use percutaneous intervention; cardiovascular or thoracic surgeons use open surgical procedures

Extensive notes throughout

Frequent changes with medical advances

Examples of categories of Heart/Pericardium subheading

- Pericardium
- Cardiac Tumor
- Pacemaker or Pacing Cardioverter-Defibrillator

Examples of services

- Pericardiocentesis: Percutaneous withdrawal of fluid from pericardial space (pericarditis)
- Cardiac Tumor: Open surgical procedure for removal of tumor on heart

Pacemakers and Cardioverter-Defibrillators (33202-33249)

Devices that assist heart in electrical function

- Differentiate between temporary and permanent devices
- Differentiate between one-chamber and dual-chamber devices

Divided by where pacer placed, approach, and type of service

Patient record indicates revision or replacement

- Pacemaker pulse generator is also called a battery
- Pacemaker leads are also called electrodes

Usual follow-up 90 days (global period)

Placed

Atrium (single chamber)

- Pulse generator and one electrode in atrium (single-chamber pacemaker)

Ventricle (single chamber)

- Pulse generator and one electrode in ventricle (single-chamber pacemaker)

Both (dual chamber)

- Pulse generator and one electrode in right ventricle and one electrode in right atrium

Biventricular, both ventricles and atrium (uses 3 leads)

- Pulse generator and one electrode in right ventricle, one electrode in right atrium, and one electrode in left ventricle via the coronary sinus

Approach

Epicardial: Open procedure to place on heart

Transvenous: Through vein to place in heart

Type of service

Initial placement or replacement of all or part of device

Number of leads placed is important in code selection

Electrophysiologic Operative Procedures (33250-33266)

Surgeon repairs defect causing abnormal rhythm

Chest opened to full view

- Cardiopulmonary (CP) bypass usually used

Endoscopy procedure

- Without cardiopulmonary bypass

Codes based on reason for procedure and if CP bypass used

Patient-Activated Event Recorder (33282, 33284)

Also known as cardiac event recorder or loop recorder

Internal surgical implantation required

Divided based on whether device is being implanted or removed

Cardiac Valves (33400-33496)

Divided by valve

- Aortic

- Mitral

- Tricuspid

- Pulmonary

Subdivided by whether replacement, repair, or excision is completed (all done with bypass machine)

Code descriptions are all similar, requiring careful reading

Coronary Artery Bypass Graft (CABG)

CABG performed for bypassing coronary arteries severely obstructed as in atherosclerosis or arteriosclerosis

Determine what was used in repair

- Vein (33510-33516)

- Artery (33533-33536)

- Both artery and vein (33517-33523 and 33533-33536)

Based on number of bypass grafts performed and if combined venous and arterial grafts are used

> *Example:* Three venous grafts

Venous Grafting Only for Coronary Artery Bypass (33510-33516)

Based on number of grafts being replaced

Combined Arterial-Venous Grafting (33517-33530)

Divided based on number of grafts and if procedure initial or reoperation

Procuring saphenous vein included, unless performed endoscopically

These codes are never used alone

- Arterial-Venous codes (33517-33523) report only **venous** graft portion of procedure

- Always used with Arterial Grafting codes (33533-33536)

> *Example:* 3 vein grafts and 2 arterial grafts = 33519 and 33534

Open procurement of saphenous vein is included in procedure (not coded separately)

Code harvesting of saphenous vein graft separately when endoscopic video-assisted procurement is performed (33508)

Code harvesting separately when of upper extremity or femoral vein

Arterial Grafting for Coronary Artery Bypass (33533-33536)
Divided based on number of grafts

Obtaining artery for grafting included in codes, except

• Procuring upper-extremity artery (e.g., radial artery), coded separately

Several codes (33542-33548) for myocardial resection, repair of ventricular septal defect (VSD), and ventricular restoration

Endovascular Repair of Descending Thoracic Aorta (33880-33891)

Reports placement of an endovascular aortic prosthesis for repair of descending thoracic aorta

• Less invasive than traditional approach of chest or abdominal incision

Synthetic aortic prosthesis is placed via catheter

• Report fluoroscopic guidance separately 75956-75959

   Includes diagnostic imaging prior to placement and intraprocedurally

Stent-graft (endoprosthesis) is deployed to reinforce weakened area

Arteries and Veins Subheading (34001-37799)

Only for noncoronary vessels

• Divided based on whether artery or vein involved

   Example: Different codes for embolectomy, depending on artery or vein

Catheters placed into vessels for monitoring, removal, repair

Using nonselective or selective catheter placement

• Nonselective: Direct placement without further manipulation

• Selective: Place and then manipulate into further order(s)

Catheter Placement Example

• Nonselective: 36000 Introduction of needle into vein

• Selective: 36012 Placement of catheter into second-order venous system

Vascular Families are Like a Tree
First-order (main) branch (tree trunk)

Second-order branch (tree limb)

Third-order branch (tree branch)

Brachiocephalic Vascular Family (Figure 3-12)

• Report farthest extent of catheter placement in a vascular family; labor intensity is increased with the extent of catheter placement

Embolectomy and Thrombectomy (34001-34490)
Embolus: Dislodged thrombus

Thrombus: Mass of material in vessel located in place of formation

• May be removed by dissection or balloon

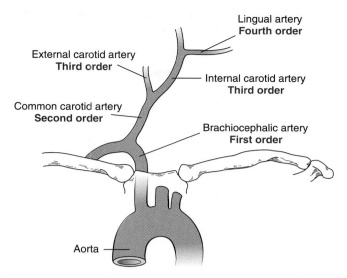

Figure **3-12** Brachiocephalic vascular family with first-, second-, third-, and fourth-order vessels.

Balloon Removal: Threaded into vessel, inflated under mass, pulled out with mass

• Codes are divided by site of incision and whether artery or vein

Venous Reconstruction—CV Repairs (34501-34530)
Types of repairs
• Valve of the femoral vein

• Vena Cava

• Saphenopopliteal vein anastomosis

Aneurysm
Aneurysm: Weakened arterial wall causing a bulge or ballooning

Repair by removal, bypass, or coil placement

Endovascular repair (34800-34834) from inside vessel

Direct (35001-35152) from outside vessel

Endovascular Repair of Abdominal Aortic Aneurysm (34800-34834)
Extensive notes preceding codes—must reading

Uses fluoroscopic guidance report Radiology 75952 or 75953

Includes access, catheter manipulation, balloon angioplasty, stent placement, site closure

Other procedures performed at same time, coded separately

Repair Arteriovenous Fistula (35180-35190)
Abnormal passage from artery or vein

Divided based on fistula type

• Congenital

- Acquired/traumatic

- By site

Repair methods

- Autogenous graft—fistula created artery to vein

- Non-auto fistula—biocompatible tube connecting artery to vein

Angioplasty and Atherectomy
Divided as open or percutaneous and by vessel

- **Transluminal:** By way of vessel

- **Transluminal Angioplasty:** Catheter passed into vessel and stretched

  - Placement of eluding or noneluding stents is coded, in addition to catheter placement

- **Transluminal Atherectomy:** Guide wire threaded into vessel and clots destroyed

Noncoronary Bypass Grafts (35500-35671)
Divided by

- Vein

- In Situ Vein (veins repaired in their original place)

- Other Than Vein

Code by type of graft and vessels being used to bypass

  Example: 35506 Bypass graft, with vein; carotid-subclavian

- Graft attached to carotid and to subclavian, bypassing defect of subclavian

Procurement of saphenous vein graft is included and not reported separately

Harvesting of upper-extremity vein or femoropopliteal vein is reported separately

Vascular Injection Procedures (36000-36550)
Divided into

- Intravenous

- Intra-arterial—Intra-aortic

- Venous

Used for many procedures, including

- Local anesthesia

- Introduction of needle

- Injection of contrast material

- Preoperative and postoperative care

  Example: Injection of opaque substance for venography (radiography of vein)

Central Venous Access (CVA) Procedures
Peripheral = long term, used for medication/chemotherapy administration

Central = short term, used for monitoring

Categories

1. Insertion

2. Repair

3. Replacement, partial or complete

4. Removal

5. Guidance for vascular access

Insertion (36555-36571)
Insertion of newly established venous access

- Tunneled under skin (e.g., Hickman, Broviac, Groshong)

- Nontunneled (e.g., Hohn catheter, triple lumen, PICC)

- Central (e.g., subclavian, intrajugular, femoral, inferior vena cava)

- Peripheral (any other type of angiocatheter)

Codes divided by tunneled/non-tunneled, central/peripheral, and age

Repair (36575, 36576)
Repair of malfunction without replacement

Repair of central venous access device

No differentiation between age of patient or central/peripheral insertion

Replacement (Partial or Complete) (36578-36585)
Partial (36578) is replacement of catheter only

Complete (36580-36585) is replacement through same venous access site

Differentiated by tunneled/non-tunneled, central/peripheral, and with or without subcutaneous port or pump

Removal (36589, 36590)
To be used for tunneled catheter

Removal of non-tunneled catheter is not reported separately

Guidance for Vascular Access
77001, Fluoroscopic guidance for central venous access device placement, replacement, or removal

- Reported in addition to primary procedure

76937, Ultrasound guidance for vascular access

- Reported in addition to primary procedure

Transcutaneous Procedures (37184-37216)
Arterial mechanical thrombectomy (37184-37186)

- Removal of thrombus by means of mechanical device

  From artery or arterial bypass graft

Venous mechanical thrombectomy (37187, 37188)

- Removal of a thrombus by means of a mechanical device

  From vein

Arterial and venous mechanical thrombectomy codes are add-on codes

- Include

  Introduction of device into thrombus

  Thrombus removal

  Injection of thrombolytic drug(s), if used

  Fluoroscopic and contrast guidance

  Follow-up angiography

- Report separately

  Diagnostic angiography

  Catheter placement(s)

  Diagnostic studies

  Pharmacologic thrombolytic infusion before or after (37201, 75894, 75898)

  Other interventions

Other Procedures (37195-37216)

- Used to report a variety of transcatheter procedures

  Example: Transcatheter biopsy, therapy, infusion, retrieval, and intravascular stents

■ Cardiovascular in Medicine Section

Services can be

- Invasive or noninvasive
- Diagnostic or therapeutic

Subheadings

- Therapeutic Services
- Cardiography
- Echocardiography
- Cardiac Catheterization
- Intracardiac Electrophysiologic (EP) Procedures
- Peripheral Arterial Disease Rehabilitation
- Other Vascular Studies

Therapeutic Services (92950-92998)

Types of services

- Cardioversion
- Infusions
- Thrombolysis
- Catheter placement

Many groups of codes divided by

- Method (e.g., balloon, blade)
- Location (e.g., aortic or mitral valve)
- Number (e.g., single or multiple vessels)

Cardiography (93000-93278)
Types of services

- Stress tests
- Holter monitor
- Electrocardiogram

Separate codes for components of study, such as

- 93000 global
- 93005 tracing only
- 93010 interpretation and report only

Echocardiography (93303-93350)
Noninvasive diagnostic procedure. Ultrasound detects presence of cardiac or vascular disease

Cardiac Catheterization (93501-93581)
Used to identify valve disorders, abnormal blood flow

Many bundled services in catheterization codes

Examples:
- Introduction
- Positioning/Repositioning of catheter
- Pressure readings inside heart or vessels
- Blood samples
- Rest/Exercise studies
- Final evaluation and report
- Many codes are -51 exempt

Three components of coding cardiac catheterization
1. Placement of catheter (93501-93533)

2. Injection (93539-93545)

3. Imaging supervision, interpretation, and report (93555 or 93556)

Intracoronary Brachytherapy
New procedure; uses radioactive substances to destroy restenosis of coronary vessel

Patients have had stent placed in coronary vessel

Stent "restenosis" (re-formation of plaque)

Cardiologist: Places guide wire and catheter

Radiation oncologist: Places radioactive elements

Intracardiac Electrophysiologic Procedures (93600-93662)
Services to diagnose and treat conditions of electrical system of heart

EP system of heart
Electrical conduction system

Electrical recording codes divided based on location of recording device

Example: Bundle of His or right ventricle

Pacing: Temporary pacing to stabilize beating of heart

Example: Intraventricular or intra-arterial pacing

Peripheral Arterial Disease (PAD) Rehabilitation (93668)
Rehabilitation sessions: 45-60 minutes

Use of motorized treadmill/track/bicycle to build patient's CV function

Supervised by exercise physiologist or nurse

If E/M is provided by physician, service is reported separately

Other Vascular Studies (93701-93790)
Category contains codes for services such as

- **Plethysmography:** Recordings of changes in size of body part when blood passes through it
- **Electronic Analysis:** Checks electronic function of devices, such as pacemakers
- **Ambulatory Blood Pressure Monitoring:** Outpatient basis over 24-hour period
- **Thermograms:** Visual recordings of body temperature

■ Cardiovascular in Radiology Section

Radiology section, Heart (75552-75556) and Aorta/Arteries (75600-75790) subsections

Prior to 1992, Radiology section contained codes for entire CV procedures

Major revision to CV radiology codes 1992

Divided complete procedures into two components: technical and professional

Example: Angiography

- Technical component angiography—remains in Radiology section
- Professional component injection—moved to Surgery section

Complete angiography requires radiology code and surgery code

Reflects common practice of cardiologist's performing injection and radiologist's performing angiography

Contrast Material
Often radiologic procedures use contrast material to improve image

Many codes have contrast material bundled into service

- "With contrast" or "with or without contrast"

Only injected contrast qualifies as with contrast

Contrast not included in description but used in procedure: Code contrast material and injection separately

• Specify site where service is received to differentiate between global, technical, and professional components of the procedure

Non-hospital-based (not employed by hospital) physician performs procedure in hospital outpatient department: Use -26 for professional component only

---

A COMPONENT CODING EXAMPLE

Two physicians (cardiologist and radiologist from same facility) perform angiography of third-order brachiocephalic artery with contrast

• Cardiologist places catheter (36217), Surgery section
• Radiologist performs angiography (75658), Radiology section
• Supply of contrast material (99070), Medicine section

HEMIC AND LYMPHATIC SYSTEM SUBSECTION (38100-38999)

Divisions

• Spleen
• General
• Lymph Nodes and Lymphatic Channels

Spleen Subheading (38100-38200)

Spleen easily ruptured, causing massive and potentially lethal hemorrhage

• May require splenectomy
• Splenectomy: Total or partial/open or laparoscopic

Often done as part of more major procedure

• Bundled into major procedure

General (38204-38242)

Codes divided based on

• Preservation
• Preparation
• Purification
• Aspiration
• Biopsy
• Harvesting
• Transplantation

Stem Cells
Immature blood cells originating in bone marrow

Used in treatment of leukemia

Types of stem cells

Allogenic: Close relative

Autologous: Patient's own

Lymph Nodes and Lymphatic Channels Subheading (38300-38999)

Two types of lymphadenectomies:

1. **Limited:** Lymph nodes only

2. **Radical:** Lymph nodes, submandibular gland, and surrounding tissue

Often bundled into more major procedure (e.g., prostatectomy)

Do not unbundle and report lymphadenectomy separately

MEDIASTINUM SUBSECTION (39000-39499)

Incision codes for foreign body removal or biopsy

Excision codes for removal of cyst or tumor

DIAPHRAGM SUBSECTION (39501-39599)

Only category: Repair

Most codes hernia or laceration repairs

DIGESTIVE SYSTEM SUBSECTION (40490-49999)

Divided by anatomic site from mouth to anus + organs that aid digestive process

> ***Example:*** Liver and gallbladder

Many bundled procedures

Endoscopy

Diagnostic procedure always bundled into surgical endoscopic

Code to furthest extent of procedure

Endoscopy Terminology

Notes define specific terminology

Code descriptions are specific regarding

- Technique and depth of scope

  Esophagoscopy: Esophagus only

  Esophagogastroscopy: Esophagus to past diaphragm

  Esophagogastroduodenoscopy: Esophagus to beyond pyloric channel

Read notes preceding 45300-45392

- Proctosigmoidoscopy: Rectum and sigmoid colon (6-25 cm)

- Sigmoidoscopy: Entire rectum, sigmoid colon, and may include part of descending colon (26-60 cm)

- Colonoscopy: Entire colon, rectum to cecum, and may include terminal ileum (greater than 60 cm)

Laparoscopy and Endoscopy

Some subheadings have both laparoscopy (outside) and endoscopy (inside) procedures

Example: Subheading Esophagus

- Endoscopy views inside
- Laparoscopy inserted through umbilicus; views from outside

New in 2006 were laparoscopic bariatric surgery codes (43770-43774)

- Use of gastric band and/or subcutaneous port components

Hemorrhoidectomy and Fistulectomy Codes (46221-46320)

Divided by

- Complexity
  - Simple: No plastic procedure involved
  - Complex: Includes plastic procedure and fissurectomy
- Anatomy
  - Subcutaneous: No muscle involvement
  - Submuscular: Splinter muscle
- Complex fistulectomy involves excision/incision of multiple fistulas

Hernia Codes (49491-49611)

Divided by

- Type of hernia

  Example: Inguinal, femoral

- Initial or subsequent repair
- Age of patient determines code choice
- Clinical presentation
  - **Strangulated:** Blood supply cut off
  - **Incarcerated:** Cannot be returned to cavity (not reducible)

Additional code is used for implantation of mesh or prosthesis

URINARY SYSTEM SUBSECTION (50010-53899)

Anatomic division

- Kidney
- Ureters
- Bladder
- Urethra

Further divided by procedure

- Incision
- Excision
- Introduction
- Repair
- Laparoscopy
- Endoscopy

Kidney Subheading (50010-50592)

Endoscopy codes are for procedure done through previously established stoma or incision

Caution: Codes may be unilateral or bilateral

Introduction Category (50382-50398)

Codes divided by renal pelvis catheter procedures or other introduction procedures

Renal pelvis catheters further divided; internal dwelling or externally accessible

Catheters for drainage and injections and for radiography

Aspirations

Insertion of guide wires

Tube changes

Usually reported with radiology component

Ureter Subheading (50600-50980)

Caution: Codes may be unilateral or bilateral

Divided by type of procedure

- Incision
- Excision
- Introduction
- Repair
- Laparoscopy codes describe surgical procedures

Bladder Subheading (51000-52700)

Includes codes for

- Incision
- Excision
- Introduction
- Urodynamics
- Repair
- Laparoscopy

- Endoscopy
- Cystoscopy
- Urethroscopy
- Cystourethroscopy
- Transurethral surgery

Many bundled codes

> *Example:* Urethral dilation is included with insertion of cystoscope

Read all descriptions carefully

Urodynamics (51725-51798)
Procedures relate to motion and flow of urine

Used to diagnose urine flow obstructions

Bundled: All usual, necessary instruments, equipment, supplies, and technical assistance

Vesical Neck and Prostate (52400-52700)
Contains codes for transurethral resection of the prostate (TURP)

> *Example:* 52601 reports a complete transurethral electrosurgical resection of the prostate and includes vasectomy, meatotomy, cystourethroscopy, urethral calibration and/or dilation, internal urethrotomy, and control of any postoperative bleeding

Other approaches are reported with 55801-55845

> *Example:* 55801 reports a removal of the prostate gland (prostatectomy) through an incision in the perineum and includes vasectomy, meatotomy, urethral calibration and/or dilation, internal urethrotomy, and control of any postoperative bleeding

MALE GENITAL SYSTEM SUBSECTION (54000-55899)

Penis (most codes)

Testis

Epididymis

Tunica Vaginalis

Scrotum

Vas Deferens

Spermatic Cord

Seminal Vesicles

Prostate

Biopsy Codes
Located in anatomical subheading to which the codes refer

> *Example:* Biopsy codes in subheadings

- Epididymis (Excision)
- Testis (Excision)

Penis (54000-54450)

Incision codes (54000-54015) differ from Integumentary System codes

- Penis incision codes for deeper structures

Destruction (54050-54065)

Codes divided by

- Extent: Simple or extensive
- Method of destruction, e.g., chemical, cryosurgery

Extensive destruction can be by any method

Excision (54100-54164)

Commonly used codes biopsy and circumcision

Introduction (54200-54250)

Many procedures for corpora cavernosa (spongy bodies of penis)

- Injection procedures for Peyronie disease (toughening of corpora cavernosa)
- Treatments for erectile dysfunction (ED)

Repair (54300-54450)

Many plastic repairs

Some repairs are staged (more than one stage)

- Stage indicated in code description

INTERSEX SURGERY SUBSECTION (55970, 55980)

There only 2 codes within subsection

1. Male to female
2. Female to male

Complicated procedures completed over extended period of time

Performed by multiple physicians with extensive specialized training

FEMALE GENITAL SYSTEM SUBSECTION (56405-58999)

Anatomic division: From vulva to ovaries

- Many bundled services

Vulva, Perineum, and Introitus (56405-56821)

Skene's gland coded with Urinary System, Incision or Excision codes

- Group of small mucous glands, lower end of urethra
  - Paraurethral duct

Incision (56405-56441)

I&D of abscess. Vulva, perineal area, or Bartholin's gland

Marsupialization
Cyst incised

Drained

Edges sutured to sides to keep cyst open creating a pouch-like repair

Destruction (56501, 56515)
Lesions destroyed by variety of methods

- Destruction = Eradication not to be confused with excision; excision is removal

Divided by simple or extensive destruction

- Complexity based on physician's judgment

- Stated in medical record

Destruction has no pathology report

Excision (56605-56740)
Biopsy includes

- Local anesthetic

- Biopsy

- Simple closure

Code based on number of lesions biopsied

Place number of lesions on CMS-1500 in Block 24-G (see Figure 3-1)

Vulvectomy. Surgical removal of portion of vulva (56620-56640)

Based on extent and size of area removed

Extent

- Simple: Skin and superficial subcutaneous tissues

- Radical: Skin and deep subcutaneous tissues

Size

- Partial: <80% vulvar area

- Complete: >80% vulvar area

Extent and size indicated in operative report

Repair (56800-56810)
Many plastic repairs

Read notes following category

- If repair procedure for wound of genitalia, use Integumentary System code

Endoscopy (56820-56825)
By means of a colposcopy

Vagina (57000-57425)
Codes divided based on service, e.g., incision, excision

Introduction (57150-57180)

Includes vaginal irrigation, insertion of devices, diaphragm, cervical caps

Report device inserted separately

- 99070 or HCPCS National Level II codes, such as A4261 (cervical cap)

Repair (57200-57335)

For nonobstetric repairs

- Obstetric repairs, use Maternity Care and Delivery codes

Manipulation (57400-57415)

Dilation: Speculum inserted into vagina, which is enlarged by dilator

Endoscopy (57420-57425)

Colposcopy codes based on purpose

- e.g., biopsy, diagnostic

Cervix Uteri (57452-57800)

Cervix uteri, narrow lower end of uterus

Services include excision, manipulation, repair

Excision (57500-57556)

Conization codes

Conization: Removal of cone of tissue from cervix

LEEP (loop electrocautery excision procedure) technology may be used for conizations or loop electrode biopsies

Corpus Uteri (58100-58579)

Many complex procedures

- Often very similar wording in code descriptions
- Requires careful reading and specific documentation in the medical record

Excision (58100-58294)

Dilation and curettage (D&C, 58120) of uterus

- After dilation, curette scrapes uterus
- Coded according to circumstances: Obstetrical or nonobstetrical

Do not report postpartum hemorrhage service with 58120

- Use 59160—Maternity and Delivery code

Many hysterectomy codes

- Based on approach (vaginal, abdominal) and extent (uterus, fallopian tubes, etc.)

Often secondary procedures performed with hysterectomy

Do not code secondary, related minor procedures separately

Introduction (58300-58356)
Common procedures

- e.g., insertion of an IUD

Report supply of device separately

Specialized services

- e.g., artificial insemination procedures

Used to report physician component of service

Component coding

- Necessary with catheter procedures for hysterosonography

- Notes following codes indicate radiology guidance component codes

Oviduct/Ovary (58600-58770)

Oviduct. Fallopian tube
Incision category contains tubal ligations

- When during same hospitalization (but not at same session as delivery), is coded separately

Laparoscopy (58660-58679)
Through abdominal wall

Codes in the laparoscopy and hysteroscopy section are divided by approach

- Then by purpose of procedure, e.g., lysis, lesion removal

Caution: If only diagnostic laparoscopy

- Do not use Female Genital System codes

- Use 49320, Digestive System

Many codes can be reported separately with appropriate modifiers

> ***Example:*** 58660 Laparoscopy, surgical, with lysis of adhesions, can be coded with any of the indented codes that follow 58660 (58661, 58662, 58670)

Ovary (58800-58960)

Two categories only: Incision and Excision

Incision: Primarily for drainage of cysts and abscesses

- Divided by surgical approach

Excision: Biopsy, wedge resection, and oophorectomy

In Vitro Fertilization (58970-58976)

Specialized codes used by physicians trained in fertilization procedures

- Codes divided by type of procedure and method used

MATERNITY CARE & DELIVERY SUBSECTION (59000-59899)

Divided by service

- Antepartum services, e.g.:

  Amniocentesis

  Fetal non-stress test

  Fetal monitoring during labor

- Type of delivery

  Vaginal delivery

  C-section

  Delivery after previous C-section

- Abortion

Gestation

Fetal gestation: Approximately 266 days (40 weeks)

EDD: Estimated Date of Delivery

- 280 days from last menstrual period (LMP)

Trimesters
First, LMP to Week 12

Second, Weeks 13-27

Third, Week 28 to EDD

Global Package and Delivery

Uncomplicated maternity care includes

- Antepartum care = Before birth

- Delivery

- Postpartum care = After birth

Antepartum Care Includes

Initial and subsequent H&P

Blood pressures

Weight

Routine urinalysis

Fetal heart tones

Monthly visits to 28 weeks

Twice-a-month visits, weeks 29 to 36

Weekly visits from week 37 to delivery

- Services not related to antepartum care are reported separately

Example: Pregnant female with complaint of suspicious mole on left shoulder

- Visits OB/GYN physician, who provides antepartum care
- Service regarding mole, not antepartum care, requires good documentation in the maternity record and a specific diagnosis relative to the treatment provided
- Listed in notes preceding 59000

Delivery Includes

Admission to hospital with admitting H&P

Management of uncomplicated labor

Vaginal or cesarean section delivery

- Complications coded separately
- Listed in notes preceding 59000

Postpartum Care Includes

Normal follow-up care for 6 weeks after delivery

- Hospital visits, office visits
- Listed in notes preceding 59000

Antepartum (59000-59076)

Amniocentesis: Insertion of needle into pregnant uterus, withdrawal of fluid (59000, 59001)

- Ultrasound guidance with this service (76946)
- Component coding often part of services in subheading

Fetal services: Include stress tests, blood sampling, monitoring, and therapeutic procedures

Excision (59100-59160)

Postpartum curettage: Removes remaining pieces of placenta or clotted blood (59160)

Nonobstetric curettage: 58120 (Corpus Uteri, Excision)

Introduction (59200)

Insertion of cervical dilator: Used to prepare and soften the cervix for an abortive procedure or delivery (for abortive procedure, see 59855)

Cervical ripening agents may be introduced to prepare cervix

- Is a separate procedure and not reported when part of more major procedure

Repair (59300-59350)

Only for repairs during pregnancy

Repairs done as a result of delivery or during pregnancy

Episiotomy or vaginal repair by other than attending

Suture repair (cerclage) of cervix or uterus (hysterorrhaphy)

Routine Global Obstetric Care

59400, Vaginal delivery

59510, Cesarean delivery

59610, Vaginal delivery after previous cesarean delivery (VBAC)

59618, Cesarean delivery following attempted vaginal delivery after previous cesarean delivery

NOTE: Take care when assigning diagnosis codes for normal versus complicated delivery. ICD-9-CM states specific guidelines for a normal delivery.

Episiotomies and Use of Forceps

Included in delivery

Not reported separately

Physician Provides Only Portion of Global Routine Care, Delivery

59409, Vaginal delivery only

59514, Cesarean delivery only

59612, Vaginal delivery only, after previous cesarean delivery

59620, Cesarean delivery only, following attempted vaginal delivery after previous cesarean delivery

Delivery of Twins

Payers differ on reporting format

- -22 (Unusual Procedural Services)
- -51 (Multiple Procedures)

Abortion Services (59812-59857)

Spontaneous: Happens naturally (for a complete spontaneous abortion, report with a code from the E/M section)

Incomplete: Requires medical intervention

Missed: Fetus dies naturally but does not abort during first half of pregnancy

Septic: Missed abortion with infection

Medical intervention

- Dilation and curettage or evacuation (suction removal)
- Intra-amniotic injections (saline or urea)
- Vaginal suppositories (prostaglandin)

ENDOCRINE SYSTEM SUBSECTION (60000-60699)

Nine glands in endocrine system; only four included in subsection

1. Thyroid
2. Parathyroid
3. Thymus
4. Adrenal

Pituitary and Pineal. *See* Nervous System subsection

Pancreas. Digestive System

Ovaries and Testes. Respective genital systems
Divided into two subheadings

• Thyroid Gland

• Parathyroid, Thymus, Adrenal Glands, and Carotid Body

Carotid Body. Refers to area adjacent to carotid artery

Can be site of tumors

Thyroid Gland, Excision Category (60001-60281)

Code descriptions often refer to

• **Partial or subtotal:** Something less than total

• **Total:** All

Thyroid, 1 gland with 2 lobes

NERVOUS SYSTEM SUBSECTION (61000-64999)

Divided anatomically

• Skull, Meninges, and Brain

• Spine and Spinal Cord

• Extracranial Nerves, Peripheral Nerves, and Autonomic Nervous System

Skull, Meninges, and Brain Subheading (61000-62258)
Categories
Injection, Drainage, or Aspiration

Twist Drills, Burr Hole(s), or Trephine

Conditions that Require Openings Into Brain to
Relieve pressure

Insert monitoring devices

Place tubing

Inject contrast material

Craniectomy or Craniotomy Category (61304-61576)
Removal of portion of skull, usually as operative site, performed emergently to prevent herniation of brain into the brainstem

Codes divided by site and condition for which procedure is performed

Surgery of Skull Base Category
Skull base: Area at base of cranium

• Lesion removal from this area very complex

Extensive category notes

Surgery of Skull Base Terminology

Approach procedure used to gain exposure of lesion

Definitive procedure is what is done to lesion

Repair/reconstruction procedure reported separately only if extensive repair

Surgery of Skull Base (61580-61619)

Approach procedure and definitive procedure coded separately

> ***Example:*** Removal of an intradural lesion using middle cranial fossa approach

- 61590 approach procedure, middle cranial fossa and

- 61608 definitive procedure of intradural resection of lesion

Cerebrospinal Fluid (CSF) Shunt Category (62180-62258)

Used to drain fluid

Codes describe placement of

- Devices

- Repair

- Replacement

- Removal of shunting devices

Spine and Spinal Cord Subheading (62263-63746)

Codes divided by condition and approach

Often used are

- Unilateral or bilateral procedures (-50)

- Multiple procedures (-51)

- Radiologic supervision and fluoroscopic guidance are coded separately

Includes codes for

- Spinal anesthetic injections 62310-62319

- Intrathecal catheter placement/implantation 62350-62355

Introduction/Injection of Anesthetic Agent, Diagnostic or Therapeutic Category (64400-64530)

Includes codes for

- Nerve blocks 64400-64450

- Facet joint injections 64470-64476

- Epidural injections 64479-64484

  - Used to provide pain relief

  - As compared with an epidural catheter placement used for anesthetic purposes

EYE AND OCULAR ADNEXA SUBSECTION (65091-68899)

Terminology extremely important

- Code descriptions often vary only slightly

Understanding of eye anatomy is necessary for proper coding in this subsection

Codes divided anatomically, e.g.,

- Eyeball
- Anterior segment
- Posterior segment
- Ocular adnexa
- Conjunctiva

Some codes specifically for patients previously operated on

Much bundling

> ***Example:*** Subheading Posterior Segment, Prophylaxis category notes indicate:

- "The following descriptors (67141, 67145) are intended to include all sessions in defined treatment period."

Cataracts

Method used depends on type of cataract and surgeon preference

Nuclear cataract: Most common, center of lens (nucleus), due to aging process

Cortical cataract: Forms in lens of cortex and extends outward; frequent in diabetics

Subcapsular cataract: Forms at back of lens

Removal and lens replacement (66830-66990)

- Extracapsular cataract extraction (ECCE) is partial removal

  Removes hard nucleus in one piece

  Removes soft cortex in multiple pieces

- Intracapsular cataract extraction (ICCE) is total removal

  Removes lens and capsule in one piece

- Phacoemulsification

  Small incision into eye and introduction of probe

  High-frequency waves fragment cataract; then suctioned out

  Lens placed through same small incision

Blepharotomy (67700)

- Incision into eyelid for drainage of abscess

Blepharoplasty

- Repair of eyelid
- Codes in Integumentary System (15820-15823)

• Codes in Eye and Ocular Adnexa (67916, 67917, 67923, 67924)

Selection of code depends on technique used to repair eyelid

AUDITORY SYSTEM SUBSECTION (69000-69990)

Codes divided by

• External Ear (69000-69399)

• Middle Ear (69400-69799)

• Internal Ear (69801-69949)

• Temporal Bone, Middle Fossa Approach (69950-69979)

• Operating Microscope (69990)

Understanding of ear anatomy is necessary for proper coding in this subsection

External, middle, and internal ear further divided by procedure

• Incision

• Excision

• Removal

• Repair

Myringotomy and tympanostomy

• Eustachian tube connects middle ear to back of throat for drainage

• Fluid collects in middle ear when tube does not function properly

• Prevents air from entering middle ear and pressure to build

• Surgical intervention

Myringotomy (incision into tympanic membrane)

Tympanostomy (incision and placement of PE tube [pressure equalization])

Operating Microscope (+69990)

Employed with procedures using microsurgical techniques

Code in addition to primary procedure performed

Do not report separately when primary procedure description includes microsurgical techniques

Example: 15758 Free fascial flap with microvascular anastomosis

Note that following 15758 is the statement:

• "(Do not report code 69990 in addition to code 15758)" indicating to the coder not to report the use of the operating microscope separately

■ RADIOLOGY SECTION (70010-79999)

Radiology: Branch of medicine that uses radiant energy to diagnose and treat patients

Specialist in radiology: Radiologist (doctor of medicine)

Radiology Subsections

1. Diagnostic Radiology
2. Diagnostic Ultrasound
3. Radiologic Guidance
4. Breast Mammography
5. Bone/Joint Studies
6. Radiation Oncology
7. Nuclear Medicine

Procedures

Fluoroscopy views inside of body, projects onto television screen

Live images by which physician can view function, structure, and defects or anomalies within an organ

> *Example:* 71034 chest x-ray with fluoroscopy

Magnetic Resonance Imaging (MRI)

MRI uses magnetic energy to view soft-tissue structures

> *Example:* 72148 MRI of spinal canal

Tomography or Computed Axial Tomography (CAT or CT Scan)

Tomography used to view single plane of body

> *Example:* 70450 tomographic scan of head or brain

Planes of Body (Figure 3-13)

Position and Projection
Position = method of positioning patients for examination

Projection path = pathway traveled by x-ray beam

Component Coding
Three component terms

1. Professional
2. Technical
3. Global

Professional Component
Physician portion of service, includes

- Supervision of technician
- Interpretation of results, including written report

Technical Component
- Technologist's services
- Equipment, film, and supplies

Global Procedure
Both professional and technical portions of radiology service

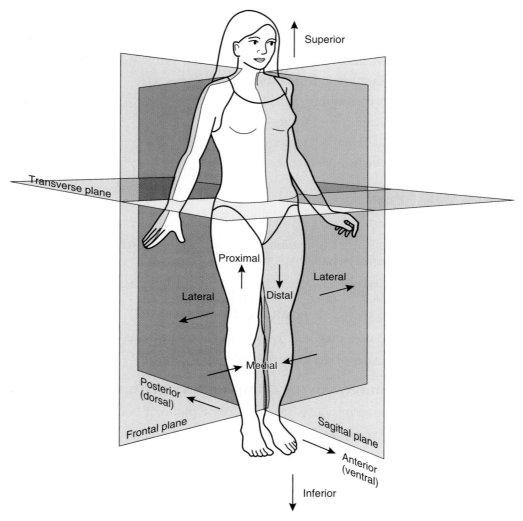

Figure **3-13** Planes of the body.

Component Modifiers

If only professional component of radiology service provided: -26 to code

If only technical component provided: -TC to code

- -TC HCPCS modifier used with CPT and HCPCS codes

If both professional and technical components of radiology service are provided (global), no modifier is needed if the service was provided in a hospital setting

>   ***Example:*** Chest x-ray

- Professional component: 71030-26 (supervision and final report)
- Technical component: 71030-TC (technician, supplies, equipment)
- Global procedure: 71030 (both professional and technical)

Third-party payers usually reimburse

- 40% professional component
- 60% technical component
- 100% global procedure

Contrast Material

Statement "with contrast" implies injection service included in code

Oral or rectal contrast does not qualify for "with contrast"

Notes indicate codes for components

> *Example:* 75801, Lymphangiography; see 38790 (Injection procedure)

Interventional Radiologist

Combination radiologist and surgeon

Provides total procedure for cystography with contrast

- Report 74430, x-ray portion
- 51600 for injection procedure
- Plus code for supply of contrast material (e.g., 99070)

DIAGNOSTIC RADIOLOGY SUBSECTION (70010-76499)

Most standard radiographic procedures

Codes often divided by whether contrast material used

Codes further divided by number of views

> *Example:* 71030, Chest x-ray, complete, minimum of 4 views

Used to:

- Diagnose disease
- Monitor disease process—progression or remission
- Therapeutic procedures (guidance)

Diagnostic Procedures Include

X-ray

Computerized axial tomography (CAT or CT scan)

Magnetic resonance imaging (MRI)

Angiography

Computed Axial Tomography (CAT or CT)

X-ray image taken in sections

Computer reconstructs and enhances image

Magnetic Resonance Imaging (MRI)

Uses magnetic fields to produce an image displayed on computer screen

Codes of same area (e.g., spine) divided by whether or not contrast material used

Angiography

Used to view vessel obstructions

Dye injected into vessel

Radiologist uses angiography to diagnose vascular conditions

Example:

- Malformation
- Stroke (cerebrovascular accident, CVA)
- Myocardial infarction (MI)

Remember
- If fewer than total number of views specified in code provided: Use -52, Reduced Service

---

DIAGNOSTIC ULTRASOUND SUBSECTION (76506-76999)

Uses high-frequency sound waves to image anatomic structures

Nine subheadings of Diagnostic Ultrasound

Primarily based on anatomy

A-mode (A = Amplitude)

Technique used to map structure outline in one-dimensional image

M-mode (M = Motion)

Technique used to display one-dimensional movement of structure

B-scan (B = Brightness)

Technique used to display two-dimensional movement of tissues and organs

Known as gray scale ultrasound

Real-Time Scan
Technique used to display both structure and motion with time of organ and tissues in a two-dimensional image

Extent of Study

Codes often divided on extent of study

Example: Extent of scan as follows

- **Complete:** Scans entire body or body region
- **Limited:** Scans part of body, e.g., one organ
- **Follow-up/repeat:** Limited study of part of body that was scanned previously

Three Locations for Ultrasound Services

76506-76999: Radiology codes for diagnostic ultrasound services

93875-93990: Medicine codes for non-invasive vascular studies

93303-93350: Medicine codes for echocardiography

RADIOLOGIC GUIDANCE SUBSECTION (77001-77032)

Guidance

- Fluoroscopic
- Computer tomography
- Magnetic resonance
- Other

BREAST MAMMOGRAPHY SUBSECTION (77051-77059)

Example: Computer-aided detection and screening

BONE/JOINT STUDIES SUBSECTION (77071-77084)

Example: Bone density, bone mineral density, and joint survey

RADIATION ONCOLOGY SUBSECTION (77261-77799)

Therapeutic use of radiation

Codes both professional and technical services

Subheading divided based on treatment

Initial consultation, prior to decision to treat, reported with E/M consultation code

- **Outpatient:** 99241-99245
- **Inpatient:** 99251-99255

Clinical Treatment Planning—Professional Component (77261-77299)

Includes

- Interpretation of special testing
- Tumor localization
- Determination of treatment volume
- Choice of treatment method
- Determination of number of treatment ports
- Selection of treatment devices
- Other necessary procedures

Clinical Treatment Planning consists of

- Planning
- Simulation

Three Levels of Planning

1. **Simple:** One treatment area, one port, or one set of parallel ports
2. **Intermediate:** Three or more ports, two separate treatment areas, multiple blocking

3. **Complex:** Complex blocking, custom shielding blocks, tangential ports, special wedges, 3+ treatment areas, special beams

Simulation

Determining placement of treatment areas/ports for radiation treatment

Does not include administration of radiation

Definitions of Simulation
1. **Simple:** 1 treatment area with 1 port or pair of ports

2. **Intermediate:** 3+ ports, 2 separate treatment areas, multiple blocking

3. **Complex:** Tangential ports, 3+ treatment areas, complex blocking

4. **Computer-generated 3-D** reconstruction of volume of tumor and critical structures

Medical Radiation, Physics, Dosimetry, Treatment Devices, and Special Services

Decision making services of physicians

- Treatment types

- Dose calculation and placement (dosimetry)

- Development of treatment device

Radiation Treatment Delivery (77401-77421)

Technical component of actual delivery of radiation

Information Needed to Code Radiation Treatment Delivery
Amount of radiation delivered

Type of radiation-electron (most common), neutron, or proton

Number of

- Areas treated (single, two, three or more)

- Ports involved (single, three or more, tangential)

- Blocks used (none, multiple, custom)

Reporting Clinical Treatment Management

Professional (physician) portion of services, including

- Review port films

- Review dosimetry, dose delivery, treatment parameters

- Treatment set-up

- Patient examination for medical E/M

Report in units of five fraction, unless last 3-4 fractions are at the end of the treatment; then you can count the last 3-4 as an additional fraction

Clinical Brachytherapy (77750-77799)

Placement of radioactive material into or around site of tumor

- Intracavitary (within body cavity)
- Interstitial (within tissues)

Source
Radioactive element delivers radiation dose over time

   Example: Seeds, ribbons, or capsules

- **Ribbons:** Seeds embedded on tape and inserted into tissue
- Tape is cut to desired length, thereby controlling amount of radiation

Clinical Brachytherapy Codes Divided Based on
Number of sources applied

- Simple 1-4
- Intermediate 5-10
- Complex 11+

NUCLEAR MEDICINE SUBSECTION (78000-79999)

Placement of radioactive material into body and measurement of emissions

Used for both diagnosis and treatment

Codes divided primarily on organ system

- Except "Therapeutic," which is for radiopharmaceutical therapies

■ PATHOLOGY AND LABORATORY SECTION (80048-89356)

Read guideline notes at beginning of each subcategory in preparation for the certification examination

Such as

- Organ or Disease Oriented Panels
- Drug Testing
- Therapeutic Drug Assays
- Evocative/Suppression Testing
- Consultation (Clinical Pathology)
- Urinalysis
- Chemistry
- Hematology and Coagulation
- Immunology
- Transfusion Medicine
- Microbiology

- Anatomic Pathology
- Cytopathology
- Cytogenetic Studies
- Surgical Pathology
- Transcutaneous Procedures
- Other Procedures
- Reproductive Medicine Procedures

Pathology and Laboratory

Codes for laboratory test only

Specimen collection coded separately

> *Example:* Venous blood draw reported 36415 (Surgery section)

Facility Indicators

Allow additional tests without physician written order

> *Example:* Urinalysis positive for bacteria, built-in indicator for culture

Pathology/Laboratory Caution

Report second or subsequent tests without -51, multiple procedures

Organ or Disease Oriented Panels (80048-80076)

Groups of tests often ordered together

> *Examples:*
> - Basic Metabolic Panel
> - General Health Panel
> - Electrolyte Panel

Rules of Panels

All tests must have been conducted

Do not use -52, Reduced Service

Additional tests, over those in panel, are reported separately

If all tests in panel not done

- List each test separately
- Do not use panel code

Drug Testing (80100-80103)

Identifies presence or absence of drug—qualitative analysis

Confirmation conducted to double-check results of positive drug test (80102)

Chromatography procedure in which multiple drugs identified

- Some machines identify all drugs present in 1 procedure
- Others require 2+ procedures to identify 2+ drugs

Code the number of procedures, not number of drugs tested for

Example:
- 2 procedures to identify 3 drugs = 80100 × 2
- 1 procedure to identify 3 drugs = 80100

Does not identify amount of drug present

- Only presence or absence

Therapeutic Drug Assays (80150-80299)

Reports the presence and amount (quantitative)

Material examined can be from any source

Drugs listed by generic names

Example: Amitriptyline, generic name for brand name Elavil

Evocative/Suppression Testing (80400-80440)

Measures stimulating (evocative) or suppressing agents

Codes report only technical component of service

Additional services reported

- Supplies and/or drugs used in testing (99070 or HCPCS code)

E/M code reported for physician monitoring of test

Consultations (Clinical Pathology) (80500, 80502)
At request of physician

Additional information about specimen

Consultant prepares written report

Levels
Limited without review of medical record

Comprehensive with review of medical record

More Consultation Codes (88321-88334)

Surgical Pathology

Used when pathologist either

- Reviews slides, material, or reports
- Provides consultation during surgery

Reported on number of specimens

Urinalysis (81000-81099)

Tests on Urine
Method of test

- e.g., tablet, reagent, or dipstick

Reason for test

- e.g., pregnancy

Constituents being tested for

- e.g., bilirubin, glucose

Equipment Used
Automated or nonautomated

Chemistry (82000-84999)
Specific tests on any bodily substances

- Urine
- Blood
- Breath
- Feces
- Sputum

Most are for quantitative (amount of) screenings only

Few report qualitative (presence of) screenings

Samples from different sources reported separately, e.g., blood, feces

Samples taken different times of day reported separately

Hematology and Coagulation (85002-85999)

Laboratory procedures on blood

   Example:
   - Complete blood count (CBC)
   - White blood cell count (WBC)

Codes divided based on method of

- Blood draw
- Test being conducted

Immunology (86000-86849)

Identifying immune system conditions caused by antibodies and antigens

   Example: Hepatitis C antibody screening

Transfusion Medicine (86850-86999)

Blood bank codes

Tests performed on blood or blood products

Do NOT identify supply of blood, but

- Collection

- Processing

- Typing

Microbiology (87001-87999)

Study of Microorganisms
Identification of organism

Sensitivities of organism to antibiotics

Microbiology Caution: Many code descriptions similar to those in Immunology (86000-86849), with only difference technique used

---

Anatomic Pathology (88000-88099)

Postmortem examinations

- Autopsies

Reports only physician service

Codes divided on extent of exam and type of examination—gross versus gross and microscopic

   Example: Gross examination without central nervous system (88000)

Cytopathology (88104-88199)

Identifies cellular changes

Common laboratory procedures, e.g., Pap smear

Codes divided by

- Type of procedure

- Technique used

Cytogenetic Studies (88230-88299)

Branch of genetics concerned with cellular abnormalities and pathologic conditions

   Example: Chromosomes

Surgical Pathology (88300-88399)

Pathology Terminology
Specimen sample of tissue of suspect area

- Basis of reporting is determined by the number of labeled specimens

Block: Frozen piece of specimen

Section is a slice of frozen block

Evaluation of Specimens to Determine Disease Pathology

All tissue removed during procedures undergoes pathology evaluation

Operative report usually coded after pathology report received

Pathology reports usually coded with operative report

Unit of measure (88300-88309), specimen

- 2 anus tags, each examined, 88304 × 2

- 1 anus tag examined in 2 different areas of tag, 88304

Types of Pathologic Examination

Microscopic: With microscope

Gross: Without microscope

- 88300, only gross exam code

- Other codes are gross and microscopic

Six levels of surgical pathology

Based on specimen examined, e.g., breast, prostate, lung, and reason for evaluation, e.g., radical procedure for suspected carcinoma

Levels divided on complexity of examination

> ***Example:***
>
> 88305, Colon, Biopsy
>
> 88307, Colon, Segmental Resection, Other than for Tumor
>
> 88309, Colon, Total Resection

Level I
- Specimen can be accurately diagnosed without microscopic examination

Level II
- Gross and microscopic examination is performed on the specimen

Levels III, IV, V, and VI
- Include gross and microscopic examination and additional ascending levels of physician work (increasing difficulty)

Based upon method of or need for removal

Same anatomical site can be listed in each level

Additional service codes 88311-88399 are not included in codes 88300-88309

> ***Example:*** Special stains (88312)

■ MEDICINE SECTION (90281-99602)

Most procedures noninvasive (not entering body)

Contains invasive procedures

> ***Example:*** 92973, Percutaneous thrombectomy

Numerous notes throughout

Many specialized tests

> **Example:** Audiology and biofeedback

New in Medicine section in 2006 was lightning bolt ($\nearrow$)

- Indicates substances pending FDA (Food and Drug Administration) approval

Immunizations

Often used

Two types of immunizations

- Active and passive

Correct coding includes

- Supply injected

- Administration of injection

Active—Bacteria or Virus

Bacteria that cause disease made nontoxic (toxoid)

- Injected to build immunity

Small dose active virus injected (vaccine)

- Injected to build immunity

> **Example:** Poliovirus

Passive Immunization

Does not cause immune response

Contains antibodies against certain diseases—immune globulins

Immune Globulins (90281-90399)

Identifies immune globulin product

> **Example:** Botulism antitoxin

Report administration separately

Immune Globulin Codes Divided by

Type
e.g., rabies, hepatitis B

Method
e.g., intramuscular, intravenous, subcutaneous

Dose
e.g., full dose, minidose

Immunization Administration (90465-90474)

Administration (giving of substance)

- Reported in addition to substance given

- 90465-90468 Patients under 8 years of age when physician counsels regarding immunization

- 90465, +90466 = Percutaneous, intradermal, subcutaneous, or intramuscular injection

- 90467, +90468 = Oral or intranasal

- 90471-90474 Patients 8 years of age or over

- 90471, +90472 = Percutaneous, intradermal, subcutaneous, or intramuscular injection

    Patients of all ages, including under 8 years of age, when physician does not counsel regarding immunization

- 90473, +90474 = Oral or intranasal

Methods of Administration

- Percutaneous

- Intradermal

- Subcutaneous

- Intramuscular

- Intranasal

- Oral

Report Administration for Each Dose—Single or Combination

Example: 10-year-old patient receives 3 separate injections

- 90471 administration tetanus

- 90472 administration rubella

- 90472 administration diphtheria

OR depending on payer:

- 90471 administration tetanus

- 90472 × 2 administration rubella and diphtheria

Vaccines, Toxoids (Vaccine Product Codes) (90476-90749)

Many codes age-specific

Example: 90658, influenza vaccine, for ages 3 and over

Codes for products for single diseases

Example: 90703, tetanus

Codes for combination diseases

Example: 90701, diphtheria, tetanus, and whole cell pertussis (DTP)

Some vaccines given on schedule

Example: 90633, 2-dose hepatitis A vaccine

- 1st dose, 1st visit

- 2nd dose, 2nd visit

Caution: There are Multiple Diphtheria Codes

- 90698-90702, 90719-90721 diphtheria and diphtheria with other substances

    Example: 90719, diphtheria for IM use

    Example: 90698, diphtheria, tetanus toxoids, and acellular pertussis (synthetic form of pertussis) (DTaP), *Haemophilus influenza* Type B (HiB), and inactivated poliovirus (IPV) for IM use

---

Remember
Do not use modifier -51 with Vaccine/Toxoid codes
Rather, depending on payer:
- List each code multiple times or
- Use times (×) symbol and indicate number

Important Reporting Rule. If vaccine administered during an office visit that was not related to the E/M

- Report E/M service (with modifier -25) + Vaccine + administration

Office visit for vaccine only: Code only vaccine and the administration (no E/M service)

Routine Vaccinations
Influenza
Substance (vaccine) 90655-90660

Administration for patients 8 or over

- G0008 HCPCS National Level II for Medicare patients
- 90471/90472

Pneumococcal
Substance (vaccine) 90732

Administration

- G0009 HCPCS National Level II for Medicare
- 90471/90472 administration

Hydration, Therapeutic, Prophylactic, or Diagnostic Injections and Infusions (90760-90779)

Infusion: Therapeutic procedure to introduce fluid into body

Hydration: Infusion for purpose of rehydration; includes prepackaged fluid

Injection: Subcutaneous (Sub-Q), intramuscular (IM), intra-arterial (IA), and intravenous (IV)

Codes report the physician work related to the infusion, hydration, or injection

- Affirmation of treatment plan
- Direct supervision of staff
- Significant separately identifiable E/M is reported with -25

Codes include

- Local anesthesia
- Intravenous start
- Access to indwelling intravenous catheter or port
- Flush at conclusion
- Standard tubing, syringes, and supplies

Multiple drug administrations in same session are reported separately

Use only one initial code to report multiple infusions or injections or combinations

> Assign initial code based on primary reason for encounter
>
> The secondary infusion/injection is reported with a subsequent or concurrent code, unless the protocol requires two separate IV sites
>
> > **Example:** If three different agents were administered in the same session, report one initial code and two additional sequential codes
>
> Determination of initial code is based on primary reason for encounter

Some codes are time based, so medical documentation must indicate time infusion begins and ends

Time is defined as the actual time used to administer the drug/substance

90760-90761 report IV infusion for hydration and includes prepackaged fluid/electrolytes

- 90760 IV infusion for hydration up to one hour
- 90761 IV infusion for hydration, each additional hour
  - Report for hydration intervals greater than 30 minutes beyond 1 hour
  - Start infusion time over if a different bag is started
  - Do not report hydration codes when the fluid is used to administer the drug

90765-90768 report therapeutic, prophylactic, or diagnostic IV infusions, other than hydration and chemotherapy

- Typically require direct physician supervision
- Special consideration for preparing, dosing, or disposing
- Trained staff who administer infusion
- Monitoring of vital signs during infusion

Therapeutic, Prophylactic, or Diagnostic Injections and Infusions (90772-90779)

Types of drug administration

- Therapeutic
- Prophylactic
- Diagnostic

Codes divided by administration method

- Subcutaneous

- Intramuscular

- Intra-arterial

- Intravenous push

A push is defined as when a health care professional is needed to administer the drug/substance and monitor the patient or an infusion that takes 15 minutes or less to administer

Also report the substance administered

Psychiatry (90801-90899)

Psychiatric treatment at same time as E/M service, report

- One code for psychotherapy with E/M

Time major billing factor

- Record indicates session time

Many services provided in partial hospital settings

- Patient in hospital during day, returns home for evenings and weekends

Codes Divided Based on
Interactive or insight-oriented psychotherapy

Inpatient or outpatient

With or without E/M service

Individual or group

Biofeedback (90901, 90911)

Used to help patients gain control over body processes

   Example: Elevated BP (blood pressure) or manage chronic pain

Patient training in biofeedback by professional

- Continues on own

Services often part psychophysiologic (mind/body) therapy

Dialysis (90918-90999)

Cleanses blood

- Temporary (non-ESRD [end-stage renal disease])

- Permanent (ESRD)

Two parts to report ESRD dialysis services

- Physician service + hemodialysis procedure

ESRD Physician Services (90918-90925)

Include

- Establishment of dialyzing cycle

- Physician services

- E/M outpatient dialysis visits

- Telephone calls

- Patient management during dialysis

Reported per month: 90918-90921
Month is defined as 30 days

Less than full month of service 90922-90925 per day

Codes divided by age

Codes are used to report outpatient dialysis services for ESRD patients

Hemodialysis Service (90935-90940)

Hemodialysis is the procedure

Used for ESRD and non-ESRD

Billed per day for inpatients receiving hemodialysis and also for outpatient non-ESRD

Includes all physician E/M services related to procedure

- Use modifier -25 if separate E/M service provided

Miscellaneous Dialysis Procedures (90945-90999)

Describes other dialysis procedures

> **Example:** Peritoneal dialysis in which toxins are passively absorbed into dialysis fluid

Peritoneal Dialysis (90945-90947)
Services billed on per-day basis for inpatient ESRD patients

Patients can receive training in self-dialysis

Codes divided by complete or partial training program

Gastroenterology (91000-91299)

For tests and treatments of esophagus, stomach, and intestine

Codes usually reported with E/M or consultation service code

- **Caution:** Many bundled services

Ophthalmology (92002-92499)

Contains E/M codes

Definitions for new and established patients same as for E/M section

Codes are for bilateral services

- If only one eye, use modifier -52 (reduced service)

Special Ophthalmologic Services (92502-92700)

For special evaluations of visual system

Goes beyond those usually provided in evaluation

May be reported in addition to basic visual service

Special Otorhinolaryngologic Services (92502-92700)

Special treatments and diagnostic services

> **Example:** Nasal function tests (rhinomanometry) or audiometric tests

All hearing tests bilateral unless one ear indicated in description

Noninvasive Vascular Diagnostic Studies (93875-93990)

Vascular codes for procedures on noncoronary veins and arteries

Include

- Patient care
- Supervision and interpretation (S&I)
- Copy of results

Pulmonary (94010-94799)

For therapies and diagnostic tests

Includes procedure and interpretation of test results

- Additional E/M service reported separately

Allergy and Clinical Immunology (95004-95199)

Divided into two suheadings

1. Allergy Testing (95004-95075)
2. Allergen Immunotherapy (95115-95199)

Allergy Testing (95004-95075)

Sensitivity testing using various types of tests

> **Example:** Percutaneous, intracutaneous, inhalation

Tests use numerous substances

> **Example:** Extracts, venoms, biologics, and foods

Type and number of tests based on physician's judgment

Coding allergy testing

Medical record will indicate

- Number of tests
- Type of test
- Method testing

Allergen Immunotherapy (95115-95199)

Codes divided into three types of services:

1. Injection only

2. Prescription and injection

3. Provision of antigen (substance) only

Physician service bundled into immunotherapy codes

If separate E/M service provided, report separately

Neurology and Neuromuscular Procedures (95805-96004)

Contains codes to report tests, such as

- Sleep tests

- Muscle tests (electromyography)

- Range-of-motion measurements

- Electroencephalogram (EEG)

Analysis and programming of neurostimulators

Many bundled services

Services usually provided in addition to E/M service

Central Nervous System (CNS) Assessments/Tests (96101-96120)

Used to report

- Psychological tests

- Speech/Language assessments

- Developmental progress assessments

- Thinking/Reasoning examinations

Codes based on per-hour basis

- Includes written report of results

Chemotherapy Administration (96401-96549)

Represents only preparation and administration of chemotherapy

- If separate E/M service provided, report E/M code + -25

Report all drugs/substances separately

Codes are not limited to patients with diagnosis of cancer

Codes also include infusion of anti-neoplastic agents, monoclonal antibody agents, and biological response modifiers for treatment of noncancer diagnoses

Chemical can be administered (injected) into

- Lesion

- Vein

- Tissue

- Muscle
- Artery
- Cavity
- Nerve

Intravenously injected chemicals: Two methods of delivery of chemical

1. IV push quickly puts into vein (15 minutes or less)

2. IV infusion delivers over longer period of time

Codes often divided by time the infusion/injection procedure takes

>   *Example:* 96413 chemotherapy administration, intravenous, infusion up to 1 hour

Report the initial code that represents the main reason why the patient was being treated, even though it might not be the first drug/substance infused

>   *Example:* Patient received 1 hour of hydration first, then 2 hours of chemotherapy intravenously. Code the initial chemotherapy infusion, 96413 for the first hour of chemo, 96415 for the second hour, then code 90760 for the hydration

Special supplies (e.g., special needles) reported separately using 99070 or HCPCS National Level II code

Report any intra-arterial catheter placement with 36620-36640

Injections with chemotherapy

- Report separately any analgesic or antiemetic (for vomiting)
- Given before or after chemotherapy

Use codes J0881 to report injection of darbepoetin alfa and J0885 to report injection of epoetin alfa

---

Photodynamic Therapy (96567-96571)

Used in addition to bronchoscopy or endoscopy codes

Injected agent remains in cancerous cells longer than normal cells

- After agent dissipates from normal cells, patient exposed to laser light
- Agent absorbs light
- Light produces oxygen and cancer cell destroyed

Special Dermatologic Procedures (96900-96999)

Usually specialized procedures provided on consultation basis

- Separate E/M consultation code would then be appropriate

Treatment of skin conditions:

Actinotherapy—with ultraviolet light

Photochemotherapy—with light-sensitive chemicals and light rays

Physical Medicine & Rehabilitation (97001-97799)

Used by physicians and therapists to report a variety of services

Treatments
Traction

Electrical stimulation (used to help heal fractures)

Patient Training
Gait training

Functional activities

Codes often have time components

> **Example:** 97761 reports prosthetic training, extremity

Active Wound Care Management (97597-97606)

Debridement
Selective debridement without anesthesia with removal of devitalized tissue by different techniques, such as sharp selective debridement with scissors, scalpel, and forceps

97597 and 97598 include total service area of all wounds

Codes based on centimeters treated

Nonselective debridement (97602): Healthy tissue removed along with necrotic tissue, with wet to moist dressings, enzymatic or abrasive type methods

Negative pressure wound therapy (NPWT) (97605, 97606)

- Vacuuming of drainage and tissue from wound
  - Then negative pressure draws the edges of the wound together
- Application of topical medications/ointments
- Assessment of wound
- Directions to patient on continued care of wound
- Each code for ongoing care reported on per-session basis

Osteopathic and Chiropractic Services (98925-98943)

Both inpatient and outpatient settings

Physician services bundled into codes

Codes divided by body area

Special Services, Procedures, and Reports (99000-99091)

Handling and conveyance of laboratory specimens

- 99000-99002

Postoperative follow-up visits included in surgical package

- 99024

Office visits after posted hours or in locations other than office

- 99050-99060

Supplies and materials

- 99070

Hospital mandated on-call services

- 99026, 99027

Moderate (Conscious) Sedation (99143-99150)

Type of sedation in which the patient can respond to verbal commands

- Appendix G contains summary of codes that include moderate (conscious) sedation

The bullseye symbol ⊙ indicates these codes in the CPT manual

Do not report sedation services with codes marked with bullseye when sedation is provided by same physician performing procedure

- Second physician provides sedation, report with 99148-99150

Included in service is:

- Patient assessment

- IV establishment

- Administration of agent

- Maintenance of sedation

- Monitoring of vital signs

- Recovery

Codes divided based on patient age (under 5 and 5 and over) and time (30 minutes and each 15 minutes over)

■ HCPCS CODING

Developed by Centers for Medicare and Medicaid Services (CMS)

- Formerly HCFA

HCPCS developed, 1983
CPT did not contain all codes necessary for Medicare services reporting

One of Two Levels of Codes

1. Level I, CPT

2. Level II, HCPCS, also known as national codes

Phased Out Level III, Local Codes
Developed by Medicare and other carriers for use at local level

Varied by locale

Discontinued October 2002 due to HIPAA code set regulations

Some codes incorporated into HCPCS Level I and Level II

Level II, National Codes

Codes for wide variety of providers

- Physicians

- Dentists

- Orthodontists

Codes for wide variety of services

- Specific drugs

- Durable medical equipment (DME)

- Ambulance services

Format

Begins with letter, followed by four digits

Example: E0605, vaporizer, room type

Each letter represents group codes

Example: "J" codes used to report drugs

Temporary Codes

Certain letters indicate temporary codes

Example: K0552, Supplies for external drug infusion pump

- K codes are temporary codes

Code book published every January, but codes are added and deleted throughout the year and providers are notified through carrier bulletins

HCPCS National Level II Index

Directs coder to specific codes

Do not code directly from index

Reference main portion of text before assigning code

Alphabetical order

Table of Drugs

Listed by generic name, not brand name

Often used when reporting immunizations or injections

■ AN OVERVIEW OF THE ICD-9-CM

INTRODUCTION

Morbidity (illness)

Mortality (death)

CM = Clinical Modification

Provides continuity of data

World Health Organization's (WHO) ICD-9 used globally; many countries already use ICD-10

1977: U.S. develops ICD-9 version

• Has more code subsets

• Data collapse back to ICD-9 for uniformity of data

Medicare

Medicare Catastrophic Act of 1988

Required use of ICD-9-CM codes for outpatient claims

Act abolished but codes still used

Uses of ICD-9-CM

Facilities track patient use through codes

Fiscal entities track health care costs

Research

• Health care quality

• Future needs

• Newer cancer center built if patient use warrants

ICD-9-CM on Insurance Forms

Diagnoses establish medical necessity

Services and diagnoses must correlate

CMS-1500 in Block 21 and 24E (Figure 3-14)

Office visit: croup, 464.4, Block 21, 1; 1 placed in Block 24E, Line 1

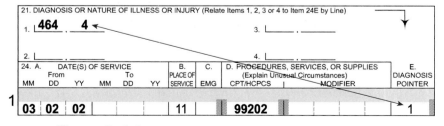

Figure **3-14** Diagnosis code and service must correlate.

> **Ethics**
> Documentation must support diagnosis and match procedures or service performed
>
> **Example:**
> - Services provided
> - Diagnosis justifies services
>
> If in doubt, check it out; don't make assumptions
>
> **Your Job:** Translate documentation into ICD-9-CM codes

FORMAT OF ICD-9-CM

Volume 1, Diseases, Tabular List

Volume 2, Diseases, Alphabetic Index

Volume 1, Diseases, Tabular List

Contains code numbers

001.0-999.9 Diagnosis codes describe condition

V & E codes = supplemental information

Volume 2, Diseases, Alphabetic Index

Appears first in book

Refers coder to code numbers in Volume 1

Never code directly from Index!

ICD-9-CM CONVENTIONS

Symbols, abbreviations, punctuation, and notations

NEC: Not elsewhere classifiable

- No more-specific code exists

NOS: Not otherwise specified

- Unspecified in documentation

[ ] Brackets

Enclose synonyms, alternative wording, or explanatory phrases

Helpful, additional information

Can affect code

Found only in Tabular List (001.0-999.9)

( ) Parentheses

Contain nonessential modifiers

- Take them or leave them

Found in Tabular List and Index

Do not affect code assignment

Colon & Brace

: **Colon:** Tabular List, completes statement with one or more modifiers

} **Brace:** Tabular List, modifying statements to right of brace

Lozenge, Section Mark, & Bold Type

□ **Lozenge:** Can indicate code unique to ICD-9-CM

§ **Section:** Can be footnote indicator

Bold type: Codes and code titles in Tabular List, Volume 1

Italicized Type

All excludes notes

Codes NOT used as principal diagnosis

Slanted Brackets [ ]

Enclose manifestations of underlying condition

Code underlying condition first

Includes, Excludes, Use Additional Code

Includes notes: In chapter, section, or category

Excludes notes: Conditions are coded elsewhere

Use Additional Code: Assignment of other code(s) is necessary

And/With

And: Means and/or

With: One condition with (in addition to) another condition

Code, if Applicable, any Causal Condition First

May be principal diagnosis if no causal condition applicable or known

>   *Example:* 707.10, Ulcer of lower limb, except decubitus; states
>   • Chronic venous hypertension with ulcer (459.31)

If ulcer caused by chronic venous hypertension

• **First:** 459.31 chronic venous hypertension

• **Second:** 707.10 ulcer of lower limb

VOLUME 2, ALPHABETIC INDEX

Nonessential Modifiers: Have no effect on code selection

Enclosed in parentheses

Clarify diagnosis

>   *Example:* Ileus (adynamic) (bowel) . . .

Terms

Main terms (bold typeface)

- Subterms
- Indented two spaces to right
- Not bold or italic

Cross References

Directs you: *see, see also*

- "*see*" directs you to specific term

  Example: Panotitis—*see* Otitis media

- "*see also*" directs you to another term for more information

  Example: Perivaginitis (*see also* Vesiculitis)

- "*see* category" Volume 1, Tabular List, specific information about use of code

  Example: Mesencephalitis (*see also* Encephalitis) 323.9; late effect—*see* category 326

Notes

Define terms

Give further coding instructions

  Example: Index: "Melanoma"

  NOTE: "Except where otherwise indicated . . ."

Mandatory fifth digits also appear as notes (one reason to never code from Index)

Eponyms

Disease or syndrome named for person

  Example: Arnold-Chiari (*see also* Spina bifida)

Etiology and Manifestation of Disease

Etiology = cause of disease

Manifestation = symptom

Combination codes = etiology and manifestation in one code

Neoplasm

In Volume 2, Index, locate Neoplasm Table under the alphabetic entry "N"

SECTIONS

Section 1, Index to Diseases

Section 2, Table of Drugs and Chemicals

Section 3, Index to External Causes of Injuries and Poisonings (E Codes)

Section 1, Index to Diseases

Largest part of Volume 2—Index

First step in coding, locate main term in Index

Subterms indented two spaces to right

May have more than one subterm

Section 2, Table of Drugs and Chemicals

Located after the Index to Diseases

Contains classification of drugs and substances to identify poisoning and adverse effects

- Adverse effect occurs when substance is taken correctly but patient has a negative reaction to substance

- Poisoning occurs when substance is incorrectly taken

   Example: Amoxicillin prescribed for bronchitis causes rash (adverse effect). Rather than one tablet of prescribed amoxicillin, patient takes 4 tablets and nausea results (poisoning)

Drug name placed alphabetically on left under heading "Substance" (Figure 3-15)

First column: "Poisoning" code for substance involved if not related to an adverse effect

E codes identify how poisoning occurred

   Example: If Alkaline antiseptic solution poisoning occurred by accident, E858.7

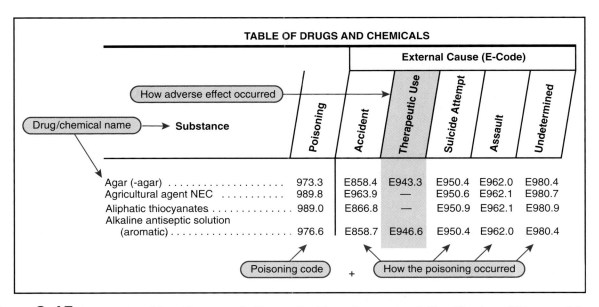

TABLE OF DRUGS AND CHEMICALS

Substance	Poisoning	External Cause (E-Code)				
		Accident	Therapeutic Use	Suicide Attempt	Assault	Undetermined
Agar (-agar)	973.3	E858.4	E943.3	E950.4	E962.0	E980.4
Agricultural agent NEC	989.8	E963.9	—	E950.6	E962.1	E980.7
Aliphatic thiocyanates	989.0	E866.8	—	E950.9	E962.1	E980.9
Alkaline antiseptic solution (aromatic)	976.6	E858.7	E946.6	E950.4	E962.0	E980.4

Figure **3-15** Section 2, Table of Drugs and Chemicals. (From *International Classification of Diseases*, 9th Revision. U.S. Department of Health and Human Services, Public Health Service, Center for Medicare and Medicaid Services.)

- Accidental poisoning by alkaline antiseptic solution: 976.6 (substance) and E858.7 (how it occurred)
- Code any resulting condition (e.g., coma)

Headings

Accident: Unintentional

Therapeutic: Correct dosage, correctly administered, with adverse effects

Suicide attempt: Self-inflicted

Assault: Intentionally inflicted by another person

Undetermined: Unknown cause

Section 3, E Codes

Alphabetic Index to External Causes of Injuries and Poisonings

Provides additional information about the nature of the injury/poisoning and locality

Never principal (inpatient), sole, or primary (outpatient) diagnosis

Separate Index to External Causes

- Alphabetical, main terms in bold
- Subterms are indented 2 spaces to right under main term

A Word of Caution about the Alphabetic Index

Some words in Index do not appear in Tabular—saves space

Exact word may not be in code description in Tabular

- But found in Alphabetic Index
- That is why you must locate the term in the Index, then locate in Tabular

VOLUME 1, TABULAR LIST

Two Major Divisions

1. Classification of Diseases and Injuries (codes 001.0-999.9)
2. Supplementary Classification (V codes and E codes)

Classification of Diseases and Injuries

Main portion of ICD-9-CM

Codes from 001.0 to 999.9

Most chapters are body systems

Example:

- Digestive System
- Respiratory System

Divisions of Classification of Diseases and Injuries

Chapters 1 through 17

- *Section:* A group of related conditions
- *Category:* Represents single disease/condition
- *Subcategory:* More specific
- *Subclassification:* Most specific

Remember
Assign to highest level of specificity, based on documentation
If 4-digit code exists, do not report 3-digit code
If 5-digit code exists, do not report 4-digit code

■ USING THE ICD-9-CM

Guidelines developed by Cooperating Parties

- American Hospital Association (AHA)
- American Health Information Management Association (AHIMA)
- Centers for Medicare and Medicaid Services (CMS)
- National Center for Health Statistics (NCHS)

GENERAL GUIDELINES

Appendix A of this text contains *Official Guidelines for Coding and Reporting*

You must know and follow the Guidelines when assigning diagnoses codes

- All certification examinations adhere to the Guidelines
- As you review this ICD-9-CM material, locate the information in the Guidelines of your ICD-9-CM
- In this way, you will become familiar with the location of Guidelines content to be able to quickly reference the Guidelines during the examination

Outpatient coders primarily use Sections I and IV

Diagnostic Coding and Reporting Guidelines do NOT cover all situations

- Outpatient coders also use many Section II and III guidelines

STEPS TO DIAGNOSIS CODING

Identify MAIN term(s) in diagnosis

Locate MAIN term(s) in Index

Review subterms

Follow cross-reference instructions (e.g., *see, see also*)

Verify code(s) in Tabular

- Read Tabular notes
- Code to highest specificity
- Never code from index!

Level of Detail in Coding

Assign diagnosis (dx) to highest level of specificity

Do NOT use 3-digit code if there is 4th

Do NOT use 4-digit code if there is 5th

Acute and Chronic Conditions

Exists alone or together

May be separate or combination codes

If two codes, code acute first

   Example: acute (577.0) and chronic (577.1) pancreatitis

When two separate codes exist, code

- Acute cystitis 595.0
- Chronic cystitis 595.2

Combination code: Both acute and chronic condition

- Diarrhea (acute) (chronic) 787.91, Acute and subacute bacterial endocarditis 421.0
- Otitis acute and subacute 382.9

Combination Code

Always use combination code if one exists

   Example: encephalomyelitis (dx) due to rubella (manifestation), 056.01

Multiple Coding for Single Condition

Etiology (cause)

Manifestation (symptom)

- Slanted brackets [ ]

   Example: Retinopathy, diabetic 250.5 *[362.01]*

- Must check Tabular notes to assign correct 5th digit for diabetes
- Tabular: 362.0, Diabetic retinopathy, instructs to "Code first diabetes 250.5"

SELECTION OF PRIMARY DIAGNOSIS

Condition for encounter

Documented in medical record

Condition that is responsible for services provided

Also list coexisting conditions

Diagnosis and procedure MUST correlate

- Medical necessity established
- No correlation = no reimbursement

Codes in Brackets

Never sequence as principal dx

Always sequence in order listed in Index

Example:

- Index lists: Diabetes, gangrene 250.7 *[785.4]*
- 785.4 = gangrene
- Tabular, 785.4 indicates "Code first any associated underlying condition: diabetes (250.7X) . . ."
- Code first diabetes, then gangrene
- 250.7X = diabetes (X = 5th digit)
- 785.4 = gangrene

Two or More Interrelated Conditions

When two or more interrelated conditions exist and either could be principal dx, either may be sequenced first

Example: Patient with mitral valve stenosis and coronary artery disease (two interrelated conditions)

- Either can be principal dx and sequenced first
- Resource intensiveness affects choice

V CODES

Located after 999.9 in Tabular

Two digits before decimal (e.g., V10.10)

Index for V codes, Alphabetic Index to Diseases

Main terms: contraception, counseling, dialysis, status, examination

Uses of V Codes

Not sick BUT receives health care (e.g., vaccination)

Services for known disease/injury (e.g., chemotherapy)

A circumstance/problem that influences patient's health BUT NOT current illness/injury

Example: Organ transplant status

Example: Birth status and outcome of delivery (newborn)

Section I.18.e of Guidelines contains the V Code Table

- Identifies how V codes can be listed (first, first/additional, additional only)

> **Special Note about "History of"**
> Index to Disease, MAIN term "History"
> Entries between "family" and "visual loss V19.0" = "Family history of"
> Entries before "family" and after "visual loss V19.0" = "Personal history of"

History V Code Categories in Tabular

V10 Personal history of malignant neoplasm

V12 Personal history of certain other diseases

V13 Personal history of other diseases

Except: V13.4 Personal history of arthritis, and V13.6, Personal history of congenital malformations. These conditions are life-long so are not true history codes

V14 Personal history of allergy to medicinal agents

V15 Other personal history presenting hazards to health

Except: V15.7 Personal history of contraception

V16 Family history of malignant neoplasm

V17 Family history of certain chronic disabling diseases

V18 Family history of certain other specific diseases

V19 Family history of other conditions

LATE EFFECTS

Late effect residual of (remaining from) previous illness/injury, e.g., burn that leaves scar

Residual coded first (scar)

Cause (burn) coded second

Late effect codes are not in a separate chapter; rather, throughout Tabular

Reference the term "Late" in the Index

There is no time limit on developing a residual

There may be more than one residual

> ***Example:*** Patient has a stroke (434.91) and develops paralysis on dominant side (hemiparesis, 438.21) and loss of ability to communicate (aphasia, 438.11)

DIAGNOSTIC CODING AND REPORTING GUIDELINES FOR OUTPATIENT SERVICES

Physician's office

Hospital-based outpatient services

Part of *Official Guidelines for Coding and Reporting*, Section IV

Guideline A

The term *first-listed diagnosis* is used rather than *principal diagnosis*

Outpatient Surgery: Reason for surgery

Observation Stay: Medical condition that occasioned admission

Guideline B

Use codes 001.0 through V84.8 to code dx, symptoms, conditions, problems, complaints, or other reason(s) for visit

Guideline C

Documentation should describe patient's condition, using terminology that includes specific diagnoses as well as symptoms, problems, or reasons for encounter

Guideline D

Selection of codes 001.0 through 999.9 (Chapters 1-17) will frequently be used to describe reason for encounter

Guideline E

Codes that describe symptoms and signs, as opposed to diagnoses, acceptable for reporting purposes when an established dx has NOT been confirmed by physician

Guideline F

V codes deal with encounters for circumstances other than disease or injury

> ***Example:*** Well-baby checkup (V20.2)

Guideline G

Codes have either three, four, or five digits

4th and/or 5th digit codes provide greater specificity

Three-digit code used ONLY if there is NO 4th or 5th digit

Where 4th and/or 5th digits provided, must be assigned

Diagnoses NOT coded to full digits available are invalid

Guideline H

List first code for dx, condition, problem, or other reason for encounter/visit shown in medical record to be chiefly responsible for services provided

List additional codes that describe any coexisting conditions

Guideline I

Do NOT code diagnoses documented as probable, suspected, questionable, ruled out, or working diagnoses

Rather, code condition(s) to highest degree of certainty for that encounter/visit, such as symptoms, signs, abnormal test results, or other reason for visit

Example: Cough and fever, probably pneumonia

- Code as cough (786.2) and fever (780.6) (in this order)

Guideline J

Chronic diseases treated on an ongoing basis may be coded and reported as many times as patient receives treatment and care for condition(s)

Guideline K

Code all documented conditions that coexist at time of visit, that require or affect patient care, treatment, or management

Do NOT code conditions previously treated, no longer existing

"History of" codes (V10-V19) may be used as secondary codes if

- Impacts current care or treatment

Guidelines L and M

For patients receiving diagnostic or therapeutic services ONLY

Sequence first

- Diagnosis,
- Condition,
- Problem, or
- Other reason shown in medical record to be chiefly responsible for encounter

Codes for other diagnoses (e.g., chronic conditions)

- May be sequenced as secondary diagnoses

Exception:

Patients receiving chemotherapy (V58.11), radiation therapy (V58.0), or rehabilitation (code depends on type)

- V code first; dx or problem for which service being performed second

Guideline N

For patients receiving preoperative evaluations ONLY

- Code from category V72.8 (Other specified examinations)
- Assign secondary code for reason for surgery
- Code also any findings related to preoperative evaluation

Guideline O

Code dx which required ambulatory surgery

If postoperative dx different

- Code postoperative dx

Guideline P

Code routine prenatal visits with no complications

- V22.0 (Supervision of normal first pregnancy)
- V22.1 (Supervision of other normal pregnancy)
- DO NOT use these codes with pregnancy complication codes

ICD-9-CM, CHAPTER 1, INFECTIOUS AND PARASITIC DISEASES

Divided based on etiology (cause of disease)

Many Combination Codes

Example: 112.0 candidiasis infection of mouth, which reports both organism and condition with one code

Multiple Codes

Sequencing must be considered

- UTI due to *Escherichia coli*
- 599.0 (UTI) etiology
- 041.4 *(E. coli)* organism (in this order)

Human Immunodeficiency Virus

Code HIV or HIV-related illness ONLY if stated as confirmed in diagnostic statement

- 042 HIV or HIV-related illness
- V08 Asymptomatic HIV status
- 795.71 Nonspecific HIV serology

Previously Diagnosed HIV-Related Illness

Code prior dx HIV-related disease 042 (HIV)

NEVER assign these patients to

- V08 (Asymptomatic) or
- 795.71 (Nonspecific serologic evidence of HIV)

HIV Sequencing

Sequence first that reason most responsible for encounter, if HIV (042)

Followed by secondary dx that affects encounter or patient care

HIV and Pregnancy

This an exception to HIV sequencing

During pregnancy, childbirth, or puerperium, code

- 647.6X (Other specified infectious and parasitic diseases), followed by 042 (HIV)

Asymptomatic HIV during pregnancy, childbirth, or puerperium

- 647.6X (Other specified infections and parasitic diseases) and

- V08 (Asymptomatic HIV infection status)

Inconclusive Laboratory Test for HIV

795.71 (Inconclusive serologic test for HIV)

HIV Screening

Code V73.89 (Screening for other specified viral disease)

- Patient in high-risk group for HIV

- V69.8 (Other problems related to lifestyle)

Patients returning for HIV screening results = V65.44 (HIV counseling)

Section I.C.1.b. Septicemia, Systemic Inflammatory Response Syndrome (SIRS) Sepsis, Severe Sepsis, and Septic Shock

Sepsis: Assign systemic infection code as first listed when sepsis is present

- Assign a sepsis code as secondary when sepsis develops during encounter

Septicemia/Sepsis: Usually a 038 septicemia code and a 995.9x SIRS code (in this order)

Septic Shock: Organ dysfunction associated with severe sepsis

- Code underlying systemic infection (e.g., 038.xx) followed by the SIRS code (995.92)

Caution
Incorrectly applying these HIV coding rules can cause patient hardship

- Insurance claims for patients with HIV usually need patient's written agreement to disclosure

---

ICD-9-CM, CHAPTER 2, NEOPLASMS

Two steps for coding neoplasms

Index

1. Locate histologic type of neoplasm (e.g., sarcoma, melanoma)
   - Review all instructions
2. Locate code identified by body site
   - Usually in Neoplasm Table in Index under "N"
   - Neoplasm Table divided into columns:
     - Malignant (primary, secondary, ca in situ)
     - Benign

- Uncertain behavior
- Unspecified

Example: Pathology report confirmed diagnosis stated in operative report of primary malignant neoplasm of the bladder neck. ICD-9-CM Index, Neoplasm Table, bladder, neck, under Primary column, 188.5. Code then referenced in Tabular to ensure accurate assignment.

Treatment directed at malignancy: Neoplasm is principal dx

Except for Chemotherapy or Radiotherapy:

- Therapy (treatment) followed by neoplasm code
  - Chemotherapy: V58.11
  - Radiotherapy: V58.0

Surgical removal of neoplasm and subsequent chemotherapy or radiotherapy

- Code malignancy as principal dx

Surgery to determine extent of malignancy

- Code malignancy as principal dx
  - V10, "Personal history of malignant neoplasm" if
    - Neoplasm was previously destroyed
    - No longer being treated

If patient receives treatment for secondary neoplasm (metastasis)

- Secondary neoplasm is principal dx
- Even though primary is known

Patient treated for anemia or dehydration due to neoplasm or therapy code

- Anemia or dehydration followed by neoplasm

Patient admitted to repair complication of surgery for an intestinal malignancy

- Complication principal dx
- Complication is reason for encounter
- Malignancy secondary dx

Patient receiving chemotherapy or radiotherapy post-op removal of neoplasm

- Code: Therapy followed by active neoplasm
- Do NOT report H/O (history of) neoplasm

ICD-9-CM, CHAPTER 3, ENDOCRINE, NUTRITIONAL, AND METABOLIC DISEASES AND IMMUNITY DISORDERS

Disorders of Other Endocrine Glands

Diabetes Mellitus 250 coded frequently

Subterms in Index often have two codes

Example:

- Diabetic iritis 250.5X for diabetes (etiology)
- *[364.42]* for iritis (manifestation)

5th digit indicates type of diabetes

0 type II or unspecified type, not stated as uncontrolled

Fifth-digit 0 is for use for type II patients, even if the patient requires insulin

1 type I [juvenile type], not stated as uncontrolled

2 type II or unspecified type, uncontrolled

Fifth-digit 2 is for use for type II, adult-onset, diabetic patients, even if the patient requires insulin

3 type I [juvenile type], uncontrolled

V58.67 used in addition to diabetes code to show long-term use if insulin

If type is not indicated, code Type II diabetes

Patient with Type II diabetes can receive insulin for periods when diabetes is uncontrolled

Type I diabetic is one who is insulin-dependent

Other Metabolic and Immunity Disorders Section

Disorders such as gout and dehydration

Disorders often have many names

Example: 242.0X Toxic diffuse goiter, also known as

- Basedow's disease
- Graves' disease
- Primary thyroid hyperplasia

ICD-9-CM, CHAPTER 4, DISEASES OF BLOOD AND BLOOD-FORMING ORGANS

Short chapter with 10 sections

Includes anemia, blood disorders, coagulation defects

Often used code, anemia

Many different types of anemia

- Hereditary hemolytic (282)
- Iron deficiency (280)
- Acquired hemolytic (283)
- Aplastic (284)
- Other and Unspecified (285)

Multiple coding often necessary

Identify underlying disease condition

ICD-9-CM, CHAPTER 5, MENTAL DISORDERS

Includes codes for

- Personality disorders
- Stress disorders
- Neuroses
- Psychoses
- Sexual deviation/dysfunction, etc.

5th digit = status of episode

Example: 304.2, cocaine dependence, is assigned the following 5th fifth digits:

- 0 unspecified (episode)
- 1 continuous
- 2 episodic
- 3 in remission

ICD-9-CM, CHAPTER 6, DISEASES OF NERVOUS SYSTEM AND SENSE ORGANS

Central Nervous System

Peripheral Nervous System

Disorders of Eye

Diseases of Ear

ICD-9-CM, CHAPTER 7, DISEASES OF CIRCULATORY SYSTEM

Three types of hypertension

1. Malignant accelerated, severe, poor prognosis
2. Benign continuous, mild (BP elevated) controllable
3. Unspecified NOT indicated as either malignant or benign

Hypertension (401-405)

Hypertension table located in Index of ICD-9-CM

- Under "H," Hypertension
- Codes divided based on type (malignant, benign, unspecified)

Hypertension, Essential, or NOS

Assign hypertension (arterial, essential, primary, systemic, NOS) to 401

4th digit indicates type

- 0 Malignant
- 1 Benign
- 9 Unspecified

Hypertension with Heart Disease

402 Category

Certain heart conditions when stated "due to hypertension" or implied ("hypertensive")

Add 4th digit for type

Use additional code to specify type of heart failure (428)

Hypertensive Kidney Disease

Cause-and-effect relationship assumed in chronic renal failure with hypertension

Category 403, Hypertensive renal disease, used when following present:

- Chronic kidney disease (585.X)
- Renal failure, unspecified (586)
- Renal sclerosis, unspecified (587)

Hypertensive Heart and Kidney Disease

Assign 404 when both hypertensive kidney disease and hypertensive heart disease stated

Assume cause-and-effect relationship

Assign 5th digit for mention of kidney and/or heart failure

- Use additional code to specify type of heart failure (428)

Hypertensive Cerebrovascular Disease

Code

- Cerebrovascular disease (430-438)
- Type of hypertension (401-405)

Hypertensive Retinopathy

Code

- Hypertensive retinopathy (362.11)
- Type of hypertension (401-405)

Hypertension, Secondary

Hypertension caused by an underlying condition

- Code
  - Underlying condition
  - Type of hypertension (405)

Hypertension, Transient

Transient hypertension: Temporary elevated BP

DO NOT assign 401-405, Hypertensive Disease

- Hypertension dx is NOT established
- Use
  - 796.2, Elevated blood pressure or
  - 642.3X, Transient hypertension of pregnancy

Hypertension, Controlled

Hypertension controlled by therapy

- Assign code from 401-405

Hypertension, Uncontrolled

Untreated or uncontrolled hypertension

- Assign code from 401-405

Documentation must state malignant hypertension to use 404

Elevated Blood Pressure

Elevated blood pressure coded 796.2

- Elevated BP reading without hypertension is dx
- Hypertension NOT stated, NOT coded to 401

ICD-9-CM, CHAPTER 8, DISEASES OF RESPIRATORY SYSTEM

Watch for "Use additional code to identify infectious organism"

Some codes indicate specific organism and do not need an additional code

Respiratory failure sequencing

If the respiratory failure is due to an acute condition (such as MI [myocardial infarction]) or acute exacerbation of a chronic condition (such as COPD [chronic obstructive pulmonary disease]), sequence the acute condition first

> **Example:** MI (acute condition) and respiratory failure

- Sequence MI first and respiratory failure second

If the respiratory failure (acute condition) is due to a chronic nonrespiratory condition (such as myasthenia gravis), sequence the respiratory failure first

> **Example:** Acute respiratory failure (acute) and myasthenia gravis (chronic)

- Sequence acute respiratory failure first and myasthenia gravis second

Acute Respiratory Infection Section

Frequently used codes, such as

- Common cold (460, acute nasopharyngitis)
- Sore throat (462, acute pharyngitis)
- Acute tonsillitis (463)
- Bronchitis (490-491)

- Acute upper respiratory infection (465, URI)
- Influenza (487, flu)

Read Guidelines for Chapter 8 for specifics on coding COPD and asthma

ICD-9-CM, CHAPTER 9, DISEASES OF DIGESTIVE SYSTEM

Mouth to anus + accessory organs

Extensive subcategories

- 574 Cholelithiasis (10 subcategories)
- Each has 5th digit subclassification

Commonly used codes

- Ulcers (531-534)
  - Gastric (531)
  - Duodenal (532)
  - Peptic (533)
  - Gastrojejunal (534)
- Hernias (550-553)

ICD-9-CM, CHAPTER 10, DISEASES OF GENITOURINARY SYSTEM

Commonly used codes

- Urinary tract infection (599.0)
- Inflammation of prostate (601.X)
- Disorders of menstruation (625-627)

Stages of kidney failure

- Stage I: Blood flow through kidney increases, kidney enlarges (585.1)
- Stage II: (mild) Small amounts of blood protein (albumin) leak into urine (microalbuminuria) (585.2)
- Stage III: (moderate) Albumin and other protein losses increase. Patient may develop high blood pressure and kidney loses ability to filter waste (585.3)
- Stage IV: (severe) Large amounts of urine pass through kidney, blood pressure increases (585.4)
- Stage V: Ability to filter waste nearly stops (585.5)
- End-stage renal failure (585.6)

  When documentation indicates chronic renal disease (CKD) and ESRD, report ESRD

- Unspecified 585.9

Status post kidney transplant, assign V42.0

ICD-9-CM, CHAPTER 11, COMPLICATIONS OF PREGNANCY, CHILDBIRTH, AND PUERPERIUM

Extensive multiple coding with many 5th digit assignments and notes

Admission for pregnancy, complication

- Obstetric complication = primary dx

Chapter 11 ICD-9-CM codes take precedence over codes from other chapters

Codes 640-676.9 share same 5th digit subclassification

- Denotes current episode of care
- 0 Unspecified as to episode of care or not applicable
- 1 Delivered, with or without mention of antepartum condition
- 2 Delivered, with mention of postpartum complication
- 3 Antepartum condition or complication
- 4 Postpartum condition or complication

General Rules

Not all encounters are pregnancy-related

   Example: Pregnant woman, broken ankle (medial malleolus, open)

   - Broken ankle (824.1)
   - V22.2 Pregnant state incidental

Complications of Pregnancy, Childbirth, and Puerperium

Chapter 11 codes (630677)

Used only on mother's medical record

Not on newborn medical record

Selection of Primary Diagnosis

Routine prenatal visits, no complications:

- V22.0, Supervision, normal **first** pregnancy or
- V22.1, Supervision, **other** normal pregnancy

Prenatal outpatient visits for high-risk pregnancies:

- V23, Supervision of high-risk pregnancy

Fifth Digit

All categories EXCEPT 650 (Normal delivery)

Requires 5th digit for

- Antepartum
- Postpartum
- If delivery has occurred

Appropriate 5th digit listed under each code

    Example: 640.0, Threatened abortion

- 0 unspecified episode

- 1 delivered with or without complication

- 3 antepartum condition or complication

Note that NOT all 5th digits are applicable (640.0, cannot assign 2 or 4)

Postpartum Period

After delivery +6 weeks

Abortions

Codes 634-637 require 5th digits

- 0 unspecified

- 1 incomplete; POC (product of conception) NOT expelled

- 2 complete; all POC expelled prior to care

Abortions with Liveborn Fetus

Attempted abortion results in liveborn fetus

- 644.21 (Early onset of delivery)

- Use V27 (Outcome of delivery)

- Attempted abortion code also assigned

ICD-9-CM, CHAPTER 12, DISEASES OF SKIN AND SUBCUTANEOUS TISSUE

Skin

Epidermis

Dermis

Subcutaneous tissue

Infectious skin/subcutaneous tissue

Scar tissue

Accessory Organs

Sweat glands

Sebaceous glands

Nails

Hair and hair follicles

Other

Multiple Codes Often Necessary

Example: Cellulitis due to *Staphylococcus,* report

- Cellulitis 682
- Staph 041

ICD-9-CM, CHAPTER 13, DISEASES OF MUSCULOSKELETAL SYSTEM AND CONNECTIVE TISSUE

Bone

Bursa

Cartilage

Fascia

Ligaments

Muscle

Synovia

Tendons

Chapter 13 Sections

Extensive notes and 5th digits

- Arthropathies (joint disease) and related disorders
- Dorsopathies (curvature of spine)
- Rheumatism, Excluding Back
- Osteopathies, Chondropathies, and Acquired Musculoskeletal Deformities

ICD-9-CM, CHAPTERS 14 AND 15, CONGENITAL ANOMALIES AND CONDITIONS ORIGINATING IN PERINATAL PERIOD

Congenital Anomalies (abnormalities at birth), 740-759

Conditions Originating in Perinatal Period

- Perinatal period through 28th day following birth
- Codes can be used after 28th day if documented that condition originated during perinatal period

Chapter 17 codes are only for the newborn record; never on the maternal record

Assign V30-V39 as first listed according to type of birth

ICD-9-CM, CHAPTER 16, SYMPTOMS, SIGNS, AND ILL-DEFINED CONDITIONS

Do NOT code a sign or symptom if

- Definitive dx made (symptoms are part of disease)

Used only if no specific dx made

ICD-9-CM, CHAPTER 17, INJURY AND POISONING

Section Examples

Fractures

Dislocations

Sprains and Strains

Intracranial Injury

Internal Injury

Crushing Injury

Foreign Body

Burns

Late Effects

Poisoning

E Codes

Provide supplemental information

Never principal diagnosis

Index and Tabular

E code Index located in Section III

Directly before the Tabular

Not in the Index to Disease, Volume 2

E codes are located after the V codes in the Tabular

Identify

- Cause of an injury or poisoning
- Intent (unintentional or intentional)
- Place it occurred

General E Code Guidelines

Use with any code in Volume 1

Initial encounter

- Use E code

Subsequent encounter

- Use late effects E codes

Intent

Unknown, Undetermined (E980-E989)

Unspecified, Undetermined (E980-E989)

Questionable, Undetermined (E980-E989)

Table of Drugs and Chemicals

Alphabetic listing with codes (see Figure 3-15)

Do NOT code directly from Table

Always reference Tabular

Two or more substances involved

If two or more substances involved

- Code each unless combination code exists

- Code substance more closely related to principal dx

- Include one code from each category (cause, intent, place)

Interaction of drug(s) and alcohol

- Use poisoning and E codes for both

Unknown or suspected intent

Unknown

Unspecified

Questionable

Undetermined cause

Intent known, cause unknown, use

- E928.9, Unspecified accident

- E958.9, Suicide and self-inflicted injury by unspecified means

- E968.9, Assault by unspecified means

Late effects of external cause

Should be used with late effect of a previous injury/poisoning

Should NOT be used with related current injury code

Coding of Burns

Multiple injuries and burns

Sequence most severe injury first (physician determined)

Current burns

Sequence highest-degree burn first

Current burns (940-948) classified by

- Depth (severity)

- Extent (% body surface)

- Agent (if necessary)

Depth of burn

1st degree: Erythema

2nd degree: Blistering

3rd degree: Full-thickness involvement

Burns classified

- According to extent of body surface involved

- Burn site NOT specified

- Additional data required

Category 948

- 4th digits = % body surface involved

- 5th digits = % body surface involved in 3rd-degree burns

- Rule of Nines applies

Burn Example: 3rd-degree burn of abdomen (10%) and 2nd-degree burn of thigh (5%) by hot water

- 942.33 Burn, abdomen, 3rd degree

- 945.26 Burn, thigh, 2nd degree

- 948.11 15% burn area

- E924.0 Burn by hot liquid

Coding for multiple injuries

Separate code for each injury

Sequence most serious injury first

Vessel and nerve damage

Code primary injury first

- Use additional code if minor nerve damage

Primary injury = nerve damage

- Code nerve damage first

Multiple fractures

Same coding principles as multiple injuries

Code multiple fractures by site

Sequenced by severity

Fractures

Not indicated as closed or open = closed

Same bone fractured AND dislocated:

- Code Fx ONLY (highest level of injury)

Coding Challenge

EXAMINATIONS

You have three opportunities to practice taking an examination:

- Pre-Examination (before study)
- Post-Examination (after study)
- Final Examination (at the end of your complete program of study)

You should have a current edition of the following texts:

- ICD-9-CM *(International Classification of Diseases, 9ᵗʰ Edition, Clinical Modification)*, Volumes 1 and 2
- HCPCS (Healthcare Common Procedure Coding System)
- CPT *(Current Procedural Terminology)*

No other reference material is allowed for any of the examinations.

- For the Pre-Examination, you will not need a computer; rather you will need paper, pencils, erasers, and the three coding references listed above (ICD-9-CM (Vols. 1 and 2), HCPCS, CPT).
- For the Post-Examination and Final Examination, you will need a computer that can use a CD-ROM.
- Each organization's certification examination has different scoring requirements, but as you take these examinations, you should strive for 80% to 90% on the Post-Examination and 70% as a minimum on the Final Examination.

NOTE: To enable the learner to calculate an examination score, minimums have been identified as "passing" within this text; however, this may or may not be the percentage identified by the American Academy of Professional Coders as a "passing" grade. It is your responsibility to review all certification information published by the American Academy of Professional Coders as they are the definitive source for information regarding the certification examination.

PRE-EXAMINATION AND POST-EXAMINATION

The Pre-Examination contains 150 questions and is located in Unit IV of the textbook. The purpose of the Pre-Examination is only to assess your beginning level of knowledge and skill—your starting place. Based on your scores, you can tailor your study to target your weakest areas and increase your scores. Take the Pre-Examination before you begin your studies, using paper and pencil. There is an answer sheet on which to place your answers; it is located directly before the examination. Remove the answer sheet from the text, and enter your answer for each of the 150 questions.

You will need to calculate your percent on each of the three sections after checking your answers. A passing score requires the following:

Section 1   **63%** or 27 of the 43 questions correct

Section 2   **73%** or 44 of the 60 questions correct

Section 3   **60%** or 28 of the 47 questions correct

Enter your scores into the software on the accompanying CD, and the software will retain this information for later use.

Immediately on completion of your study, you should complete the Post-Examination on the CD. After you are finished, the CD will automatically compare your Pre-Examination scores with your Post-Examination scores, and will store the results for when you take the Final Examination. By comparing the results of the Pre-Examination and the Post-Examination (the same examination will be taken twice), the software illustrates the improvements you have achieved.

Rationales for each question are available for review after you complete the Post-Examination. Study the questions for which you did not choose the right response. Did you misread the question, did you not know the material well enough to answer correctly, or did you run out of time? Knowing why you missed a question is an important step toward improving your skill level.

Ideally, you should complete each examination in one sitting (5 hours or 300 minutes); if time does not allow, spread the examination times over several periods. There are no time extensions during an actual examination setting, and learning how to judge the amount of time you to spend on each question is an important part of this learning experience to prepare you for the real certification examination.

FINAL EXAMINATION

If you scored well on all areas of the Post-Examination (80% to 90%), you are ready to move on to the Final Examination, which is on the CD. The real certification examination is currently paper and pencil, but in the future will be computer-based. Once you have completed the Final Examination, the software will compare all your scores to illustrate your improvement.

If you did not attain a minimum score on each section, you should develop a plan to restudy those particular areas where the examination indicates you are having difficulties. There are rationales for each question in the Final Examination, and you should review that information as well as material in the text. You can take any of the practice examinations again after your additional study.

PRE-EXAMINATION ANSWER SHEET

SECTION 1

Medical terminology

1. Ⓐ Ⓑ Ⓒ Ⓓ
2. Ⓐ Ⓑ Ⓒ Ⓓ
3. Ⓐ Ⓑ Ⓒ Ⓓ
4. Ⓐ Ⓑ Ⓒ Ⓓ
5. Ⓐ Ⓑ Ⓒ Ⓓ
6. Ⓐ Ⓑ Ⓒ Ⓓ
7. Ⓐ Ⓑ Ⓒ Ⓓ
8. Ⓐ Ⓑ Ⓒ Ⓓ
9. Ⓐ Ⓑ Ⓒ Ⓓ
10. Ⓐ Ⓑ Ⓒ Ⓓ
11. Ⓐ Ⓑ Ⓒ Ⓓ
12. Ⓐ Ⓑ Ⓒ Ⓓ
13. Ⓐ Ⓑ Ⓒ Ⓓ

Anatomy

14. Ⓐ Ⓑ Ⓒ Ⓓ
15. Ⓐ Ⓑ Ⓒ Ⓓ
16. Ⓐ Ⓑ Ⓒ Ⓓ
17. Ⓐ Ⓑ Ⓒ Ⓓ
18. Ⓐ Ⓑ Ⓒ Ⓓ
19. Ⓐ Ⓑ Ⓒ Ⓓ
20. Ⓐ Ⓑ Ⓒ Ⓓ
21. Ⓐ Ⓑ Ⓒ Ⓓ
22. Ⓐ Ⓑ Ⓒ Ⓓ

ICD-9-CM

23. Ⓐ Ⓑ Ⓒ Ⓓ
24. Ⓐ Ⓑ Ⓒ Ⓓ
25. Ⓐ Ⓑ Ⓒ Ⓓ
26. Ⓐ Ⓑ Ⓒ Ⓓ
27. Ⓐ Ⓑ Ⓒ Ⓓ
28. Ⓐ Ⓑ Ⓒ Ⓓ
29. Ⓐ Ⓑ Ⓒ Ⓓ
30. Ⓐ Ⓑ Ⓒ Ⓓ
31. Ⓐ Ⓑ Ⓒ Ⓓ
32. Ⓐ Ⓑ Ⓒ Ⓓ
33. Ⓐ Ⓑ Ⓒ Ⓓ

HCPCS

34. Ⓐ Ⓑ Ⓒ Ⓓ
35. Ⓐ Ⓑ Ⓒ Ⓓ
36. Ⓐ Ⓑ Ⓒ Ⓓ
37. Ⓐ Ⓑ Ⓒ Ⓓ
38. Ⓐ Ⓑ Ⓒ Ⓓ

Concepts of coding

39. Ⓐ Ⓑ Ⓒ Ⓓ
40. Ⓐ Ⓑ Ⓒ Ⓓ
41. Ⓐ Ⓑ Ⓒ Ⓓ
42. Ⓐ Ⓑ Ⓒ Ⓓ
43. Ⓐ Ⓑ Ⓒ Ⓓ

SECTION 2

10000

44. Ⓐ Ⓑ Ⓒ Ⓓ
45. Ⓐ Ⓑ Ⓒ Ⓓ
46. Ⓐ Ⓑ Ⓒ Ⓓ
47. Ⓐ Ⓑ Ⓒ Ⓓ
48. Ⓐ Ⓑ Ⓒ Ⓓ
49. Ⓐ Ⓑ Ⓒ Ⓓ
50. Ⓐ Ⓑ Ⓒ Ⓓ
51. Ⓐ Ⓑ Ⓒ Ⓓ
52. Ⓐ Ⓑ Ⓒ Ⓓ

20000

53. Ⓐ Ⓑ Ⓒ Ⓓ
54. Ⓐ Ⓑ Ⓒ Ⓓ
55. Ⓐ Ⓑ Ⓒ Ⓓ
56. Ⓐ Ⓑ Ⓒ Ⓓ
57. Ⓐ Ⓑ Ⓒ Ⓓ
58. Ⓐ Ⓑ Ⓒ Ⓓ
59. Ⓐ Ⓑ Ⓒ Ⓓ
60. Ⓐ Ⓑ Ⓒ Ⓓ
61. Ⓐ Ⓑ Ⓒ Ⓓ
62. Ⓐ Ⓑ Ⓒ Ⓓ

30000

63. Ⓐ Ⓑ Ⓒ Ⓓ
64. Ⓐ Ⓑ Ⓒ Ⓓ
65. Ⓐ Ⓑ Ⓒ Ⓓ
66. Ⓐ Ⓑ Ⓒ Ⓓ
67. Ⓐ Ⓑ Ⓒ Ⓓ
68. Ⓐ Ⓑ Ⓒ Ⓓ
69. Ⓐ Ⓑ Ⓒ Ⓓ
70. Ⓐ Ⓑ Ⓒ Ⓓ
71. Ⓐ Ⓑ Ⓒ Ⓓ
72. Ⓐ Ⓑ Ⓒ Ⓓ

40000

73. Ⓐ Ⓑ Ⓒ Ⓓ
74. Ⓐ Ⓑ Ⓒ Ⓓ
75. Ⓐ Ⓑ Ⓒ Ⓓ
76. Ⓐ Ⓑ Ⓒ Ⓓ
77. Ⓐ Ⓑ Ⓒ Ⓓ
78. Ⓐ Ⓑ Ⓒ Ⓓ
79. Ⓐ Ⓑ Ⓒ Ⓓ
80. Ⓐ Ⓑ Ⓒ Ⓓ
81. Ⓐ Ⓑ Ⓒ Ⓓ
82. Ⓐ Ⓑ Ⓒ Ⓓ

50000

83. Ⓐ Ⓑ Ⓒ Ⓓ
84. Ⓐ Ⓑ Ⓒ Ⓓ
85. Ⓐ Ⓑ Ⓒ Ⓓ
86. Ⓐ Ⓑ Ⓒ Ⓓ
87. Ⓐ Ⓑ Ⓒ Ⓓ
88. Ⓐ Ⓑ Ⓒ Ⓓ
89. Ⓐ Ⓑ Ⓒ Ⓓ
90. Ⓐ Ⓑ Ⓒ Ⓓ
91. Ⓐ Ⓑ Ⓒ Ⓓ
92. Ⓐ Ⓑ Ⓒ Ⓓ
93. Ⓐ Ⓑ Ⓒ Ⓓ

60000

94. Ⓐ Ⓑ Ⓒ Ⓓ
95. Ⓐ Ⓑ Ⓒ Ⓓ
96. Ⓐ Ⓑ Ⓒ Ⓓ
97. Ⓐ Ⓑ Ⓒ Ⓓ
98. Ⓐ Ⓑ Ⓒ Ⓓ
99. Ⓐ Ⓑ Ⓒ Ⓓ
100. Ⓐ Ⓑ Ⓒ Ⓓ
101. Ⓐ Ⓑ Ⓒ Ⓓ
102. Ⓐ Ⓑ Ⓒ Ⓓ
103. Ⓐ Ⓑ Ⓒ Ⓓ

SECTION 3

E/M

104. Ⓐ Ⓑ Ⓒ Ⓓ
105. Ⓐ Ⓑ Ⓒ Ⓓ
106. Ⓐ Ⓑ Ⓒ Ⓓ
107. Ⓐ Ⓑ Ⓒ Ⓓ
108. Ⓐ Ⓑ Ⓒ Ⓓ
109. Ⓐ Ⓑ Ⓒ Ⓓ
110. Ⓐ Ⓑ Ⓒ Ⓓ
111. Ⓐ Ⓑ Ⓒ Ⓓ
112. Ⓐ Ⓑ Ⓒ Ⓓ
113. Ⓐ Ⓑ Ⓒ Ⓓ
114. Ⓐ Ⓑ Ⓒ Ⓓ
115. Ⓐ Ⓑ Ⓒ Ⓓ

Anesthesia

116. Ⓐ Ⓑ Ⓒ Ⓓ
117. Ⓐ Ⓑ Ⓒ Ⓓ
118. Ⓐ Ⓑ Ⓒ Ⓓ
119. Ⓐ Ⓑ Ⓒ Ⓓ
120. Ⓐ Ⓑ Ⓒ Ⓓ
121. Ⓐ Ⓑ Ⓒ Ⓓ

70000

122. Ⓐ Ⓑ Ⓒ Ⓓ
123. Ⓐ Ⓑ Ⓒ Ⓓ
124. Ⓐ Ⓑ Ⓒ Ⓓ
125. Ⓐ Ⓑ Ⓒ Ⓓ
126. Ⓐ Ⓑ Ⓒ Ⓓ
127. Ⓐ Ⓑ Ⓒ Ⓓ
128. Ⓐ Ⓑ Ⓒ Ⓓ
129. Ⓐ Ⓑ Ⓒ Ⓓ
130. Ⓐ Ⓑ Ⓒ Ⓓ

80000

131. Ⓐ Ⓑ Ⓒ Ⓓ
132. Ⓐ Ⓑ Ⓒ Ⓓ
133. Ⓐ Ⓑ Ⓒ Ⓓ
134. Ⓐ Ⓑ Ⓒ Ⓓ
135. Ⓐ Ⓑ Ⓒ Ⓓ
136. Ⓐ Ⓑ Ⓒ Ⓓ
137. Ⓐ Ⓑ Ⓒ Ⓓ
138. Ⓐ Ⓑ Ⓒ Ⓓ
139. Ⓐ Ⓑ Ⓒ Ⓓ
140. Ⓐ Ⓑ Ⓒ Ⓓ

90000

141. Ⓐ Ⓑ Ⓒ Ⓓ
142. Ⓐ Ⓑ Ⓒ Ⓓ
143. Ⓐ Ⓑ Ⓒ Ⓓ
144. Ⓐ Ⓑ Ⓒ Ⓓ
145. Ⓐ Ⓑ Ⓒ Ⓓ
146. Ⓐ Ⓑ Ⓒ Ⓓ
147. Ⓐ Ⓑ Ⓒ Ⓓ
148. Ⓐ Ⓑ Ⓒ Ⓓ
149. Ⓐ Ⓑ Ⓒ Ⓓ
150. Ⓐ Ⓑ Ⓒ Ⓓ

Pre-Examination Results

Section 1: _____

*Section 2: _____

*Section 3: _____

*Please note that for Sections 2 and 3, each question is worth 2 points. This will make a difference in the initial scoring on the CD-ROM.

■ PRE-EXAMINATION
SECTION 1

Questions 1-43

Medical Terminology

1. The cup-shaped depression on the hip joint that receives the head of the femur is the:
   A. acetabulum
   B. calcaneus
   C. trochlea
   D. medial malleolus

2. The lower third of the small intestine is the:
   A. jejunum
   B. tenue
   C. ileum
   D. duodenum

3. This term means to divert or make an artificial passage:
   A. burr
   B. occipital
   C. shunt
   D. catheter

4. This term means to identify the presence of and the amount of:
   A. qualitative
   B. definitive
   C. authoritative
   D. quantitative

5. The term that means the expansion of:
   A. dilation
   B. curettage
   C. tocolysis
   D. manipulation

6. This term means the outermost covering of the eyeball:
   A. sclera
   B. lacrimal
   C. ciliary
   D. chorea

7. This term means the soft tissue around the nail border:
   A. sebaceous
   B. dermis
   C. lunula
   D. perionychium

8. This term means to turn downward:
   A. flexion
   B. adduction
   C. circumduction
   D. pronation

9. This combining form means artery:
   A. angi/o
   B. aort/o
   C. arteri/o
   D. atri/o

10. This abbreviation means that the neonate has a lower than normal weight:
    A. VLBW
    B. LNBW
    C. BWLN
    D. LBWV

11. This muscle is used to chew:
    A. temporal
    B. masseter
    C. trapezius
    D. sternocleidomastoid

12. This term means flat plate:
    A. lamina
    B. lysis
    C. chondral
    D. scoliosis

13. The combining form that means nerve root:
    A. rhiz/o
    B. poli/o
    C. phas/o
    D. myel/o

Anatomy

14. This gland is located at the base of the brain in a depression in the skull:
    A. thymus
    B. hypothalamus
    C. pituitary
    D. pineal

15. Which of the following is not a part of the kidney?
    A. cortex
    B. trigone
    C. medulla
    D. pyramids

16. Which of the following is an endocrine gland?
    A. spleen
    B. bone marrow
    C. tonsils
    D. adrenal

17. This is nature's pacemaker:
    A. atrioventricular node
    B. bundle of His
    C. septum
    D. sinoatrial node

18. This is divided into the medulla oblongata, pons, and midbrain:
    A. brainstem
    B. diencephalon
    C. cerebellum
    D. cerebrum

19. This is located in the middle ear:
    A. vestibule
    B. cochlea
    C. auricle
    D. stapes

20. This is located in the pharynx and contains the adenoids:
    A. oropharynx
    B. laryngopharynx
    C. nasopharynx
    D. sphenoidal

21. This is another name for the bulbourethral gland:
    A. tunica albuginea
    B. seminal vesicles
    C. prostate
    D. Cowper's

22. The approximate number of days of gestation of the fetus:
    A. 240
    B. 255
    C. 266
    D. 277

ICD-9-CM

23. A patient is diagnosed with bilateral otitis media:
    A. 382.9
    B. 382.4
    C. 381.6
    D. 382.02

24. A patient is diagnosed with bacterial endocarditis due to AIDS:
    A. 421.0, 042
    B. 042, 421.9
    C. 421.1, 042
    D. 042, 421.0

25. **HOLTER REPORT**

   LOCATION: Outpatient, Clinic.

   INDICATION: Patient with atrial fibrillation on Lanoxin. Patient with known cardiomyopathy.

   BASELINE DATA: An 86-year-old man with congestive heart failure on Elavil, Vasotec, Lanoxin, and Lasix. The patient was monitored for the 24 hours in which the analysis was performed.

   INTERPRETATION:

   1. The predominant rhythm is atrial fibrillation. The average ventricular rate is 74 beats per minute, minimum 49 beats per minute, and maximum 114 beats per minute.

   2. A total of 4948 ventricular ectopic beats were detected. There were four forms. There were 146 couplets with one triplet and five runs of bigeminy. There were two runs of ventricular tachycardia, the longest for 5 beats at a rate of 150 beats per minute. There was no ventricular fibrillation.

   3. There were no prolonged pauses.

   CONCLUSION:

   4. Predominant rhythm is atrial fibrillation with well-controlled ventricular rate.

   5. There are no prolonged pauses.

   6. Asymptomatic, nonsustained, ventricular tachycardia.

   A. 427.3, 425.4
   B. 425.4, 427.3
   C. 427.31, 425.4
   D. 427.32, 425.4

26. A 51-year-old male patient had surgery to remove two separate carbuncles of the left axilla. Pathology report indicated staphylococcal infection.
   A. 680.3, 041.10
   B. 680.9, 041.01
   C. 680.3, 041.19
   D. 680.9, 041.09

27. The discharge diagnoses for a patient who was admitted for dyspnea were as follows: pneumonia, *Klebsiella pneumoniae*, COPD with emphysema, multifocal atrial tachycardia, mild dementia.
   A. 482, 492.8, 427.5, 294.8
   B. 486, 492.8, 427.89, 294.8
   C. 486, 492.0, 427.89, 294.11
   D. 482.0, 492.8, 427.89, 294.8

28. A patient with spinal stenosis of cervical disk C4-5 and C5-6 with intervertebral disk displacement had a cervical diskectomy, corpectomy, allograft from C4 to C6, and placement of arthrodesis (a 34-mm plate from C4 to C6).
   A. 722.90
   B. 723.0, 722.1
   C. 723.0, 722.0
   D. 723.1, 722.51

29. A patient presents for an influenza vaccination and pneumococcal vaccination.
   A. V04.8, V03.89
   B. V04.7, V03.82
   C. V04.81, V03.82
   D. V06.6

30. A patient with a family history of malignant neoplasm of the breast receives a screening mammography, bilaterally (77057).
   A. V76.11
   B. V76.11, V16.3
   C. V16.3
   D. V10.3, V76.11

31. A patient with unstable angina, hypertension, diabetes with hypoglycemia, and a history of myocardial infarction is admitted for cardiac catheterization.
   A. 413.9, 401.9, 250.80, 412
   B. 411.1, 401.9, 250.80, 412
   C. 411.1, 401.0, 250.80, 412
   D. 411.1, 401.9, 250.00, 410.9

32. A 4-year-old patient is seen by the physician in the outpatient clinic setting for chronic lymphoid leukemia that is currently in remission.
   A. 204.11
   B. 204.21
   C. 203.11
   D. 204.81

33. A patient has staphylococcal septicemia with systemic inflammatory response syndrome (SIRS) with respiratory and hepatic failure.
   A. 995.92, 038.10, 518.81, 570
   B. 038.10, 995.92, 518.81, 570
   C. 518.81, 570, 038.10, 995.92
   D. 038.10, 518.81, 570, 995.92

HCPCS

34. All third-party payers require the use of HCPCS codes in submissions for service provided to any patient.
   A. True
   B. False

35. A 62-year-old male Medicare patient presents for a digital rectal examination and a total prostate-specific antigen test (PSA).
   A. G0102
   B. G0103
   C. G0102, G0107
   D. G0102, G0103

36. An 82-year-old female Medicare patient has a single energy x-ray absorp-
    tiometry (SEXA) bone density study of two sites of the wrist.
    A. 77079
    B. 77080
    C. G0130
    D. 77078

37. A 72-year-old male Medicare patient receives 30 minutes of individual dia-
    betes outpatient self-management training session.
    A. G0109
    B. G0176
    C. 99213
    D. G0108

38. A Medicare patient presents for an influenza vaccination and pneumococcal
    vaccination.
    A. G0008
    B. G0009
    C. G0008, G0009
    D. G0010, G0008

Concepts of Coding

39. The term OIG stands for the Office of the:
    A. Information Group
    B. Insurance Group
    C. Inspector General
    D. Insurance General

40. This part of Medicare is the non-hospital portion:
    A. Part A
    B. Part B
    C. Part C
    D. Part D

41. This is the group to which the CMS delegates the daily operation of the
    Medicare and Medicaid programs:
    A. FI
    B. OG
    C. PRO
    D. HEW

42. This physician receives reimbursements for Medicare directly from the fiscal
    intermediary:
    A. PIB
    B. PRA
    C. PAR
    D. PEER

43. Which of the following is NOT true about the Outpatient Prospective
    Payment System?
    A. Known as the APC
    B. Was implemented in 2000
    C. Payment rates for each APC are published in the *Federal Register*
    D. Is applicable to non-Medicare and Medicare patients

SECTION 2

Questions 44-103

10000 Integumentary

44. A 24-year-old female is seen in the office for a single subcutaneous cyst that needs to be incised and drained.
    A. 10061
    B. 10080
    C. 10060
    D. 11400

45. A 10-year-old boy presents for injuries caused by falling off his bike. All wounds were superficial. He has a 2-cm wound to his nose and a 1-cm wound to his cheek. He also has a 2.5-cm wound to his elbow. All injuries were simple repair by means of suture.
    A. 12011, 12001
    B. 12013, 12001
    C. 12013, 12002
    D. 12011, 12002

46. Dr. Smith performed a bilateral radical mastectomy, including the pectoral muscles and axillary lymph nodes, on a 63-year-old female with breast cancer.
    A. 19305, 174.9
    B. 19306-50, 174.9
    C. 19305-50, 174.9
    D. 19307-50, 174.9

47. What code(s) would you use to report chemosurgery, Mohs' micrographic technique, with five tissue blocks, first stage of the genitalia?
    A. 17311
    B. 17312
    C. 17311, 17312
    D. 17313

48. A 40-year-old male is in for layered closure of wounds due to a motor vehicle accident. The patient sustained injuries to the forehead, 1.5 cm, and a 1-cm wound to the eyebrow when his head hit the steering wheel. Code the service only.
    A. 12011
    B. 12051
    C. 13131
    D. 12001

49. Which code would the surgeon use to report the shaving of an epidermal lesion of the arm when a lesion diameter is greater than 2 cm?
    A. 11402
    B. 11200
    C. 11303
    D. 11602

50. A 73-year-old male is admitted by Dr. Smith for an excision of a nail and nail matrix, complete, for permanent removal with amputation of a tuft of distal phalanx. A 1.8-cm single pinch skin graft was needed to cover the tip of the digit.
    A. 11752
    B. 11750
    C. 11750, 15050
    D. 11752, 15050

51. What code would you use for an initial 11% debridement of both arms resulting from burns, without general anesthesia?
    A. 16020
    B. 16025
    C. 16030-50
    D. 16030

52. Donna, a 41-year-old female, presents for biopsies of both breasts. Dr. Smith will be doing the biopsies using fine-needle aspiration with imaging guidance.
    A. 19102-50
    B. 10022-50
    C. 10021
    D. 19103-50

53. Katie is seen in the clinic by Dr. Smith for several scars on her face caused by acne. Dr. Smith decides to do an epidermal chemical peel of the face.
    A. 15780
    B. 15781
    C. 15789
    D. 15788

20000 Musculoskeletal System

54. Richard, a 34-year-old male, fell from a 4-foot scaffolding and hit his heel on the bottom rung of the support, fracturing his calcaneus in several locations. The orthopedic surgeon manipulated the bone pieces back into position and secured the fracture sites by means of percutaneous fixation.
    A. 28415
    B. 28405
    C. 28406
    D. 28456

55. Sammy, a 5-year-old male, tumbled down the stairs at daycare, striking and fracturing his coccygeal bone. The physician manually manipulated the bone into proper alignment and told Sammy's mother to have the child sit on a rubber ring to alleviate the pain.
    A. 27510
    B. 28445
    C. 27202
    D. 27200

56. Alice, a 42-year-old female, is a carpenter at the local college. While on a ladder repairing a window frame, the weld on the rung of the metal ladder loosened and she fell backward and down a distance of 8 feet. She landed on her left hip, resulting in a dislocation. With the patient under general anesthesia, the Allis maneuver is used to repair an anterior dislocation of the right hip. The pelvis is stabilized and pressure applied to the thigh to reduce the hip and bring it into proper alignment.
   A. 27250
   B. 27252
   C. 27253
   D. 27254

57. A 13-year-old female sustained multiple tibial tuberosity fractures of the left knee while playing soccer at her local track meet. The physician extended the left leg and manipulated several fragments back into place. The knee was then aspirated. A long-leg knee brace was then placed on the knee.
   A. 27334
   B. 27550
   C. 27538
   D. 27330

58. Under general anesthesia, 5-year-old Michael's tarsal dislocation was reduced by means of manipulation. Two-view intraoperative x-rays demonstrated that the tarsus was in correct alignment, and a short-leg cast was then applied. (Code only the reduction service.)
   A. 28545, 29405
   B. 28545, 29405, 73620
   C. 28540, 73620
   D. 28545

59. Dr. Clark applied a cranial halo to Gordon to stabilize the cervical spine in preparation for x-rays and subsequent surgery. The scalp was sterilized and local anesthesia injected over the pin insertion sites. Posterior and anterior cranial pins are inserted and the halo device attached.
   A. 20664
   B. 20661, 90772
   C. 20661
   D. 20664, 90772

60. Samantha was playing in the back yard when her brother fired a pellet gun at her leg at close range. The pellet penetrated the skin and lodged in the muscle underlying the area. The physician removed the pellet without complication or incident.
   A. 20520
   B. 20525
   C. 10120
   D. 10121

61. Kevin comes in with a deep hematoma on his shoulder that he has had for some time. After an exam was performed of the shoulder area, the physician decides that the hematoma needs to be incised and drained.
   A. 23030
   B. 10140
   C. 10060
   D. 10160

62. Marsha is admitted to same-day surgery after having an abnormal shoulder x-ray in the clinic yesterday. The physician decides to do a diagnostic arthroscopy.
    A. 29806
    B. 29805
    C. 23066
    D. 23100

63. Cole comes into the orthopedic department today with his mother after falling from the top bunk bed, where he and his brother were wrestling. Cole is having pain in his left lower leg and is unable to bear weight on it. Cole is taken to the x-ray department. After the physician talks with the radiologist regarding the diagnosis of sprained ankle, the physician decides to apply a walking short leg cast from just below Cole's knee to his toes.
    A. 29405, 845.00, E884.4
    B. 29515, 845.00, E888.9
    C. 29355, 959.7, E884.4
    D. 29425, 845.00, E884.4

30000 Respiratory System and Cardiovascular System

64. **PREOPERATIVE DIAGNOSIS:** Deviated septum.

    PROCEDURE PERFORMED:

    1. Septoplasty

    2. Reduction of inferior turbinates

    The patient was taken to the operating room and placed under general anesthesia. The fracture of the inferior turbinates was first performed to do the septoplasty. Once this was done, the septoplasty was completed and the turbinates were placed back in their original position. The patient was taken to recovery in satisfactory condition. Code the procedure(s) and the diagnosis:
    A. 30520, 30130, 470
    B. 30520, 30130-51, 470
    C. 30520, 30140-51, 802.0
    D. 30520, 30140-52, 470

65. The patient is seen in the clinic for chronic sinusitis. The physician decides to schedule an endoscopic sinus surgery for the next day. The patient arrives to same-day surgery, and the physician performs an endoscopic total ethmoidectomy with an endoscopic maxillary antrostomy with removal of maxillary tissue. Code the procedure(s) and diagnosis.
    A. 31254, 31256-51, 473.9
    B. 31255, 31267-51, 461.9
    C. 31255, 31267-51, 473.9
    D. 31200, 31225-51, 473.9

66. Faye, an 88-year-old female, is taken to same-day surgery for a possible small chicken bone stuck in her larynx. The physician does a direct laryngoscopy to check the larynx. On inspection, a small bone fragment is seen obstructing the larynx. The physician using an operating microscope removes the bone fragment. The patient is sent home in satisfactory condition.
A. 31526, 933.1, E915
B. 31531, 933.1, E912
C. 31530, 935.0, E912
D. 31511, 933.1, E912

67. **OPERATIVE REPORT**

PREOPERATIVE DIAGNOSIS: Ventilator dependency, aspiration pneumonia.

PROCEDURE PERFORMED: Tracheostomy.

DESCRIPTION OF PROCEDURE: After consent was obtained, the patient was taken to the operating room and placed on the operating room table in the supine position. After an adequate level of general endotracheal anesthesia was obtained, the patient was positioned for tracheostomy. The patient's neck was prepped with Betadine and then draped in a sterile manner. A curvilinear incision was marked approximately a fingerbreadth above the sternal notch in the area just below the cricoid cartilage. This area was then infiltrated with 1% Xylocaine with 1:100,000 units of epinephrine. After several minutes, sharp dissection was carried down through the skin and subcutaneous tissue. The subcutaneous fat was removed down to the strap muscles. Strap muscles were divided in the midline and retracted laterally. The cricoid cartilage was then identified. The thyroid gland was divided in the midline with the Bovie, and then the two lobes were retracted laterally, exposing the anterior wall of the trachea. The space between the second and third tracheal rings was then identified. This was infiltrated with local solution. A cut was then made through the anterior wall. The endotracheal tube was then advanced superiorly. An inferior cut into the third tracheal ring was then done to make a flap. This was secured to the skin with 4-0 Vicryl suture. A no. 6 Shiley cuffed tracheostomy tube was then placed and secured to the skin with ties as well as the tracheostomy strap. The patient tolerated the procedure well and was taken to the critical care unit in stable condition. Report the procedure(s) and diagnosis(es).

A. 94002, 60220, 31600-51, 507.0
B. 31500, 31600-51, 507.8
C. 31600, 507.0
D. 94002, 31502-51, 31600-51, 518.81, 507.0

68. Carl, a 58-year-old male, is taken to the operating room to remove his permanent pacemaker after successfully getting his heart back to normal sinus rhythm.
A. 33236
B. 33238
C. 33243
D. 33233

69. This 70-year-old male is admitted for coronary ASHD. A prior cardiac catheterization showed numerous native vessels to be 70% to 100% blocked. The patient was taken to the operating room. After opening the chest and separating the rib cage, a coronary artery bypass was performed using five venous grafts and four coronary arterial grafts. Code the graft procedure(s) and the diagnosis:
   A. 33536, 33517-51, 414.9
   B. 33533, 33522, 414.05
   C. 33536, 33522, 414.01
   D. 33514, 414

70. What code(s) would be used to report an arterial catheterization?
   A. 36600
   B. 36620, 36625
   C. 36620
   D. 36640

71. This patient is taken to the operating room for a ruptured spleen. Repair of the ruptured spleen with a partial splenectomy is done.
   A. 38101-58, 38115-51-58, 289.59
   B. 38115, 289.59
   C. 38120, 865.04
   D. 38129, 865.14

72. This 60-year-old female was seen previously for a laparoscopic biopsy of her cervical lymph nodes. The biopsy came back showing abnormal cells. The decision was made to do a lymphadenectomy. The patient was brought to the operating room and put under general anesthesia. After completing a radical neck dissection, the lymph nodes were excised. The patient was returned to recovery in satisfactory condition. Code the lymphadenectomy only.
   A. 38720, 38570-51
   B. 38720, 38500-51
   C. 38571
   D. 38724

73. A 58-year-old patient has a PICC line with a port placed for chemotherapy infusion. Fluoroscopic guidance was used to gain access and check placement.
   A. 36568, 77001
   B. 36570, 77002
   C. 36571, 77001
   D. 36556, 77001

40000 Digestive System

74. **OPERATIVE REPORT**

    PROCEDURE: Excision of parotid tumor or gland or both. Once the patient was successfully under general anesthesia, Dr. Green, assisted by Dr. Smith, opened the area in which the parotid gland is located. After carefully inspecting the gland, the decision was made to excise the total gland because of the size of the tumor (5 cm). With careful dissection and preservation of the facial nerve, the parotid gland was removed. The wound was cleaned and closed, and the patient was brought to recovery in satisfactory condition. Report only Dr. Smith's service.
    A. 42410-80, 11041, 142.0
    B. 42426-62, 210.2
    C. 42420-80, 239.8
    D. 11426, 239.8

75. A 9-year-old boy is in for a tonsillectomy because of chronic tonsillitis and possible adenoidectomy. On inspection of the adenoids they were found not to be inflamed; then we did a tonsillectomy only.
    A. 42820, 474.10
    B. 42825, 474.00
    C. 42830, 42825-51, 474.10
    D. 42826, 42835-51, 474.02

76. What code would you use to report a rigid proctosigmoidoscopy with guide wire?
    A. 52260
    B. 45386
    C. 45339
    D. 45303

77. A 62-year-old female presents to Acute Surgical Care for a sigmoidoscopy. The physician inserts a flexible scope into the patient's rectum and determines the rectum is clear of any polyps. The scope is advanced to the sigmoid colon, and a total of three polyps are found. Using the snare technique, the polyps are removed. The remainder of the colon is free of polyps. The flexible scope is withdrawn. The polyps were benign.
    A. 45383, 211.3
    B. 44110, 153.9
    C. 45338, 211.3
    D. 44111, 153.3

78. This patient is in for multiple external hemorrhoids. After inspection of the hemorrhoids, the physician decides to excise all the hemorrhoids.
    A. 46250, 455.3
    B. 46615, 455.0
    C. 46255, 455.3
    D. 46083, 455.5

79. **OPERATIVE REPORT**

PREOPERATIVE DIAGNOSIS: Barrett's esophagus with severe dysplasia, possible carcinoma.

POSTOPERATIVE DIAGNOSIS: Same.

PROCEDURE PERFORMED: Exploratory laparotomy, biopsy of liver lesion, immobilization of stomach with pyloroplasty and placement of feeding tube.

OPERATIVE NOTE: With the patient under general anesthesia, the abdomen was prepped and draped in a sterile manner. Midline incision was made from the xiphoid to below the pubis. Sharp dissection was carried down into the peritoneal cavity, and hemostasis was maintained with electrocautery. We began by exploring the abdominal cavity. The liver was carefully palpated. The area that had been identified on CT was at the very apex of the right lobe of the liver. We could feel this area, and it did not have a thickened feel to it but was more consistent with an area of hemangioma. There was a small secondary lesion on the undersurface of the right lobe. A biopsy was taken, and it did return a diagnosis of hemangioma. The rest of the liver appeared normal, and in my opinion we did not need to proceed with anything further. We thus began with mobilization of the stomach, taking down the greater curvature vessels, preserving the gastroepiploica. We carried our dissection all the way up into the hiatal hernia, preserving the blood supply to the spleen and not injuring it. We were then able to detach the left gastric artery such that the stomach was tethered on its other vasculature but appeared completely viable. All these vessels were taken down with clamps and ligatures of 2-0 silk. We then circumferentially went around the esophagus and carried our dissection all the way back toward the pylorus. We then had the entire stomach freed up from the pylorus all the way up to the diaphragm. The stomach appeared viable with reasonable circulation. A Heineke-Mikulicz pyloroplasty then was performed to open the pylorus in one direction and close it in another using interrupted 3-0 silk sutures to complete the pyloroplasty. With this accomplished, we then picked up the jejunum approximately 40 or 50 cm beyond the ligament of Treitz and placed a red rubber feeding tube using a Witzel technique; this was a number 18-2. This was attached to the skin and brought out through a separate stab incision. The abdominal cavity was then checked for hemostasis, and everything appeared to be intact. We then closed the incision using running 0 loop nylon. We closed the skin with staples. A sterile dressing was applied. Code the biopsy of the liver lesion and pyloroplasty only.

A. 49000, 43830-51, 47001-51, 228.00, 150.9
B. 43800, 47001-51, 150.9
C. 43800, 47001
D. 43800, 47001-51

80. **OPERATIVE REPORT**

PREOPERATIVE DIAGNOSIS: Upper gastrointestinal bleeding.

POSTOPERATIVE DIAGNOSIS: Multiple serpiginous ulcers in the gastric antrum and body, not bleeding.

FINDINGS: The video therapeutic double-channel endoscope was passed without difficulty into the oropharynx. The gastroesophageal junction was seen at 42 cm. Inspection of the esophagus revealed no erythema, ulceration, exudates, stricture, or other mucosal abnormalities. The stomach proper was entered. The endoscope was advanced to the second duodenum. Inspection of the second duodenum, first duodenum, duodenal bulb, and pylorus revealed no abnormalities. Retroflexion revealed no lesion along the cardia or lesser curvature. Inspection of the antrum, body, and fundus of the stomach revealed no abnormality except there were multiple serpiginous ulcerations in the gastric antrum and body. They were not bleeding. They had no recent stigmata of bleeding. Photographs and biopsies were obtained. The patient tolerated the procedure well.

A. 43258, 531.9
B. 43234, 531.30
C. 43239, 531.90
D. 43239, 532.9

81. How would you code an excision of a ruptured appendix with generalized peritonitis?
A. 44970
B. 44950
C. 44960
D. 44960-22

82. Kevin is admitted to same-day surgery today for a laparoscopic cholecystectomy.
A. 47600
B. 47562, 47550
C. 47560
D. 47562

83. **INDICATION:** Sean is a 2-year-old boy who was born with a cleft lip.

PROCEDURE: This 2-year-old male was taken to the operating room for plastic repair of a unilateral cleft lip.

A. 40702-52, 749.10
B. 40700, 749.10
C. 30460, 749.20
D. 40525, 749.20

50000 Urinary, Male Genital System, Female Genital System, and Maternity Care and Delivery

84. **OPERATIVE REPORT**

   DIAGNOSIS: Acute renal insufficiency.

   PROCEDURE: Renal biopsy.

   The patient was taken to the operating room for a percutaneous needle biopsy of the right and left kidneys.
   A. 49000-50
   B. 50555-50
   C. 50542-LT, 50542-RT
   D. 50200-50

85. What code would you use to report a cystourethroscopic biopsy of the bladder?
   A. 52354
   B. 52204
   C. 52224
   D. 52250

86. **OPERATIVE REPORT**

   DIAGNOSIS: Large bladder neck obstruction.

   PROCEDURE PERFORMED: Cystoscopy and transurethral resection of the prostate.

   The patient is a 78-year-old male with obstructive symptoms and subsequent urinary retention. The patient underwent the usual spinal anesthetic, was put in the dorsolithotomy position, prepped, and draped in the usual fashion. Cystoscopic visualization showed a marked high-riding bladder. Median lobe enlargement was such that it was difficult even to get the cystoscope over. Inside the bladder, marked trabeculation was noted. No stones were present.

   The urethra was well lubricated and dilated. The resectoscopic sheath was passed with the aid of an obturator with some difficulty because of the median lobe. TURP of the median lobe was performed, getting several big loops of tissue, which helped to improve visualization. Anterior resection of the roof was carried out from the bladder neck. Bladder-wall resection was taken from the 10 to 8 o'clock position. This eliminated the rest of the median lobe tissue as well. The patient tolerated the procedure well. Code the procedure(s) performed and the diagnosis.
   A. 52450, 52001-51, 596.0
   B. 52450, 52001-51, 753.6
   C. 52450, 52000-59, 596.0
   D. 52450, 52000, 753.6

87. What code would you use to code reconstruction of the penis for straightening of chordee?
   A. 54435
   B. 54328
   C. 54360
   D. 54300

88. Clamp circumcision.
   A. 54160
   B. 54150
   C. 54150-52
   D. 54161

89. Jim is a 42-year-old male in for a bilateral vasectomy that will include three postoperative semen examinations.
   A. 52402
   B. 52648
   C. 55250
   D. 55250 × 3

90. Patient is seen for a Bartholin's gland abscess. The physician incised and drained the abscess.
   A. 56420
   B. 50600
   C. 53060
   D. 56405

91. This 21-year-old female is seen at the clinic today for a colposcopy. The physician will take multiple biopsies of the cervix uteri.
   A. 56821
   B. 57421
   C. 57455
   D. 57456

92. Sarah is a 37-year-old female diagnosed with an ectopic pregnancy. The patient was taken to the operating room for treatment of a tubal ectopic pregnancy, abdominal approach.
   A. 59130
   B. 59150
   C. 59120
   D. 59121

93. What code(s) would you use to report a cesarean delivery including the postpartum care?
   A. 58611, 59430
   B. 59400
   C. 59515
   D. 59622

60000 Endocrine System, Nervous System, Eye and Ocular Adnexa

94. **OPERATIVE REPORT**

   DIAGNOSIS: Malignant tumor, thyroid.

   PROCEDURE: Thyroidectomy, total.

   The patient was prepped and draped. The neck area was opened. With careful radical dissection of the neck completed, one could visualize the size of the tumor. The decision was made to do a total thyroidectomy.
   The pathology report later indicated that the tumor was malignant.
   A. 60240, 193
   B. 60271, 193
   C. 60220, 164.0
   D. 60254, 193

95. What code would you use to report burr hole(s) to drain an abscess of the brain?
   A. 61253
   B. 61150
   C. 61156
   D. 61151

96. The patient was brought to the operating room to repair an aneurysm of the intracranial artery by balloon catheter.
   A. 61698
   B. 61697
   C. 61710
   D. 61700

97. **OPERATIVE REPORT**

PREOPERATIVE DIAGNOSIS: Obstructed ventriculoperitoneal shunt.

PROCEDURE PERFORMED: Revision of shunt. Replacement of ventricular valve and peritoneal end. Entire shunt replacement.

PROCEDURE: Under general anesthesia, the patient's head, neck, and abdomen were prepped and draped in the usual manner. An incision was made over the previous site where the shunt had been inserted in the posterior right occipital area. This shunt was found to be nonfunctioning and was removed. The problem was that we could not get the ventricular catheter out without probably producing bleeding, so it was left inside. The peritoneal end of the shunt was then pulled out through the same incision. Having done this, I placed a new ventricular catheter into the ventricle. I then attached this to a medium pressure bulb valve and secured this with 3-0 silk to the subcutaneous tissue. We then went to the abdomen and made an incision below the previous site, and we were able to trocar the peritoneal end of the shunt by making a stab wound in the neck and then connecting it up to the shunt. This was then connected to the shunt. Pumping on the shunt, we got fluid coming out the other end. I then inserted this end of the shunt into the abdomen by dividing the rectus fascia, splitting the muscle, and dividing the peritoneum and placing the shunt into the abdomen. One 2-0 chromic suture was used around the peritoneum. The wound was then closed with 2-0 Vicryl, 2-0 plain in the subcutaneous tissue, and surgical staples on the skin. The stab wound on the neck was closed with surgical staples. The head wound was closed with 2-0 Vicryl on the galea and surgical staples on the skin. A dressing was applied. The patient was discharged to the recovery room.

A. 63740, 996.2
B. 62256, 996.56
C. 62160, 996.2
D. 62230, 996.2

98. **OPERATIVE REPORT**

DIAGNOSIS: Herniated disk.

PROCEDURE: Hemilaminectomy L4–5 and L5–S1.

The patient was taken to the operating room prepped and draped in the usual fashion. Once the lower back area was opened, after decompression of the nerve roots, the interspace at L4–5 disk was excised. Next the interspace at L5–S1 disk was excised. The patient tolerated the procedure well.
A. 63045, 63048, 722.2
B. 63040, 63043, 839.00
C. 63030, 63035, 722.10
D. 63040, 63043, 722.10

99. Delores, a 67-year-old female, is seen today for destruction of a lesion of her cornea. The lesion is removed by thermocauterization.
A. 65400
B. 65450
C. 65435
D. 65410

100. What code would you use to code the removal of a foreign body embedded in the eyelid?
   A. 67830
   B. 67413
   C. 67801
   D. 67938

101. Kristie is a 14-year-old female with a diagnosis of chronic otitis media. The patient was taken to same-day surgery and placed under general anesthesia. Dr. White performed a bilateral tympanostomy with the insertion of ventilating tubes. The patient tolerated the procedure well.
   A. 69421-50, 69433-51, 382.1
   B. 69420-50, 382.4
   C. 69436-50, 382.9
   D. 69436-50, 382.02

102. Kristie, a 15-year-old female, is seen today for removal of bilateral ventilating tubes that Dr. White inserted 1 year ago. Patient required general anesthesia.
   A. 69205-50
   B. 69424-79
   C. 69424-50
   D. 69424-50-78

103. What code would you use for a revision mastoidectomy resulting in a radical mastoidectomy?
   A. 69502
   B. 69511
   C. 69602
   D. 69603

SECTION 3

Questions 104-150

Evaluation and Management (E/M)

104. A second opinion is requested by a 90-year-old patient whose ophthalmologist recently diagnosed the patient with bilateral senile cataracts. Her regular ophthalmologist has recommended surgical removal of the cataracts and implantation of lenses. The patient presents to the clinic stating that she is concerned about the necessity of the procedure at this time. During the detailed history, the patient states that she has had decreasing vision over the last year or two but has always had excellent vision. She cannot recall any eye trauma in the past. The physician conducted a detailed visual examination and confirmed the diagnosis of the patient's ophthalmologist. The medical decision making was of low complexity.
   A. 99253
   B. 92002
   C. 99245
   D. 99243

105. The attending physician requests a consultation for an inpatient from an interventional radiologist for a second opinion about a 63-year-old male with abnormal areas within the liver. The recommendation for a CT-guided biopsy is requested, which the attending has recommended be performed. During the comprehensive history, the patient reported right upper quadrant pain. His liver enzymes were elevated. Previous CT study revealed multiple low attenuation areas within the liver (infection versus tumor). The laboratory studies were creatinine, 0.9; hemoglobin, 9.5; PT and PTT, 13.0/31.5 with an INR of 1.2. The comprehensive physical examination showed that the lungs were clear to auscultation and the heart had regular rate and rhythm. The mental status was oriented times three. Temperature, intermittent low-grade fever, up to 101°F, usually occurred at night. The CT-guided biopsy was considered appropriate for this patient. The medical decision making was of high complexity.
    A. 99245
    B. 99254
    C. 99223
    D. 99255

106. A cardiology consultation is requested for a 71-year-old inpatient for recent onset of dyspnea on exertion and chest pain. The comprehensive history reveals that the patient cannot walk three blocks without exhibiting retrosternal squeezing sensation with shortness of breath. She relates that she had the first episode 3 months ago, which she attributed to indigestion. Her medical history is negative for stroke, tuberculosis, cancer, or rheumatic fever but includes seborrheic keratosis and benign positional vertigo. She has no known allergies. A comprehensive physical examination reveals a pleasant, elderly female in no apparent distress. She has a blood pressure of 150/70 with a heart rate of 76. Weight is 131 pounds, and she is 5 foot 4 inches. Head and neck reveal JBP less than 5 cm. Normal carotid volume and upstroke without bruit. Chest examination shows clear to auscultation with no rales, crackles, crepitations, or wheezing. Cardiovascular examination reveals a normal PMI without RV lift. Normal S1 and S2 with an S3, without murmur, are noted. The medical decision making complexity is high based on the various diagnosis options.
    A. 99223
    B. 99245
    C. 99255
    D. 99254

107. A new patient presents to the emergency department with an ankle sprain received when he fell while Rollerblading. The patient is in apparent pain, and the ankle has begun to swell. He is unable to flex the ankle. The patient reports that he did strike his head on the sidewalk as a result of the fall. The physician completes an expanded problem focused history and examination. The medical decision making complexity is low.
    A. 99232
    B. 99282
    C. 99202
    D. 99284

108. An 89-year-old female patient is admitted to the skilled nursing facility after being seen in the office earlier today. The daughter brought the patient to the office. As a part of the detailed history, conducted with the patient's daughter, it is found that the patient was diagnosed with dementia last year. The patient was moved to this city from Anytown so that the daughter could care for her mother. The patient is noncontributory, and the physician relies on medical record documentation brought in by the daughter from her mother's previous physician. Of late, the patient has become more and more withdrawn and noncommunicative. She has wandered away from the daughter's home twice in the last week and on the last occasion was found walking on the street. After a comprehensive examination, it was decided that the patient would be admitted to the nursing facility today. The physician spent 45 minutes with the patient and in preparation of the medical documentation for admittance to the nursing facility. The medical decision making was of high complexity.
    A. 99310
    B. 99327
    C. 99305
    D. 99306

109. The physician provides a service to a new patient in a custodial care center. The patient is a paraplegic who has pneumonia of moderate severity. The physician performed an expanded problem-focused history and examination. The examination focused on the respiratory and cardiovascular systems, based on the patient's current complaint and past history of tachycardia. The medical decision making was of low complexity.
    A. 99326
    B. 99325
    C. 99342
    D. 99308

110. A 66-year-old male presents for a complete physical. There are no new complaints since my previous examination on 06/09 of last year. The patient spends 6 hours a week golfing and reports a brisk and active retirement. He does not smoke and has only an occasional glass of wine. He sleeps well but has been having nocturia times three. On physical examination, the patient is a well-developed, well-nourished male. The physician continues and provides a complete examination of the patient lasting 45 minutes.
    A. 99387
    B. 99403
    C. 99450
    D. 99397

111. A new patient is seen in the office with complaints of a fever, chills, and difficulty breathing. The patient states that he has not been well for several weeks now and has progressively gotten weaker. He has not been able to work for the past week and before that was frequently absent from work over the course of 2 weeks. He is uncertain how long fever has been present but believes that it has been approximately 4 days. He does not have a thermometer at home and does not know what his temperature has been. He has been sleeping in a living room recliner because when he lies down, he has increased difficulty breathing. The detailed history and examination centered around the respiratory and cardiovascular systems. The upper respiratory findings included conjunctival injection, nasal discharge, and pharyngeal erythema. A rapid test pack was used to diagnose the viral infection. Chest x-ray showed patchy bilateral infiltrates. The physician diagnosed the patient with influenza A. The medical decision making complexity was low.
    A. 99203
    B. 99213
    C. 99205
    D. 99215

112. A new patient is admitted to the observation unit of the local hospital after a 10-foot fall from a ladder. The patient struck his head on the side of the garage as he fell into a hedge that somewhat broke his fall. He has significant bruising on the left side of his body and complains of a 5/10 pain under his left arm. A series of x-rays has been ordered in addition to an MRI. The physician completed a comprehensive history and physical examination. It was decided to admit the patient to observation based on some evidence that he may have hit the left side of his head during the fall. The medical decision making is moderately complex. The patient was discharged the following day.
    A. 99222
    B. 99219
    C. 99235
    D. 99220

113. An established patient is admitted to the hospital by his attending physician after a car accident in which the patient hit the steering wheel of the automobile with significant enough force to fold the wheel backward. The patient complains of significant pain in the right shoulder. After a detailed history and physical examination, the physician believed the patient may have sustained a right rotator cuff injury. The medical decision making was straightforward in complexity.
    A. 99283
    B. 99243
    C. 99221
    D. 99253

114. An established patient is seen in a nursing facility by the physician because the patient, who is a diabetic, has developed a Stage II decubitus ulcer with cellulitis. The physician performs a detailed history and examination. The medical decision making complexity is moderate. The physician revises the patient's medical care plan.
    A. 99310
    B. 99309
    C. 99315
    D. 99214

115. The attending physician for an inpatient requests a subsequent consultation from another physician who earlier in the week had provided an initial inpatient consultation. The consultant provides a detailed interval history and examination. The medical decision making was of high complexity.
     A. 99253
     B. 99243
     C. 99233
     D. 99221

Anesthesia

116. If anesthesia service were provided to a patient who had mild systemic disease, what would the physical status modifier be?
     A. P1
     B. P2
     C. P3
     D. P4

117. The qualifying circumstances code indicates a 72-year-old female.
     A. 99100
     B. 99116
     C. 99135
     D. 99140

118. This type of sedation decreases the level of the patient's alertness but allows the patient to cooperate during the procedure.
     A. topical
     B. local
     C. regional
     D. moderate

119. The national unit values for anesthesia services are listed in this publication:
     A. BVR by AS
     B. RVG by ASA
     C. ASA by RVG
     D. RVP by ASA

120. When reporting anesthesia services for two procedures performed on the same patient during the same operative procedure, you would do the following to calculate the unit value of the services:
     A. Add the units of the two procedures together.
     B. Subtract the procedure with the lowest unit value from the procedure with the highest unit value.
     C. Report only the units for the lowest unit value procedure.
     D. Report only the units for the highest unit value procedure.

121. Anesthesia provided for an anterior cervical diskectomy with decompression of a single interspace of the spinal cord and nerve roots and including osteophytectomy (63075).
     A. 00620
     B. 00630
     C. 00600
     D. 00640

70000 Radiology

122. A 62-year-old male comes into the clinic complaining of shortness of breath. The physician orders a chest x-ray, frontal and lateral. The x-ray results were nonconclusive.
    A. 71015, 786.09
    B. 71020, 786.05
    C. 71035, 786.9
    D. 71020 × 2, 786.05

123. A patient is in for an MRI (magnetic resonance imaging) of the pelvis with contrast material(s).
    A. 72125
    B. 72198
    C. 72196
    D. 72159

124. What code(s) would you use for an endoscopic catheterization of the biliary ductal system for the professional radiology component?
    A. 43271, 74328
    B. 74328-26
    C. 74300-26
    D. 74330-26

125. Jennifer is a 29-year-old pregnant female in for a follow-up ultrasound with image documentation of the uterus.
    A. 74740
    B. 76816
    C. 74710
    D. 76856

126. What codes would you use for complex brachytherapy isodose calculation for a patient with prostate cancer?
    A. 77776, 184
    B. 77300, 185
    C. 77327-22, 186
    D. 77328, 185

127. Therapeutic radiology treatment planning is the "prescription" for a patient who will start radiation therapy for a cancerous neoplasm of the adrenal gland. What code would you use for a complex treatment planning?
    A. 60540
    B. 77315
    C. 77263
    D. 77401

128. Because of the number of headaches this 50-year-old female had been experiencing, her physician ordered a CT of her head, without contrast materials.
    A. 70450
    B. 70460
    C. 70470
    D. 70496

129. A patient presents to the clinic for a barium enema that was ordered by his physician. Once the patient drinks the barium, the patient will be taken to radiology for a colon x-ray, including KUB.
    A. 74000
    B. 74241
    C. 74270
    D. 74247

130. A woman has a bilateral screening mammogram. The film is digitized (CAD, computer aided detection) for the physician's further review. Assign the appropriate service and diagnosis codes.
    A. 77056, 77051, V76.11
    B. 77057, 77051, V76.12
    C. 77057, V76.12
    D. 77057, 77052, V76.12

80000 Pathology and Laboratory

131. A patient presents to the laboratory at the clinic for the following tests: thyroid stimulating hormone, comprehensive metabolic panel, and an automated hemogram with manual differential WBC count (CBC). How would you code this lab?
    A. 84443, 80053, 85027, 85007
    B. 80050
    C. 84443
    D. 84445, 80051, 85025

132. An 80-year-old female patient presented to the laboratory for a lipid panel that includes measurement of total serum cholesterol, lipoprotein (direct measurement, HDL), and triglycerides.
    A. 82465, 83718, 84478
    B. 82465-52, 83718, 84478
    C. 80061-52
    D. 80061

133. Philip has end-stage renal failure and comes to the clinic lab today for his monthly urinalysis (qualitative, microscopic only).
    A. 81015, 586
    B. 81001, 584.9
    C. 81015, 585.6
    D. 81003, 585.6

134. This 33-year-old male has been suffering from chronic fatigue. His physician has ordered a TSH test.
    A. 80418, 780.71
    B. 80438, 780.79
    C. 80440, 780.71
    D. 84443, 780.79

135. Surgical pathology, gross examination, or microscopic examination is most often required when a sample of an organ, tissue, or body fluid is taken from the body. What codes would you use to report biopsy of the colon, hematoma, pancreas, and a tumor of the testis?
 A. 88304, 88304, 88309, 88309
 B. 88305, 88303, 88307, 88309
 C. 88305, 88304, 88307, 88309
 D. 88307, 88304, 88309

136. A patient presents to the clinic laboratory for a prothrombin time measurement because of long-term use of Coumadin.
 A. 85210, V58.62
 B. 85610, V58.61
 C. 85230, V58
 D. 85210, V58.61

137. The patient presented to the laboratory at the clinic for the following blood tests ordered by her physician: albumin (serum), bilirubin (total), and BUN (quantitative):
 A. 82044, 82248, 84520
 B. 82040, 82252, 84525
 C. 82040, 82247, 84520
 D. 82044, 82247, 84540

138. A 70-year-old male who suffers from atrial fibrillation has been on long-term use of digoxin. He comes into the lab today to have a quantitative drug assay performed for digoxin:
 A. 80100
 B. 80102
 C. 80299
 D. 80162

139. This 68-year-old female suffers from chronic liver disease and needs a hepatic function panel performed every 6 months. Tests include total bilirubin (82247), direct bilirubin (82248), total protein (84155), alanine aminotransferases (ALT and SGPT) (84460), aspartate aminotransferases (AST and SGOT) (84450), and what other lab tests?
 A. 80061, 83718
 B. 82040, 82247
 C. 84295, 84450
 D. 82040, 84075

140. Edgar is status post kidney transplant and comes into the clinic lab for a follow-up creatinine clearance.
 A. 82540, V42.0
 B. 82575, V42.0
 C. 82565, 586
 D. 82570, 585.6

90000 Medicine

141. An elderly male comes in for his flu (split virus, IM) and pneumonia (23-valent, IM) vaccines. Code only the immunization administration and diagnoses for the vaccines.
    A. 90471, 90658, 90472, 90732, V04.81, V03.82
    B. 90471 × 2, 90658, 90732, V04.81
    C. 90471, 90472, V04.81, V03.82
    D. 90658, 90732, V05.8, V04.81

142. Code the substance of DTP given intramuscularly to a 10-year-old.
    A. 90700, 90471
    B. 90702
    C. 90701, 90471
    D. 90701

143. Katie is a 9-year-old female who comes into the clinic to have her first ophthalmologic exam. The exam was intermediate.
    A. 99203
    B. 92002
    C. 92002, 99203
    D. 92004

144. Katie is back for a 2-year follow-up comprehensive ophthalmologic exam. The physician provides a gas-permeable, extended wear contact lens for the right eye. She is to follow up in 1 week to see how her contact is working. Code the exam and the supply of contact lenses.
    A. 92014, V2513-RT
    B. V2513-RT
    C. 92014, V2530-RT
    D. 92014, V2512-RT

145. This 70-year-old male is taken to the emergency room with severe chest pain. The physician provided an expanded problem-focused history and examination. While the physician is examining the patient, his pressures drop and he goes into cardiac arrest. Cardiopulmonary resuscitation is given to the patient, and his pressure returns to normal; he is transferred to the intensive care unit in critical condition. Code the cardiopulmonary resuscitation and the diagnosis. The medical decision making was of low complexity.
    A. 99282, 92950, 427.5
    B. 99238, 92970, 427.5
    C. 92950, 427.5
    D. 92960, 427.5

146. The patient is taken to the operating room for insertion of a Swan-Ganz catheter. The physician inserts the catheter for monitoring cardiac output measurements and blood gases.
    A. 36013, 93503
    B. 36013
    C. 93508
    D. 93503

147. Dr. Green orders a sleep study for Dan, a 51-year-old male who has been diagnosed with obstructive sleep apnea. The sleep study will be done with C-PAP (continuous positive airway pressure), included 6 parameters, and was attended by the technologist.
    A. 95806, 786.03
    B. 95807, 780.53
    C. 95811, 327.23
    D. 95806, 780.57

148. Ann is a 58-year-old female with end-stage renal failure. She receives dialysis Tuesdays, Thursdays, and Saturdays each week. Code a full month of dialysis for the month of December.
    A. 90918, 593.9
    B. 90921, 585
    C. 90921-52, 585
    D. 90935, 586

149. **OPERATIVE REPORT**

    PROCEDURE PERFORMED: Primary stenting of 70% proximal posterior descending artery stenosis.

    INDICATIONS: Atherosclerotic heart disease.

    DESCRIPTION OF PROCEDURE: Please see the computer report. Please note that a 2.5 × 13-mm pixel stent was deployed.

    COMPLICATIONS: None

    RESULTS: Successful primary stenting of 70% proximal posterior descending artery stenosis with no residual stenosis at the end of the procedure.

    A. 92980-RC, 92981, 414.01
    B. 92982-RC, 414.9
    C. 92980-RC, 413.9
    D. 92980-RC, 414.01

150. Dr. Barrette is a neuroradiologist who has taken Betty, a 42-year-old female, with a diagnosis of carotid stenosis, to the operating room to perform a thromboendarterectomy, unilateral with a patch graft. During the surgery, the patient is monitored by electroencephalogram (EEG). Code the monitoring only.
    A. 35301, 95955, 433.10
    B. 35301-50, 433.30
    C. 95955, 433.10
    D. 95955

ANSWERS TO THE PRE-EXAMINATION

Section 1

1. A	16. D	31. B
2. C	17. D	32. A
3. C	18. A	33. B
4. D	19. D	34. B
5. A	20. C	35. D
6. A	21. D	36. C
7. D	22. C	37. D
8. D	23. A	38. C
9. C	24. D	39. C
10. A	25. C	40. B
11. B	26. A	41. A
12. A	27. D	42. C
13. A	28. C	43. D
14. C	29. C	
15. B	30. B	

Section 2

44. C	64. D	84. D
45. B	65. C	85. B
46. C	66. B	86. C
47. A	67. C	87. D
48. B	68. D	88. B
49. C	69. C	89. C
50. D	70. C	90. A
51. D	71. B	91. C
52. B	72. D	92. D
53. D	73. C	93. C
54. C	74. C	94. D
55. D	75. B	95. B
56. B	76. D	96. C
57. C	77. C	97. D
58. D	78. A	98. C
59. C	79. C	99. B
60. A	80. C	100. D
61. A	81. C	101. C
62. B	82. D	102. C
63. D	83. B	103. D

Section 3

104. D	120. D	136. B
105. D	121. C	137. C
106. C	122. B	138. D
107. B	123. C	139. D
108. C	124. B	140. B
109. B	125. B	141. C
110. D	126. D	142. D
111. A	127. C	143. B
112. B	128. A	144. A
113. C	129. C	145. C
114. B	130. D	146. D
115. C	131. B	147. C
116. B	132. D	148. B
117. A	133. C	149. D
118. D	134. D	150. D
119. B	135. C	

Appendix A

ICD-9-CM Official Guidelines for Coding and Reporting

Effective December 1, 2005
Narrative changes appear in bold text
Items underlined have been moved within the guidelines
since April 2005
The guidelines include the updated V Code Table

The Centers for Medicare and Medicaid Services (CMS) and the National Center for Health Statistics (NCHS), two departments within the U. S. Federal Government's Department of Health and Human Services (DHHS) provide the following guidelines for coding and reporting using the International Classification of Diseases, 9th Revision, Clinical Modification (ICD-9-CM). These guidelines should be used as a companion document to the official version of the ICD-9-CM as published on CD-ROM by the U.S. Government Printing Office (GPO).

These guidelines have been approved by the four organizations that make up the Cooperating Parties for the ICD-9-CM: the American Hospital Association (AHA), the American Health Information Management Association (AHIMA), CMS, and NCHS. These guidelines are included on the official government version of the ICD-9-CM, and also appear in *"Coding Clinic for ICD-9-CM"* published by the AHA.

These guidelines are a set of rules that have been developed to accompany and complement the official conventions and instructions provided within the ICD-9-CM itself. These guidelines are based on the coding and sequencing instructions in Volumes I, II and III of ICD-9-CM, but provide additional instruction. Adherence to these guidelines when assigning ICD-9-CM diagnosis and procedure codes is required under the Health Insurance Portability and Accountability Act (HIPAA). The diagnosis codes (Volumes 1–2) have been adopted under HIPAA for all healthcare settings. Volume 3 procedure codes have been adopted for inpatient procedures reported by hospitals. A joint effort between the healthcare provider and the coder is essential to achieve complete and accurate documentation, code assignment, and reporting of diagnoses and procedures. These guidelines have been developed to assist both the healthcare provider and the coder in identifying those diagnoses and procedures that are to be reported. The importance of consistent, complete documentation in the medical record cannot be overemphasized. Without such documentation accurate coding cannot be achieved. The entire record should be reviewed to determine the specific reason for the encounter and the conditions treated.

The term encounter is used for all settings, including hospital admissions. In the context of these guidelines, the term provider is used throughout the guidelines to mean physician or any qualified health care practitioner who is legally accountable for establishing the patient's diagnosis. Only this set of guidelines, approved by the Cooperating Parties, is official.

The guidelines are organized into sections. Section I includes the structure and conventions of the classification and general guidelines that apply to the entire classification, and chapter-specific guidelines that correspond to the chapters as they are arranged in the classification. Section II includes guidelines for selection of principal diagnosis for non-outpatient settings. Section III includes guidelines for reporting additional diagnoses in non-outpatient settings. Section IV is for outpatient coding and reporting.

ICD-9-CM Official Guidelines for Coding and Reporting

Section I.   Conventions, general coding guidelines and chapter specific guidelines

   A. Conventions for the ICD-9-CM

    1. Format:

    2. Abbreviations

       a. Index abbreviations

       b. Tabular abbreviations

    3. Punctuation

    4. Includes and Excludes Notes and Inclusion terms

    5. Other and Unspecified codes

       a. "Other" code

       b. "Unspecified" codes

    6. Etiology/manifestation convention ("code first", "use additional code" and "in diseases classified elsewhere" notes)

    7. "And"

    8. "With"

    9. "See" and "See Also"

   B. General Coding Guidelines

    1. Use of Both Alphabetic Index and Tabular List

    2. Locate each term in the Alphabetic Index

    3. Level of Detail in Coding

    4. Code or codes from 001.0 through V84.8

    5. Selection of codes 001.0 through 999.9

    6. Signs and symptoms

    7. Conditions that are an integral part of a disease process

    8. Conditions that are not an integral part of a disease process

    9. Multiple coding for a single condition

    10. Acute and Chronic Conditions

    11. Combination Code

16. Chapter 16: Signs, Symptoms and Ill-Defined Conditions (780-799)

Reserved for future guideline expansion

17. Chapter 17: Injury and Poisoning (800-999)

   a. Coding of Injuries

   b. Coding of Fractures

   c. Coding of Burns

   d. Coding of Debridement of Wound, Infection, or Burn

   e. Adverse Effects, Poisoning and Toxic Effects

   f. Complications of care

18. Classification of Factors Influencing Health Status and Contact with Health Service (Supplemental V01-V84)

   a. Introduction

   b. V codes use in any healthcare setting

   c. V Codes indicate a reason for an encounter

   d. Categories of V Codes

   e. V Code Table

19. Supplemental Classification of External Causes of Injury and Poisoning (E-codes, E800-E999)

   a. General E Code Coding Guidelines

   b. Place of Occurrence Guideline

   c. Adverse Effects of Drugs, Medicinal and Biological Substances Guidelines

   d. Multiple Cause E Code Coding Guidelines

   e. Child and Adult Abuse Guidelines

   f. Unknown or Suspected Intent Guideline

   g. Undetermined Cause

   h. Late Effects of External Cause Guidelines

   i. Misadventures and Complications of Care Guidelines

   j. Terrorism Guidelines

Section II. Selection of Principal Diagnosis

   A. Codes for symptoms, signs, and ill-defined conditions

   B. Two or more interrelated conditions, each potentially meeting the definition for principal diagnosis

   C. Two or more diagnoses that equally meet the definition for principal diagnosis

   D. Two or more comparative or contrasting conditions

   E. A symptom(s) followed by contrasting/comparative diagnoses

   F. Original treatment plan not carried out

G. Complications of surgery and other medical care

H. Uncertain Diagnosis

I. Admission from Observation Unit

   1. Admission Following Medical Observation

   2. Admission Following Post-Operative Observation

J. Admission from Outpatient Surgery

Section III. Reporting Additional Diagnoses

A. Previous condition

B. Abnormal findings

C. Uncertain Diagnosis

Section IV. Diagnostic Coding and Reporting Guidelines for Outpatient Services

A. Selection of first-listed condition

   1. Outpatient Surgery

   2. Observation Stay

B. Codes from 001.0 through V84.8

C. Accurate reporting of ICD-9-CM diagnosis codes

D. Selection of codes 001.0 through 999.9

E. Codes that describe symptoms and signs

F. Encounters for circumstances other than a disease or injury

G. Level of Detail in Coding

   1. ICD-9-CM codes with 3, 4, or 5 digits

   2. Use of full number of digits required for a code

H. ICD-9-CM code for the diagnosis, condition, problem, or other reason for encounter/visit

I. "Probable", "suspected", "questionable", "rule out", or "working diagnosis"

J. Chronic diseases

K. Code all documented conditions that coexis

L. Patients receiving diagnostic services only

M. Patients receiving therapeutic services only

N. Patients receiving preoperative evaluations only

O. Ambulatory surgery

P. Routine outpatient prenatal visits

SECTION I. CONVENTIONS, GENERAL CODING GUIDELINES AND CHAPTER SPECIFIC GUIDELINES

The conventions, general guidelines and chapter-specific guidelines are applicable to all health care settings unless otherwise indicated.

A. Conventions for the ICD-9-CM

The conventions for the ICD-9-CM are the general rules for use of the classification independent of the guidelines. These conventions are incorporated within the index and tabular of the ICD-9-CM as instructional notes. The conventions are as follows:

1. Format:

The ICD-9-CM uses an indented format for ease in reference

2. Abbreviations

a. Index abbreviations

NEC   "Not elsewhere classifiable"

This abbreviation in the index represents "other specified" when a specific code is not available for a condition the index directs the coder to the "other specified" code in the tabular.

b. Tabular abbreviations

NEC   "Not elsewhere classifiable"

This abbreviation in the tabular represents "other specified". When a specific code is not available for a condition the tabular includes an NEC entry under a code to identify the code as the "other specified" code (See Section I.A.5.a. "Other" codes").

NOS   "Not otherwise specified"

This abbreviation is the equivalent of unspecified. (See Section I.A.5.b., "Unspecified" codes)

3. Punctuation

[ ]   Brackets are used in the tabular list to enclose synonyms, alternative wording or explanatory phrases. Brackets are used in the index to identify manifestation codes. (See Section I.A.6. "Etiology/ manifestations")

( )   Parentheses are used in both the index and tabular to enclose supplementary words that may be present or absent in the statement of a disease or procedure without affecting the code number to which it is assigned. The terms within the parentheses are referred to as nonessential modifiers.

:   Colons are used in the Tabular list after an incomplete term which needs one or more of the modifiers following the colon to make it assignable to a given category.

4. Includes and Excludes Notes and Inclusion terms

Includes: This note appears immediately under a three-digit code title to further define, or give examples of, the content of the category.

Excludes: An excludes note under a code indicates that the terms excluded from the code are to be coded elsewhere. In some cases the codes for the excluded terms should not be used in conjunction with the code from which it is excluded. An example of this is a congenital condition excluded from an acquired form of the same condition. The congenital and acquired codes should not be used together. In other cases, the excluded terms may be used together with an excluded code. An example of this is when fractures of different bones are coded to different codes. Both codes may be used together if both types of fractures are present.

Inclusion terms: List of terms is included under certain four and five digit codes. These terms are the conditions for which that code number is to be used. The terms may be synonyms of the code title, or, in the case of "other specified" codes, the terms are a list of the various conditions assigned to that code. The inclusion terms are not necessarily exhaustive. Additional terms found only in the index may also be assigned to a code.

5. Other and Unspecified codes

a. "Other" codes

Codes titled "other" or "other specified" (usually a code with a 4th digit 8 or fifth-digit 9 for diagnosis codes) are for use when the information in the medical record provides detail for which a specific code does not exist. Index entries with NEC in the line designate "other" codes in the tabular. These index entries represent specific disease entities for which no specific code exists so the term is included within an "other" code.

b. "Unspecified" codes

Codes (usually a code with a 4th digit 9 or 5th digit 0 for diagnosis codes) titled "unspecified" are for use when the information in the medical record is insufficient to assign a more specific code.

6. Etiology/manifestation convention ("code first", "use additional code" and "in diseases classified elsewhere" notes)

Certain conditions have both an underlying etiology and multiple body system manifestations due to the underlying etiology. For such conditions, the ICD-9-CM has a coding convention that requires the underlying condition be sequenced first followed by the manifestation. Wherever such a combination exists, there is a "use additional code" note at the etiology code, and a "code first" note at the manifestation code. These instructional notes indicate the proper sequencing order of the codes, etiology followed by manifestation.

In most cases the manifestation codes will have in the code title, "in diseases classified elsewhere." Codes with this title are a component of the etiology/manifestation convention. The code title indicates that it is a manifestation code. "In diseases classified elsewhere" codes are never permitted to be used as first listed or principal diagnosis codes. They must be used in conjunction with an underlying condition code and they must be listed following the underlying condition.

There are manifestation codes that do not have "in diseases classified elsewhere" in the title. For such codes a "use additional code" note will still be present and the rules for sequencing apply.

In addition to the notes in the tabular, these conditions also have a specific index entry structure. In the index both conditions are listed together with the etiology code first followed by the manifestation codes in brackets. The code in brackets is always to be sequenced second.

The most commonly used etiology/manifestation combinations are the codes for Diabetes mellitus, category 250. For each code under category 250 there is a use additional code note for the manifestation that is specific for that particular diabetic manifestation. Should a patient have more than one manifestation of diabetes, more than one code from category 250 may be used with as many manifestation codes as are needed to fully describe the patient's complete diabetic condition. The **category** 250 diabetes codes should be sequenced first, followed by the manifestation codes.

"Code first" and "Use additional code" notes are also used as sequencing rules in the classification for certain codes that are not part of an etiology/manifestation combination. See - Section I.B.9. "Multiple coding for a single condition".

7. "And"

The word "and" should be interpreted to mean either "and" or "or" when it appears in a title.

8. "With"

The word "with" in the alphabetic index is sequenced immediately following the main term, not in alphabetical order.

9. "See" and "See Also"

The "see" instruction following a main term in the index indicates that another term should be referenced. It is necessary to go to the main term referenced with the "see" note to locate the correct code.

A "see also" instruction following a main term in the index instructs that there is another main term that may also be referenced that may provide additional index entries that may be useful. It is not necessary to follow the "see also" note when the original main term provides the necessary code.

B. General Coding Guidelines

1. Use of Both Alphabetic Index and Tabular List

Use both the Alphabetic Index and the Tabular List when locating and assigning a code. Reliance on only the Alphabetic Index or the Tabular List leads to errors in code assignments and less specificity in code selection.

2. Locate each term in the Alphabetic Index

Locate each term in the Alphabetic Index and verify the code selected in the Tabular List. Read and be guided by instructional notations that appear in both the Alphabetic Index and the Tabular List.

3. Level of Detail in Coding

Diagnosis and procedure codes are to be used at their highest number of digits available.

ICD-9-CM diagnosis codes are composed of codes with either 3, 4, or 5 digits. Codes with three digits are included in ICD-9-CM as the heading of a category of codes that may be further subdivided by the use of fourth and/or fifth digits, which provide greater detail.

A three-digit code is to be used only if it is not further subdivided. Where fourth-digit subcategories and/or fifth-digit subclassifications are provided, they must be assigned. A code is invalid if it has not been coded to the full number of digits required for that code. For example, Acute myocardial infarction, code 410, has fourth digits that describe the location of the infarction (e.g., 410.2, Of inferolateral wall), and fifth digits that identify the episode of care. It would be incorrect to report a code in category 410 without a fourth and fifth digit.

ICD-9-CM Volume 3 procedure codes are composed of codes with either 3 or 4 digits. Codes with two digits are included in ICD-9-CM as the heading of a category of codes that may be further subdivided by the use of third and/or fourth digits, which provide greater detail.

4. Code or codes from 001.0 through V84.8

The appropriate code or codes from 001.0 through V84.8 must be used to identify diagnoses, symptoms, conditions, problems, complaints or other reason(s) for the encounter/visit.

5. Selection of codes 001.0 through 999.9

The selection of codes 001.0 through 999.9 will frequently be used to describe the reason for the admission/encounter. These codes are from the section of ICD-9-CM for the classification of diseases and injuries (e.g., infectious and parasitic diseases; neoplasms; symptoms, signs, and ill-defined conditions, etc.).

6. Signs and symptoms

Codes that describe symptoms and signs, as opposed to diagnoses, are acceptable for reporting purposes when a related definitive diagnosis has not been established (confirmed) by the provider. Chapter 16 of ICD-9-CM, Symptoms, Signs, and Ill-defined conditions (codes 780.0-799.9) contain many, but not all codes for symptoms.

7. Conditions that are an integral part of a disease process

Signs and symptoms that are integral to the disease process should not be assigned as additional codes.

8. Conditions that are not an integral part of a disease process

Additional signs and symptoms that may not be associated routinely with a disease process should be coded when present.

9. Multiple coding for a single condition

In addition to the etiology/manifestation convention that requires two codes to fully describe a single condition that affects multiple body systems, there are other single conditions that also require more than one code. "Use additional code" notes are found in the tabular at codes that are not part of an etiology/manifestation pair where a secondary code is useful to fully describe a condition. The sequencing rule is the same as the etiology/manifestation pair - , "use additional code" indicates that a secondary code should be added.

For example, for infections that are not included in chapter 1, a secondary code from category 041, Bacterial infection in conditions classified elsewhere and of unspecified site, may be required to identify the bacterial organism causing the infection. A "use additional code" note will normally be found at the infectious disease code, indicating a need for the organism code to be added as a secondary code.

"Code first" notes are also under certain codes that are not specifically manifestation codes but may be due to an underlying cause. When a "code first" note is present and an underlying condition is present the underlying condition should be sequenced first.

"Code, if applicable, any causal condition first", notes indicate that this code may be assigned as a principal diagnosis when the causal condition is unknown or not applicable. If a causal condition is known, then the code for that condition should be sequenced as the principal or first-listed diagnosis.

Multiple codes may be needed for late effects, complication codes and obstetric codes to more fully describe a condition. See the specific guidelines for these conditions for further instruction.

10. Acute and Chronic Conditions

If the same condition is described as both acute (subacute) and chronic, and separate subentries exist in the Alphabetic Index at the same indentation level, code both and sequence the acute (subacute) code first.

11. Combination Code

A combination code is a single code used to classify:

Two diagnoses, or

A diagnosis with an associated secondary process (manifestation)

A diagnosis with an associated complication

Combination codes are identified by referring to subterm entries in the Alphabetic Index and by reading the inclusion and exclusion notes in the Tabular List.

Assign only the combination code when that code fully identifies the diagnostic conditions involved or when the Alphabetic Index so directs. Multiple coding should not be used when the classification provides a combination code that clearly identifies all of the elements documented in the diagnosis. When the combination code lacks necessary specificity in describing the manifestation or complication, an additional code should be used as a secondary code.

12. Late Effects

A late effect is the residual effect (condition produced) after the acute phase of an illness or injury has terminated. There is no time limit on when a late effect code can be used. The residual may be apparent early, such as in cerebrovascular accident cases, or it may occur months or years later, such as that due to a previous injury. Coding of late effects generally requires two codes sequenced in the following order: The condition or nature of the late effect is sequenced first. The late effect code is sequenced second.

An exception to the above guidelines are those instances where the code for late effect is followed by a manifestation code identified in the Tabular List and title, or the late effect code has been expanded (at the fourth and fifth-digit levels) to include the manifestation(s). The code for the acute phase of an illness or injury that led to the late effect is never used with a code for the late effect.

13. Impending or Threatened Condition

Code any condition described at the time of discharge as "impending" or "threatened" as follows:

If it did occur, code as confirmed diagnosis.

If it did not occur, reference the Alphabetic Index to determine if the condition has a subentry term for "impending" or "threatened" and also reference main term entries for "Impending" and for "Threatened."

If the subterms are listed, assign the given code.

If the subterms are not listed, code the existing underlying condition(s) and not the condition described as impending or threatened.

C. Chapter-Specific Coding Guidelines

In addition to general coding guidelines, there are guidelines for specific diagnoses and/or conditions in the classification. Unless otherwise indicated, these guidelines apply to all health care settings. Please refer to Section II for guidelines on the selection of principal diagnosis.

1. Chapter 1: Infectious and Parasitic Diseases (001-139)

a. Human Immunodeficiency Virus (HIV) Infections

1) Code only confirmed cases

Code only confirmed cases of HIV infection/illness. This is an exception to the hospital inpatient guideline Section II, H.

In this context, "confirmation" does not require documentation of positive serology or culture for HIV; the provider's diagnostic statement that the patient is HIV positive, or has an HIV-related illness is sufficient.

2) Selection and sequencing of HIV codes

(a) Patient admitted for HIV-related condition

If a patient is admitted for an HIV-related condition, the principal diagnosis should be 042, followed by additional diagnosis codes for all reported HIV-related conditions.

(b) Patient with HIV disease admitted for unrelated condition

If a patient with HIV disease is admitted for an unrelated condition (such as a traumatic injury), the code for the unrelated condition (e.g., the nature of injury code) should be the principal diagnosis. Other diagnoses would be 042 followed by additional diagnosis codes for all reported HIV-related conditions.

(c) Whether the patient is newly diagnosed

Whether the patient is newly diagnosed or has had previous admissions/encounters for HIV conditions is irrelevant to the sequencing decision.

(d) Asymptomatic human immunodeficiency virus

V08 Asymptomatic human immunodeficiency virus [HIV] infection, is to be applied when the patient without any documentation of symptoms is listed as being "HIV positive," "known HIV," "HIV test positive," or similar terminology. Do not use this code if the term "AIDS" is used or if the patient is treated for any HIV-related illness or is described as having any condition(s) resulting from his/her HIV positive status; use 042 in these cases.

(e) Patients with inconclusive HIV serology

Patients with inconclusive HIV serology, but no definitive diagnosis or manifestations of the illness, may be assigned code 795.71, Inconclusive serologic test for Human Immunodeficiency Virus [HIV].

(f) Previously diagnosed HIV-related illness

Patients with any known prior diagnosis of an HIV-related illness should be coded to 042. Once a patient has developed an HIV-related illness, the patient should always be assigned code 042 on every subsequent admission/encounter. Patients previously diagnosed with any HIV illness (042) should never be assigned to 795.71 or V08.

(g) HIV Infection in Pregnancy, Childbirth and the Puerperium

During pregnancy, childbirth or the puerperium, a patient admitted (or presenting for a health care encounter) because of an HIV-related illness should receive a principal diagnosis code of 647.6X, Other specified infectious and parasitic diseases in the mother classifiable elsewhere, but complicating the pregnancy, childbirth or the puerperium, followed by 042 and the code(s) for the HIV-related illness(es). Codes from Chapter 15 always take sequencing priority.

Patients with asymptomatic HIV infection status admitted (or presenting for a health care encounter) during pregnancy, childbirth, or the puerperium should receive codes of 647.6X and V08.

(h) Encounters for testing for HIV

If a patient is being seen to determine his/her HIV status, use code V73.89, Screening for other specified viral disease. Use code V69.8, Other problems related to lifestyle, as a secondary code if an asymptomatic patient is in a known high risk group for HIV. Should a patient with signs or symptoms or illness, or a confirmed HIV related diagnosis be tested for HIV, code the signs and symptoms or the diagnosis. An additional counseling code V65.44 may be used if counseling is provided during the encounter for the test.

When a patient returns to be informed of his/her HIV test results use code V65.44, HIV counseling, if the results of the test are negative.

If the results are positive but the patient is asymptomatic use code V08, Asymptomatic HIV infection. If the results are positive and the patient is symptomatic use code 042, HIV infection, with codes for the HIV related symptoms or diagnosis. The HIV counseling code may also be used if counseling is provided for patients with positive test results.

b. Septicemia, Systemic Inflammatory Response Syndrome (SIRS), Sepsis, Severe Sepsis, and Septic Shock

1) Sepsis as principal diagnosis or secondary diagnosis

(a) Sepsis as principal diagnosis

If sepsis is present on admission, and meets the definition of principal diagnosis, the underlying systemic infection code (e.g., 038.xx, 112.5, etc) should be assigned as the principal diagnosis, followed by code 995.91, Systemic inflammatory response syndrome due to infectious process without organ dysfunction, as required by the sequencing rules in the Tabular List. Codes from subcategory 995.9 can never be assigned as a principal diagnosis.

(b) Sepsis as secondary diagnoses

When sepsis develops during the encounter (it was not present on admission), the sepsis codes may be assigned as secondary diagnoses, following the sequencing rules provided in the Tabular List.

(c) Documentation unclear as to whether sepsis present on admission

If the documentation is not clear whether the sepsis was present on admission, the provider should be queried. After provider query, if sepsis is determined at that point to have met the definition of principal diagnosis, the underlying systemic infection (038.xx, 112.5, etc) may be used as principal diagnosis along with code 995.91, Systemic inflammatory response syndrome due to infectious process without organ dysfunction.

2) Septicemia/Sepsis

In most cases, it will be a code from category 038, Septicemia, that will be used in conjunction with a code from subcategory 995.9 such as the following:

(a) Streptococcal sepsis

If the documentation in the record states streptococcal sepsis, codes 038.0 and code 995.91 should be used, in that sequence.

(b) Streptococcal septicemia

If the documentation states streptococcal septicemia, only code 038.0 should be assigned, however, the provider should be queried whether the patient has sepsis, an infection with SIRS.

(c) Sepsis or SIRS must be documented

Either the term sepsis or SIRS must be documented, to assign a code from subcategory 995.9.

3) Terms sepsis, severe sepsis, or SIRS

If the terms sepsis, severe sepsis, or SIRS are used with an underlying infection other than septicemia, such as pneumonia, cellulitis or a nonspecified urinary tract infection, a code from category 038 should be assigned first, then code 995.91, followed by the code for the initial infection. The use of the terms sepsis or SIRS indicates that the patient's infection has advanced to the point of a systemic infection so the systemic infection should be sequenced before the localized infection. The instructional note under subcategory 995.9 instructs to assign the underlying systemic infection first.

Note: The term urosepsis is a nonspecific term. If that is the only term documented then only code 599.0 should be assigned based on the default for the term in the ICD-9-CM index, in addition to the code for the causal organism if known.

4) Severe sepsis

For patients with severe sepsis, the code for the systemic infection (e.g., 038.xx, 112.5, etc) or trauma should be sequenced first, followed by either code 995.92, Systemic inflammatory response syndrome due to infectious process with organ dysfunction, or code 995.94, Systemic inflammatory response syndrome due to noninfectious process with organ dysfunction. Codes for the specific organ dysfunctions should also be assigned.

5) Septic shock

(a) Sequencing of septic shock

Septic shock is a form of organ dysfunction associated with severe sepsis. A code for the initiating underlying systemic infection followed by a code for SIRS (code 995.92) must be assigned before the code for septic shock. As noted in the sequencing instructions in the Tabular List, the code for septic shock cannot be assigned as a principal diagnosis.

(b) Septic Shock without documentation of severe sepsis

Septic shock cannot occur in the absence of severe sepsis. A code from subcategory 995.9 must be sequenced before the code for septic shock. The use additional code notes and the code first note provide sequencing instructions.

6) Sepsis and septic shock associated with abortion

Sepsis and septic shock associated with abortion, ectopic pregnancy, and molar pregnancy are classified to category codes in Chapter 11 (630-639).

7) Negative or inconclusive blood cultures

Negative or inconclusive blood cultures do not preclude a diagnosis of septicemia or sepsis in patients with clinical evidence of the condition, however, the provider should be queried.

8) Newborn sepsis

See Section I.C.15.j for information on the coding of newborn sepsis.

9) Sepsis due to a Postprocedural Infection

Sepsis resulting from a postprocedural infection is a complication of care. For such cases code 998.59, Other postoperative infections, should be coded first followed by the appropriate codes for the sepsis. The other guidelines for coding sepsis should then be followed for the assignment of additional codes.

10) External cause of injury codes with SIRS

An external cause code is not needed with codes 995.91, Systemic inflammatory response syndrome due to infectious process without organ dysfunction, or code 995.92, Systemic inflammatory response syndrome due to infectious process with organ dysfunction.

Refer to Section I.C.19.a.7 for instruction on the use of external cause of injury codes with codes for SIRS resulting from trauma.

2. Chapter 2: Neoplasms (140-239)

General guidelines

Chapter 2 of the ICD-9-CM contains the codes for most benign and all malignant neoplasms. Certain benign neoplasms, such as prostatic adenomas, may be found in the specific body system chapters. To properly code a neoplasm it is necessary to determine from the record if the neoplasm is benign, in-situ, malignant, or of uncertain histologic behavior. If malignant, any secondary (metastatic) sites should also be determined.

The neoplasm table in the Alphabetic Index should be referenced first. However, if the histological term is documented, that term should be referenced first, rather than going immediately to the Neoplasm Table, in order to determine which column in the Neoplasm Table is appropriate. For example, if the documentation indicates "adenoma," refer to the term in the Alphabetic Index to review the entries under this term and the instructional note to "see also neoplasm, by site, benign." The table provides the proper code based on the type of neoplasm and the site. It is important to select the proper column in the table that corresponds to the type of neoplasm. The tabular should then be referenced to verify that the correct code has been selected from the table and that a more specific site code does not exist.

See Section I. C. 18.d.4. for information regarding V codes for genetic susceptibility to cancer.

a. Treatment directed at the malignancy

If the treatment is directed at the malignancy, designate the malignancy as the principal diagnosis.

b. Treatment of secondary site

When a patient is admitted because of a primary neoplasm with metastasis and treatment is directed toward the secondary site only, the secondary neoplasm is designated as the principal diagnosis even though the primary malignancy is still present.

c. Coding and sequencing of complications

Coding and sequencing of complications associated with the malignancies or with the therapy thereof are subject to the following guidelines:

1) Anemia associated with malignancy

When admission/encounter is for management of an anemia associated with the malignancy, and the treatment is only for anemia, the **appropriate** anemia **code (such as code 285.22, Anemia in neoplastic disease)** is designated as the principal diagnosis and is followed by the appropriate code(s) for the malignancy.

Code 285.22 may also be used as a secondary code if the patient suffers from anemia and is being treated for the malignancy.

2) Anemia associated with chemotherapy, <u>immunotherapy and radiation therapy</u>

When the admission/encounter is for management of an anemia associated with chemotherapy, **immunotherapy** or radiotherapy and the only treatment is for the anemia, the anemia is sequenced first followed by **code E933.1. The appropriate neoplasm code should be assigned as an additional code.**

3) Management of dehydration due to the malignancy

When the admission/encounter is for management of dehydration due to the malignancy or the therapy, or a combination of both, and only the dehydration is being treated (intravenous rehydration), the dehydration is sequenced first, followed by the code(s) for the malignancy.

4) Treatment of a complication resulting from a surgical procedure

When the admission/encounter is for treatment of a complication resulting from a surgical procedure, designate the complication as the principal or first-listed diagnosis if treatment is directed at resolving the complication.

d. Primary malignancy previously excised

When a primary malignancy has been previously excised or eradicated from its site and there is no further treatment directed to that site and there is no evidence of any existing primary malignancy, a code from category V10, Personal history of malignant neoplasm, should be used to indicate the former site of the malignancy. Any mention of extension, invasion, or metastasis to another site is coded as a secondary malignant neoplasm to that site. The secondary site may be the principal or first-listed with the V10 code used as a secondary code.

e. Admissions/Encounters involving chemotherapy, <u>immunotherapy</u> and radiation therapy

1) Episode of care involves surgical removal of neoplasm

When an episode of care involves the surgical removal of a neoplasm, primary or secondary site, followed by adjunct chemotherapy or radiation treatment **during the same episode of care**, the neoplasm code should be assigned as principal or first-listed diagnosis, using codes in the 140-198 series or where appropriate in the 200-203 series.

2) Patient admission/encounter solely for administration of chemotherapy, immunotherapy and radiation therapy

If a patient admission/encounter is solely for the administration of chemotherapy, **immunotherapy** or radiation therapy **assign** code V58.0, Encounter for radiation therapy, or **V58.11**, Encounter for **antineoplastic** chemotherapy, **or V58.12, Encounter for antineoplastic immunotherapy as** the first-listed or principal diagnosis. If a patient receives **more than one of these therapies during the same admission more than one of these codes may be assigned, in any sequence.**

3) Patient admitted for radiotherapy/chemotherapy and immunotherapy and develops complications

When a patient is admitted for the purpose of radiotherapy, **immunotherapy** or chemotherapy and develops complications such as uncontrolled nausea and vomiting or dehydration, the principal or first-listed diagnosis is V58.0, Encounter for radiotherapy, or V58.1**1**, **Encounter for antineoplastic chemotherapy, or V58.12, Encounter for antineoplastic immunotherapy** followed by any codes for the complications.

See Section I.C.18.d.7. for additional information regarding after-care V codes.

f. Admission/encounter to determine extent of malignancy

When the reason for admission/encounter is to determine the extent of the malignancy, or for a procedure such as paracentesis or thoracentesis, the primary malignancy or appropriate metastatic site is designated as the principal or first-listed diagnosis, even though chemotherapy or radiotherapy is administered.

g. Symptoms, signs, and ill-defined conditions listed in Chapter 16

Symptoms, signs, and ill-defined conditions listed in Chapter 16 characteristic of, or associated with, an existing primary or secondary site malignancy cannot be used to replace the malignancy as principal or first-listed diagnosis, regardless of the number of admissions or encounters for treatment and care of the neoplasm.

See section I.C.18.d.14, Encounter for prophylactic organ removal

3. Chapter 3: Endocrine, Nutritional, and Metabolic Diseases and Immunity Disorders (240-279)

a. Diabetes mellitus

Codes under category 250, Diabetes mellitus, identify complications/manifestations associated with diabetes mellitus. A fifth-digit is required for all category 250 codes to identify the type of diabetes mellitus and whether the diabetes is controlled or uncontrolled.

1) Fifth-digits for category 250:

The following are the fifth-digits for the codes under category 250:

0   type II or unspecified type, not stated as uncontrolled

1   type I, [juvenile type], not stated as uncontrolled

2   type II or unspecified type, uncontrolled

3   type I, [juvenile type], uncontrolled

The age of a patient is not the sole determining factor, though most type I diabetics develop the condition before reaching puberty. For this reason type I diabetes mellitus is also referred to as juvenile diabetes.

2) Type of diabetes mellitus not documented

If the type of diabetes mellitus is not documented in the medical record the default is type II.

3) Diabetes mellitus and the use of insulin

All type I diabetics must use insulin to replace what their bodies do not produce. However, the use of insulin does not mean that a patient is a type I diabetic. Some patients with type II diabetes mellitus are unable to control their blood sugar through diet and oral medication alone and do require insulin. If the documentation in a medical record does not indicate the type of diabetes but does indicate that the patient uses insulin, the appropriate fifth-digit for type II must be used. For type II patients who routinely use insulin, code V58.67, Long-term (current) use of insulin, should also be assigned to indicate that the patient uses insulin. Code V58.67 should not be assigned if insulin is given temporarily to bring a type II patient's blood sugar under control during an encounter.

4) Assigning and sequencing diabetes codes and associated conditions

When assigning codes for diabetes and its associated conditions, the code(s) from category 250 must be sequenced before the codes for the associated conditions. The diabetes codes and the secondary codes that correspond to them are paired codes that follow the etiology/manifestation convention of the classification (See Section I.A.6., Etiology/manifestation convention). Assign as many codes from category 250 as needed to identify all of the associated conditions that the patient has. The corresponding secondary codes are listed under each of the diabetes codes.

(a) Diabetic retinopathy/diabetic macular edema Diabetic macular edema, code 362.07, is only present with diabetic retinopathy. Another code from subcategory 362.0, Diabetic retinopathy, must be used with code 362.07. Codes under subcategory 362.0 are diabetes manifestation codes, so they must be used following the appropriate diabetes code.

5) Diabetes mellitus in pregnancy and gestational diabetes

(a) For diabetes mellitus complicating pregnancy, see Section I.C.11.f., Diabetes mellitus in pregnancy.

(b) For gestational diabetes, see Section I.C.11, g., Gestational diabetes.

6) Insulin pump malfunction

(a) Underdose of insulin due insulin pump failure

An underdose of insulin due to an insulin pump failure should be assigned 996.57, Mechanical complication due to insulin pump, as the principal or first listed code, followed by the appropriate diabetes mellitus code based on documentation.

(b) Overdose of insulin due to insulin pump failure

The principal or first listed code for an encounter due to an insulin pump malfunction resulting in an overdose of insulin, should also be 996.57, Mechanical complication due to insulin pump, followed by code 962.3, Poisoning by insulins and antidiabetic agents, and the appropriate diabetes mellitus code based on documentation.

4. Chapter 4: Diseases of Blood and Blood Forming Organs (280-289)

a. Anemia of chronic disease

Subcategory 285.2, Anemia in chronic illness, has codes for anemia in chronic kidney disease, code 285.21; anemia in neoplastic disease, code 285.22; and anemia in other chronic illness, code 285.29. These codes can be used as the principal/first listed code if the reason for the encounter is to treat the anemia. They may also be used as secondary codes if treatment of the anemia is a component of an encounter, but not the primary reason for the encounter. When using a code from subcategory 285 it is also necessary to use the code for the chronic condition causing the anemia.

1) Anemia in chronic kidney disease

When assigning code 285.21, Anemia in chronic kidney disease. It is also necessary to assign a code from category 585, Chronic kidney disease, to indicate the stage of chronic kidney disease.

See I.C.10.a. Chronic kidney disease (CKD)

2) Anemia in neoplastic disease

When assigning code 285.22, Anemia in neoplastic disease, it is also necessary to assign the neoplasm code that is responsible for the anemia. Code 285.22 is for use for anemia that is due to the malignancy, not for anemia due to antineoplastic chemotherapy drugs, which is an adverse effect.

See I.C.2.c.1 Anemia associated with malignancy

See I.C.2.c.2 Anemia associated with chemotherapy, immunotherapy and radiation therapy

See I.C.17.e.1. Adverse effects

5. Chapter 5: Mental Disorders (290-319)

Reserved for future guideline expansion

6. Chapter 6: Diseases of Nervous System and Sense Organs (320-389)

Reserved for future guideline expansion

7. Chapter 7: Diseases of Circulatory System (390-459)

a. Hypertension

Hypertension Table

The Hypertension Table, found under the main term, "Hypertension", in the Alphabetic Index, contains a complete listing of all conditions due to or associated with hypertension and classifies them according to malignant, benign, and unspecified.

1) Hypertension, Essential, or NOS

Assign hypertension (arterial) (essential) (primary) (systemic) (NOS) to category code 401 with the appropriate fourth digit to indicate malignant (.0), benign (.1), or unspecified (.9). Do not use either .0 malignant or .1 benign unless medical record documentation supports such a designation.

2) Hypertension with Heart Disease

Heart conditions (425.8, 429.0-429.3, 429.8, 429.9) are assigned to a code from category 402 when a causal relationship is stated (due to hypertension) or implied (hypertensive). Use an additional code from category 428 to identify the type of heart failure in those patients with heart failure. More than one code from category 428 may be assigned if the patient has systolic or diastolic failure and congestive heart failure.

The same heart conditions (425.8, 429.0-429.3, 429.8, 429.9) with hypertension, but without a stated causal relationship, are coded separately. Sequence according to the circumstances of the admission/encounter.

3) Hypertensive Kidney Disease

Assign codes from category 403, Hypertensive **kidney** disease, when conditions classified to categories 585-587 are present. Unlike hypertension with heart disease, ICD-9-CM presumes a cause-and-effect relationship and classifies renal failure with hypertension as hypertensive **kidney** disease.

4) Hypertensive Heart and Kidney Disease

Assign codes from combination category 404, Hypertensive heart and **kidney** disease, when both hypertensive **kidney** disease and hypertensive heart disease are stated in the diagnosis. Assume a relationship between the hypertension and the **kidney** disease, whether or not the condition is so designated. Assign an additional code from category 428, to identify the type of heart failure. More than one code from category 428 may be assigned if the patient has systolic or diastolic failure and congestive heart failure.

5) Hypertensive Cerebrovascular Disease

First assign codes from 430-438, Cerebrovascular disease, then the appropriate hypertension code from categories 401-405.

6) Hypertensive Retinopathy

Two codes are necessary to identify the condition. First assign the code from subcategory 362.11, Hypertensive retinopathy, then the appropriate code from categories 401-405 to indicate the type of hypertension.

7) Hypertension, Secondary

Two codes are required: one to identify the underlying etiology and one from category 405 to identify the hypertension. Sequencing of codes is determined by the reason for admission/encounter.

8) Hypertension, Transient

Assign code 796.2, Elevated blood pressure reading without diagnosis of hypertension, unless patient has an established diagnosis of hypertension. Assign code 642.3x for transient hypertension of pregnancy.

9) Hypertension, Controlled

Assign appropriate code from categories 401-405. This diagnostic statement usually refers to an existing state of hypertension under control by therapy.

10) Hypertension, Uncontrolled

Uncontrolled hypertension may refer to untreated hypertension or hypertension not responding to current therapeutic regimen. In either case, assign the appropriate code from categories 401-405 to designate the stage and type of hypertension. Code to the type of hypertension.

11) Elevated Blood Pressure

For a statement of elevated blood pressure without further specificity, assign code 796.2, Elevated blood pressure reading without diagnosis of hypertension, rather than a code from category 401.

b. Cerebral infarction/stroke/cerebrovascular accident (CVA)

The terms stroke and CVA are often used interchangeably to refer to a cerebral infarction. The terms stroke, CVA, and cerebral infarction NOS are all indexed to the default code 434.91, Cerebral artery occlusion, unspecified, with infarction. Code 436, Acute, but ill-defined, cerebrovascular disease, should not be used when the documentation states stroke or CVA.

c. Postoperative cerebrovascular accident

A cerebrovascular hemorrhage or infarction that occurs as a result of medical intervention is coded to 997.02, Iatrogenic cerebrovascular infarction or hemorrhage. Medical record documentation should clearly specify the cause- and-effect relationship between the medical intervention and the cerebrovascular accident in order to assign this code. A secondary code from the code range 430-432 or from a code from subcategories 433 or 434 with a fifth digit of "1" should also be used to identify the type of hemorrhage or infarct.

This guideline conforms to the use additional code note instruction at category 997. Code 436, Acute, but ill-defined, cerebrovascular disease, should not be used as a secondary code with code 997.02.

d. Late Effects of Cerebrovascular Disease

1) Category 438, Late Effects of Cerebrovascular disease

Category 438 is used to indicate conditions classifiable to categories 430-437 as the causes of late effects (neurologic deficits), themselves classified elsewhere. These "late effects" include neurologic deficits that persist after initial onset of conditions classifiable to 430-437. The neurologic deficits caused by cerebrovascular disease may be present from the onset or may arise at any time after the onset of the condition classifiable to 430-437.

2) Codes from category 438 with codes from 430-437

Codes from category 438 may be assigned on a health care record with codes from 430-437, if the patient has a current cerebrovascular accident (CVA) and deficits from an old CVA.

3) Code V12.59

Assign code V12.59 (and not a code from category 438) as an additional code for history of cerebrovascular disease when no neurologic deficits are present.

e. Acute myocardial infarction (AMI)

1) ST elevation myocardial infarction (STEMI) and non ST elevation myocardial infarction (NSTEMI)

The ICD-9-CM codes for acute myocardial infarction (AMI) identify the site, such as anterolateral wall or true posterior wall. Subcategories 410.0-410.6 and 410.8 are used for ST elevation myocardial infarction (STEMI). Subcategory 410.7, Subendocardial infarction, is used for non ST elevation myocardial infarction (NSTEMI) and nontransmural MIs.

2) Acute myocardial infarction, unspecified

Subcategory 410.9 is the default for the unspecified term acute myocardial infarction. If only STEMI or transmural MI without the site is documented, query the provider as to the site, or assign a code from subcategory 410.9.

3) AMI documented as nontransmural or subendocardial but site provided

If an AMI is documented as nontransmural or subendocardial, but the site is provided, it is still coded as a subendocardial AMI. If NSTEMI evolves to STEMI, assign the STEMI code. If STEMI converts to NSTEMI due to thrombolytic therapy, it is still coded as STEMI.

8. **Chapter 8: Diseases of Respiratory System (460–519)**

a. **Chronic Obstructive Pulmonary Disease [COPD] and Asthma**

1) **Conditions that comprise COPD and Asthma**

The conditions that comprise COPD are obstructive chronic bronchitis, subcategory 491.2, and emphysema, category 492. All asthma codes are under category 493, Asthma. Code 496, Chronic airway obstruction, not elsewhere classified, is a nonspecific code that should only be used when the documentation in a medical record does not specify the type of COPD being treated.

2) **Acute exacerbation of chronic obstructive bronchitis and asthma**

The codes for chronic obstructive bronchitis and asthma distinguish between uncomplicated cases and those in acute exacerbation. An acute exacerbation is a worsening or a decompensation of a chronic condition. An acute exacerbation is not equivalent to an infection superimposed on a chronic condition, though an exacerbation may be triggered by an infection.

3) **Overlapping nature of the conditions that comprise COPD and asthma**

Due to the overlapping nature of the conditions that make up COPD and asthma, there are many variations in the way these conditions are documented. Code selection must be based on the terms as documented. When selecting the correct code for the documented type of COPD and asthma, it is essential to first review the index, and then verify the code in the tabular list. There are many instructional notes under the different COPD subcategories and codes. It is important that all such notes be reviewed to assure correct code assignment.

4) **Acute exacerbation of asthma and status asthmaticus**

An acute exacerbation of asthma is an increased severity of the asthma symptoms, such as wheezing and shortness of breath. Status asthmaticus refers to a patient's failure to respond to therapy administered during an asthmatic episode and is a life threatening complication that requires emergency care. If status asthmaticus is documented by the provider with any type of COPD or with acute bronchitis, the status asthmaticus should be sequenced first. It supersedes any type of COPD including that with acute exacerbation or acute bronchitis. It is inappropriate to assign an asthma code with 5th digit 2, with acute exacerbation, together with an asthma code with 5th digit 1, with status asthmatics. Only the 5th digit 1 should be assigned.

b. **Chronic Obstructive Pulmonary Disease [COPD] and Bronchitis**

1) **Acute bronchitis with COPD**

Acute bronchitis, code 466.0, is due to an infectious organism. When acute bronchitis is documented with COPD, code 491.22, Obstructive chronic bronchitis with acute bronchitis, should be assigned. It is not necessary to also assign code 466.0. If a medical

c. Coding of Burns

Current burns (940-948) are classified by depth, extent and by agent (E code). Burns are classified by depth as first degree (erythema), second degree (blistering), and third degree (full-thickness involvement).

1) Sequencing of burn <u>and related condition</u> codes

Sequence first the code that reflects the highest degree of burn when more than one burn is present.

    a. When the reason for the admission or encounter is for treatment of external multiple burns, sequence first the code that reflects the burn of the highest degree.

    b. When a patient has both internal and external burns, the circumstances of admission govern the selection of the principal diagnosis or first-listed diagnosis.

    c. When a patient is admitted for burn injuries and other related conditions such as smoke inhalation and/or respiratory failure, the circumstances of admission govern the selection of the principal or first-listed diagnosis.

2) Burns of the same local site

Classify burns of the same local site (three-digit category level, 940-947) but of different degrees to the subcategory identifying the highest degree recorded in the diagnosis.

3) Non-healing burns

Non-healing burns are coded as acute burns.

Necrosis of burned skin should be coded as a non-healed burn.

4) Code 958.3, Posttraumatic wound infection

Assign code 958.3, Posttraumatic wound infection, not elsewhere classified, as an additional code for any documented infected burn site.

5) Assign separate codes for each burn site

When coding burns, assign separate codes for each burn site. Category 946 Burns of Multiple specified sites, should only be used if the location of the burns are not documented. Category 949, Burn, unspecified, is extremely vague and should rarely be used.

6) Assign codes from category 948, Burns

Burns classified according to extent of body surface involved, when the site of the burn is not specified or when there is a need for additional data. It is advisable to use category 948 as additional coding when needed to provide data for evaluating burn mortality, such as that needed by burn units. It is also advisable to use category 948 as an additional code for reporting purposes when there is mention of a third-degree burn involving 20 percent or more of the body surface.

In assigning a code from category 948:

> Fourth-digit codes are used to identify the percentage of total body surface involved in a burn (all degree).
>
> Fifth-digits are assigned to identify the percentage of body surface involved in third-degree burn.
>
> Fifth-digit zero (0) is assigned when less than 10 percent or when no body surface is involved in a third-degree burn.
>
> Category 948 is based on the classic "rule of nines" in estimating body surface involved: head and neck are assigned nine percent, each arm nine percent, each leg 18 percent, the anterior trunk 18 percent, posterior trunk 18 percent, and genitalia one percent. Providers may change these percentage assignments where necessary to accommodate infants and children who have proportionately larger heads than adults and patients who have large buttocks, thighs, or abdomen that involve burns.

7) Encounters for treatment of late effects of burns

Encounters for the treatment of the late effects of burns (i.e., scars or joint contractures) should be coded to the residual condition (sequelae) followed by the appropriate late effect code (906.5-906.9). A late effect E code may also be used, if desired.

8) Sequelae with a late effect code and current burn

When appropriate, both a sequelae with a late effect code, and a current burn code may be assigned on the same record (when both a current burn and sequelae of an old burn exist).

d. Coding of Debridement of Wound, Infection, or Burn

Excisional debridement involves surgical removal or cutting away, as opposed to a mechanical (brushing, scrubbing, washing) debridement.

For coding purposes, excisional debridement is assigned to code 86.22.

Nonexcisional debridement is assigned to code 86.28.

e. Adverse Effects, Poisoning and Toxic Effects

The properties of certain drugs, medicinal and biological substances or combinations of such substances, may cause toxic reactions. The occurrence of drug toxicity is classified in ICD-9-CM as follows:

1) Adverse Effect

When the drug was correctly prescribed and properly administered, code the reaction plus the appropriate code from the E930-E949 series. Codes from the E930-E949 series must be used to identify the causative substance for an adverse effect of drug, medicinal and biological substances, correctly prescribed and properly administered. The effect, such as tachycardia, delirium, gastrointestinal hemorrhaging, vomiting, hypokalemia, hepatitis, renal failure, or respiratory failure, is coded and followed by the appropriate code from the E930-E949 series.

Adverse effects of therapeutic substances correctly prescribed and properly administered (toxicity, synergistic reaction, side effect, and idiosyncratic reaction) may be due to (1) differences among patients, such as age, sex, disease, and genetic factors, and (2) drug-related factors, such as type of drug, route of administration, duration of therapy, dosage, and bioavailability.

2) Poisoning

(a) Error was made in drug prescription

Errors made in drug prescription or in the administration of the drug by provider, nurse, patient, or other person, use the appropriate poisoning code from the 960-979 series.

(b) Overdose of a drug intentionally taken

If an overdose of a drug was intentionally taken or administered and resulted in drug toxicity, it would be coded as a poisoning (960-979 series).

(c) Nonprescribed drug taken with correctly prescribed and properly administered drug

If a nonprescribed drug or medicinal agent was taken in combination with a correctly prescribed and properly administered drug, any drug toxicity or other reaction resulting from the interaction of the two drugs would be classified as a poisoning.

(d) Sequencing of poisoning

When coding a poisoning or reaction to the improper use of a medication (e.g., wrong dose, wrong substance, wrong route of administration) the poisoning code is sequenced first, followed by a code for the manifestation. If there is also a diagnosis of drug abuse or dependence to the substance, the abuse or dependence is coded as an additional code.

See Section I.C.3.a.6.b. if poisoning is the result of insulin pump malfunctions and Section I.C.19 for general use of E-codes.

3) Toxic Effects

(a) Toxic effect codes

When a harmful substance is ingested or comes in contact with a person, this is classified as a toxic effect. The toxic effect codes are in categories 980-989.

(b) Sequencing toxic effect codes

A toxic effect code should be sequenced first, followed by the code(s) that identify the result of the toxic effect.

(c) External cause codes for toxic effects

An external cause code from categories E860-E869 for accidental exposure, codes E950.6 or E950.7 for intentional self-harm, category E962 for assault, or categories E980-E982, for undetermined, should also be assigned to indicate intent.

f. Complications of care

1) Transplant complications

(a) Transplant complications other than kidney

Codes under subcategory 996.8, Complications of transplanted organ, are for use for both complications and rejection of transplanted organs. A transplant complication code is only assigned if the complication affects the function of the transplanted organ. Two codes are required to fully describe a transplant complication, the appropriate code from subcategory 996.8 and a secondary code that identifies the complication.

Pre-existing conditions or conditions that develop after the transplant are not coded as complications unless they affect the function of the transplanted organs.

Post-transplants surgical complications that do not relate to the function of the transplanted organ are classified to the specific complication. For example, a surgical wound dehiscence would be coded to the wound dehiscence, not as a transplant complication.

Post-transplant patients who are seen for treatment unrelated to the transplanted organ should be assigned a code from category V42, Organ or tissue replaced by transplant, to identify the transplant status of the patient. A code from category V42 should never be used with a code from subcategory 996.8.

(b) Kidney transplant and chronic kidney disease

Patients with chronic kidney disease (CKD) following a transplant should not be assumed to have transplant failure or rejection unless it is documented by the provider. If documentation supports the presence of failure or rejection, then it is appropriate to assign code 996.81, Complications of transplanted organs, kidney followed by the appropriate CKD code.

18. Classification of Factors Influencing Health Status and Contact with Health Service (Supplemental V01-V84)

Note: The chapter specific guidelines provide additional information about the use of V codes for specified encounters.

a. Introduction

ICD-9-CM provides codes to deal with encounters for circumstances other than a disease or injury. The Supplementary Classification of Factors Influencing Health Status and Contact with Health Services (V01.0-V84.8) is provided to deal with occasions when circumstances other than a disease or injury (codes 001-999) are recorded as a diagnosis or problem.

There are four primary circumstances for the use of V codes:

1) A person who is not currently sick encounters the health services for some specific reason, such as to act as an organ donor, to receive prophylactic care, such as inoculations or health screenings, or to receive counseling on health related issues.

2) A person with a resolving disease or injury, or a chronic, long-term condition requiring continuous care, encounters the health care system for specific aftercare of that disease or injury (e.g., dialysis for renal disease; chemotherapy for malignancy; cast change). A diagnosis/symptom code should be used whenever a current, acute, diagnosis is being treated or a sign or symptom is being studied.

3) Circumstances or problems influence a person's health status but are not in themselves a current illness or injury.

4) Newborns, to indicate birth status.

b. V codes use in any healthcare setting

V codes are for use in any healthcare setting. V codes may be used as either a first listed (principal diagnosis code in the inpatient setting) or secondary code, depending on the circumstances of the encounter. Certain V codes may only be used as first listed, others only as secondary codes. See Section I.C.18.e, **V Code Table.**

c. V Codes indicate a reason for an encounter

They are not procedure codes. A corresponding procedure code must accompany a V code to describe the procedure performed.

d. Categories of V Codes

1) Contact/Exposure

Category V01 indicates contact with or exposure to communicable diseases. These codes are for patients who do not show any sign or symptom of a disease but have been exposed to it by close personal contact with an infected individual or are in an area where a disease is epidemic. These codes may be used as a first listed code to explain an encounter for testing, or, more commonly, as a secondary code to identify a potential risk.

2) Inoculations and vaccinations

Categories V03-V06 are for encounters for inoculations and vaccinations. They indicate that a patient is being seen to receive a prophylactic inoculation against a disease. The injection itself must be represented by the appropriate procedure code. A code from V03-V06 may be used as a secondary code if the inoculation is given as a routine part of preventive health care, such as a well-baby visit.

3) Status

Status codes indicate that a patient is either a carrier of a disease or has the sequelae or residual of a past disease or condition. This includes such things as the presence of prosthetic or mechanical devices resulting from past treatment. A status code is informative, because the status may affect the course of treatment and its outcome. A status code is distinct from a history code. The history code indicates that the patient no longer has the condition.

A status code should not be used with a diagnosis code from one of the body system chapters, if the diagnosis code includes the information provided by the status code. For example, code V42.1, Heart transplant status, should not be used with code 996.83, Complications of transplanted heart. The status code does not provide additional information. The complication code indicates that the patient is a heart transplant patient.

The status V codes/categories are:

V02   Carrier or suspected carrier of infectious diseases

> Carrier status indicates that a person harbors the specific organisms of a disease without manifest symptoms and is capable of transmitting the infection.

V08   Asymptomatic HIV infection status

> This code indicates that a patient has tested positive for HIV but has manifested no signs or symptoms of the disease.

V09   Infection with drug-resistant microorganisms

> This category indicates that a patient has an infection that is resistant to drug treatment. Sequence the infection code first.

V21   Constitutional states in development

V22.2   Pregnant state, incidental

> This code is a secondary code only for use when the pregnancy is in no way complicating the reason for visit. Otherwise, a code from the obstetric chapter is required.

V26.5x   Sterilization status

V42   Organ or tissue replaced by transplant

V43   Organ or tissue replaced by other means

V44   Artificial opening status

V45   Other postsurgical states

V46   Other dependence on machines

V49.6   Upper limb amputation status

V49.7   Lower limb amputation status

V49.81   Postmenopausal status

V49.82   Dental sealant status

V49.83   Awaiting organ transplant status

V58.6   Long-term (current) drug use

> This subcategory indicates a patient's continuous use of a prescribed drug (including such things as aspirin

therapy) for the long-term treatment of a condition or for prophylactic use. It is not for use for patients who have addictions to drugs.

Assign a code from subcategory V58.6, Long-term (current) drug use, if the patient is receiving a medication for an extended period as a prophylactic measure (such as for the prevention of deep vein thrombosis) or as treatment of a chronic condition (such as arthritis) or a disease requiring a lengthy course of treatment (such as cancer). Do not assign a code from subcategory V58.6 for medication being administered for a brief period of time to treat an acute illness or injury (such as a course of antibiotics to treat acute bronchitis).

V83   Genetic carrier status

Genetic carrier status indicates that a person carries a gene, associated with a particular disease, which may be passed to offspring who may develop that disease. The person does not have the disease and is not at risk of developing the disease.

V84   Genetic susceptibility status

Genetic susceptibility indicates that a person has a gene that increases the risk of that person developing the disease.

Codes from category V84, Genetic susceptibility to disease, should not be used as principal or first-listed codes. If the patient has the condition to which he/she is susceptible, and that condition is the reason for the encounter, the code for the current condition should be sequenced first. If the patient is being seen for follow-up after completed treatment for this condition, and the condition no longer exists, a follow-up code should be sequenced first, followed by the appropriate personal history and genetic susceptibility codes. If the purpose of the encounter is genetic counseling associated with procreative management, a code from subcategory V26.3, Genetic counseling and testing, should be assigned as the first-listed code, followed by a code from category V84.

Additional codes should be assigned for any applicable family or personal history.

See Section I.C. 18.d.14 for information on prophylactic organ removal due to a genetic susceptibility.

Note: Categories V42-V46, and subcategories V49.6, V49.7 are for use only if there are no complications or malfunctions of the organ or tissue replaced, the amputation site or the equipment on which the patient is dependent. These are always secondary codes.

4) History (of)

There are two types of history V codes, personal and family. Personal history codes explain a patient's past medical condition that no longer exists and is not receiving any treatment, but that has the potential for recurrence, and therefore may require continued monitoring. The exceptions to this general rule are category V14, Personal history of allergy to medicinal agents, and subcategory V15.0, Allergy, other than to medicinal agents. A person who has had an allergic episode to a substance or food in the past should always be considered allergic to the substance.

Family history codes are for use when a patient has a family member(s) who has had a particular disease that causes the patient to be at higher risk of also contracting the disease.

Personal history codes may be used in conjunction with follow-up codes and family history codes may be used in conjunction with screening codes to explain the need for a test or procedure. History codes are also acceptable on any medical record regardless of the reason for visit. A history of an illness, even if no longer present, is important information that may alter the type of treatment ordered.

The history V code categories are:

V10   Personal history of malignant neoplasm

V12   Personal history of certain other diseases

V13   Personal history of other diseases

> Except: V13.4, Personal history of arthritis, and V13.6, Personal history of congenital malformations. These conditions are life-long so are not true history codes.

V14   Personal history of allergy to medicinal agents

V15   Other personal history presenting hazards to health

> Except: V15.7, Personal history of contraception.

V16   Family history of malignant neoplasm

V17   Family history of certain chronic disabling diseases

V18   Family history of certain other specific diseases

V19   Family history of other conditions

5) Screening

Screening is the testing for disease or disease precursors in seemingly well individuals so that early detection and treatment can be provided for those who test positive for the disease. Screenings that are recommended for many subgroups in a population include: routine mammograms for women over 40, a fecal occult blood test for everyone over 50, an amniocentesis to rule out a fetal anomaly for pregnant women over 35, because the incidence of breast cancer and colon cancer in these subgroups is higher than in the general population, as is the incidence of Down's syndrome in older mothers.

The testing of a person to rule out or confirm a suspected diagnosis because the patient has some sign or symptom is a diagnostic examination, not a screening. In these cases, the sign or symptom is used to explain the reason for the test.

A screening code may be a first listed code if the reason for the visit is specifically the screening exam. It may also be used as an additional code if the screening is done during an office visit for other health problems. A screening code is not necessary if the screening is inherent to a routine examination, such as a pap smear done during a routine pelvic examination.

Should a condition be discovered during the screening then the code for the condition may be assigned as an additional diagnosis.

The V code indicates that a screening exam is planned. A procedure code is required to confirm that the screening was performed.

The screening V code categories:

V28   Antenatal screening

V73-V82 Special screening examinations

6) Observation

There are two observation V code categories. They are for use in very limited circumstances when a person is being observed for a suspected condition that is ruled out. The observation codes are not for use if an injury or illness or any signs or symptoms related to the suspected condition are present. In such cases the diagnosis/symptom code is used with the corresponding E code to identify any external cause.

The observation codes are to be used as principal diagnosis only. The only exception to this is when the principal diagnosis is required to be a code from the V30, Live born infant, category. Then the V29 observation code is sequenced after the V30 code. Additional codes may be used in addition to the observation code but only if they are unrelated to the suspected condition being observed.

The observation V code categories:

V29   Observation and evaluation of newborns for suspected condition not found

> For the birth encounter, a code from category V30 should be sequenced before the V29 code.

V71   Observation and evaluation for suspected condition not found

7) Aftercare

Aftercare visit codes cover situations when the initial treatment of a disease or injury has been performed and the patient requires continued care during the healing or recovery phase, or for the long-term consequences of the disease. The aftercare V code should not be used if treatment is directed at a current, acute disease or injury. The diagnosis code is to be used in these cases. Exceptions to this rule are codes V58.0, Radiotherapy, and **codes from subcategory** V58.1, **Encounter for c**hemotherapy **and immunotherapy for neoplastic conditions**. These codes are to be first listed, followed by the diagnosis code when a patient's encounter is solely to receive radiation therapy or chemotherapy for the treatment of a neoplasm. Should a patient receive both chemotherapy and radiation therapy during the same encounter code V58.0 and V58.1 may be used together on a record with either one being sequenced first.

The aftercare codes are generally first listed to explain the specific reason for the encounter. An aftercare code may be used as an additional code when some type of aftercare is provided in addition to the reason for admission and no diagnosis code is applicable. An example of this would be the closure of a colostomy during an encounter for treatment of another condition.

Certain aftercare V code categories need a secondary diagnosis code to describe the resolving condition or sequelae, for others, the condition is inherent in the code title.

Additional V code aftercare category terms include, fitting and adjustment, and attention to artificial openings.

Status V codes may be used with aftercare V codes to indicate the nature of the aftercare. For example code V45.81, Aortocoronary bypass status, may be used with code V58.73, Aftercare following surgery of the circulatory system, NEC, to indicate the surgery for which the aftercare is being performed. Also, a transplant status code may be used following code V58.44, Aftercare following organ transplant, to identify the organ transplanted. A status code should not be used when the aftercare code indicates the type of status, such as using V55.0, Attention to tracheostomy with V44.0, Tracheostomy status.

The aftercare V category/codes:

V52	Fitting and adjustment of prosthetic device and implant
V53	Fitting and adjustment of other device
V54	Other orthopedic aftercare
V55	Attention to artificial openings
V56	Encounter for dialysis and dialysis catheter care
V57	Care involving the use of rehabilitation procedures
V58.0	Radiotherapy
V58.11	**Encounter for antineoplastic chemotherapy**
V58.12	**Encounter for antineoplastic immunotherapy**
V58.3	Attention to surgical dressings and sutures
V58.41	Encounter for planned post-operative wound closure
V58.42	Aftercare, surgery, neoplasm
V58.43	Aftercare, surgery, trauma

V58.44   Aftercare involving organ transplant

V58.49   Other specified aftercare following surgery

V58.7x   Aftercare following surgery

V58.81   Fitting and adjustment of vascular catheter

V58.82   Fitting and adjustment of non-vascular catheter

V58.83   Monitoring therapeutic drug

V58.89   Other specified aftercare

8) Follow-up

The follow-up codes are used to explain continuing surveillance following completed treatment of a disease, condition, or injury. They imply that the condition has been fully treated and no longer exists. They should not be confused with aftercare codes that explain current treatment for a healing condition or its sequelae. Follow-up codes may be used in conjunction with history codes to provide the full picture of the healed condition and its treatment. The follow-up code is sequenced first, followed by the history code.

A follow-up code may be used to explain repeated visits. Should a condition be found to have recurred on the follow-up visit, then the diagnosis code should be used in place of the follow-up code.

The follow-up V code categories:

V24   Postpartum care and evaluation

V67   Follow-up examination

9) Donor

Category V59 is the donor codes. They are used for living individuals who are donating blood or other body tissue. These codes are only for individuals donating for others, not for self donations. They are not for use to identify cadaveric donations.

10) Counseling

Counseling V codes are used when a patient or family member receives assistance in the aftermath of an illness or injury, or when support is required in coping with family or social problems. They are not necessary for use in conjunction with a diagnosis code when the counseling component of care is considered integral to standard treatment.

The counseling V categories/codes:

V25.0   General counseling and advice for contraceptive management

V26.3   Genetic counseling

V26.4   General counseling and advice for procreative management

V61   Other family circumstances

V65.1   Person consulted on behalf of another person

V65.3   Dietary surveillance and counseling

V65.4   Other counseling, not elsewhere classified

11) Obstetrics and related conditions

See Section I.C.11, the Obstetrics guidelines for further instruction on the use of these codes.

V codes for pregnancy are for use in those circumstances when none of the problems or complications included in the codes from the Obstetrics chapter exist (a routine prenatal visit or postpartum care). Codes V22.0, Supervision of normal first pregnancy, and V22.1, Supervision of other normal pregnancy, are always first listed and are not to be used with any other code from the OB chapter.

The outcome of delivery, category V27, should be included on all maternal delivery records. It is always a secondary code.

V codes for family planning (contraceptive) or procreative management and counseling should be included on an obstetric record either during the pregnancy or the postpartum stage, if applicable.

Obstetrics and related conditions V code categories:

V22   Normal pregnancy

V23   Supervision of high-risk pregnancy

> Except: V23.2, Pregnancy with history of abortion.
>
> Code 646.3, Habitual aborter, from the OB chapter is required to indicate a history of abortion during a pregnancy.

V24   Postpartum care and evaluation

V25   Encounter for contraceptive management

> Except V25.0x (See Section I.C.18.d.11, Counseling)

V26   Procreative management

> Except V26.5x, Sterilization status, V26.3 and V26.4 (See Section I.C.18.d.11, Counseling)

V27   Outcome of delivery

V28   Antenatal screening

> (See Section I.C.18.d.6, Screening)

12) Newborn, infant and child

See Section I.C.15, the Newborn guidelines for further instruction on the use of these codes.

Newborn V code categories:

V20   Health supervision of infant or child

V29   Observation and evaluation of newborns for suspected condition not found (See Section I.C.18.d.7, Observation).

V30-V39 Liveborn infant according to type of birth

13) Routine and administrative examinations

The V codes allow for the description of encounters for routine examinations, such as, a general check-up, or, examinations for administrative purposes, such as, a pre-employment physical. The codes are for use as first listed codes only, and are not to be used if the examination is for diagnosis of a suspected condition or for treatment purposes. In such cases the diagnosis code is used. During a routine exam, should a diagnosis or condition be discovered, it should be coded as an additional code. Pre-existing and chronic conditions and history codes may also be included as additional codes as long as the examination is for administrative purposes and not focused on any particular condition.

Pre-operative examination V codes are for use only in those situations when a patient is being cleared for surgery and no treatment is given.

The V codes categories/code for routine and administrative examinations:

V20.2   Routine infant or child health check

> Any injections given should have a corresponding procedure code.

V70   General medical examination

V72   Special investigations and examinations

> Except V72.5 and V72.6

14) Miscellaneous V codes

The miscellaneous V codes capture a number of other health care encounters that do not fall into one of the other categories. Certain of these codes identify the reason for the encounter, others are for use as additional codes that provide useful information on circumstances that may affect a patient's care and treatment.

Prophylactic Organ Removal

For encounters specifically for prophylactic removal of breasts, ovaries, or another organ due to a genetic susceptibility to cancer or a family history of cancer, the principal or first listed code should be a code from subcategory V50.4, Prophylactic organ removal, followed by the appropriate genetic susceptibility code and the appropriate family history code.

If the patient has a malignancy of one site and is having prophylactic removal at another site to prevent either a new primary malignancy or metastatic disease, a code for the malignancy should also be assigned in addition to a code from subcategory V50.4. A V50.4 code should not be assigned if the patient is having organ removal for treatment of a malignancy, such as the removal of the testes for the treatment of prostate cancer.

Miscellaneous V code categories/codes:

V07   Need for isolation and other prophylactic measures

V50   Elective surgery for purposes other than remedying health states

V58.5	Orthodontics
V60	Housing, household, and economic circumstances
V62	Other psychosocial circumstances
V63	Unavailability of other medical facilities for care
V64	Persons encountering health services for specific procedures, not carried out
V66	Convalescence and Palliative Care
V68	Encounters for administrative purposes
V69	Problems related to lifestyle

15) Nonspecific V codes

Certain V codes are so non-specific, or potentially redundant with other codes in the classification, that there can be little justification for their use in the inpatient setting. Their use in the outpatient setting should be limited to those instances when there is no further documentation to permit more precise coding. Otherwise, any sign or symptom or any other reason for visit that is captured in another code should be used.

Nonspecific V code categories/codes:

V11	Personal history of mental disorder
	A code from the mental disorders chapter, with an in remission fifth-digit, should be used.
V13.4	Personal history of arthritis
V13.6	Personal history of congenital malformations
V15.7	Personal history of contraception
V23.2	Pregnancy with history of abortion
V40	Mental and behavioral problems
V41	Problems with special senses and other special functions
V47	Other problems with internal organs
V48	Problems with head, neck, and trunk
V49	Problems with limbs and other problems

Exceptions:

V49.6	Upper limb amputation status
V49.7	Lower limb amputation status
V49.81	Postmenopausal status
V49.82	Dental sealant status
V49.83	Awaiting organ transplant status

V51	Aftercare involving the use of plastic surgery
V58.2	Blood transfusion, without reported diagnosis
V58.9	Unspecified aftercare

V72.5   Radiological examination, NEC

V72.6   Laboratory examination

Codes V72.5 and V72.6 are not to be used if any sign or symptoms, or reason for a test is documented. See Section IV.K. and Section IV.L. of the Outpatient guidelines.

V Code Table
Items in bold indicate a change from the April 2005 table
Items underlined have been moved within the table since April 2005

FIRST LISTED: V codes/categories/subcategories which are only acceptable as principal/first listed.

Codes:

V22.0	Supervision of normal first pregnancy
V22.1	Supervision of other normal pregnancy
V46.12	Encounter for respirator dependence during power failure
V46.13	**Encounter for weaning from respirator [ventilator]**
V56.0	Extracorporeal dialysis
V58.0	Radiotherapy

V58.0 and V58.11 may be used together on a record with either one being sequenced first, when a patient receives both chemotherapy and radiation therapy during the same encounter code.

V58.11   **Encounter for antineoplastic chemotherapy**

V58.0 and **V58.11** may be used together on a record with either one being sequenced first, when a patient receives both chemotherapy and radiation therapy during the same encounter code.

V58.12   **Encounter for antineoplastic immunotherapy**

Categories/Subcategories:

V20	Health supervision of infant or child
V24	Postpartum care and examination
V29	Observation and evaluation of newborns for suspected condition not found

> Exception: A code from the V30-V39 may be sequenced before the V29 if it is the newborn record.

V30-V39	Liveborn infants according to type of birth
<u>V57</u>	<u>Care involving use of rehabilitation procedures</u>
V59	Donors
V66	Convalescence and palliative care

> Exception: V66.7 Palliative care

V68	Encounters for administrative purposes
V70	General medical examination

> Exception: V70.7 Examination of participant in clinical trial

V71	Observation and evaluation for suspected conditions not found
V72	Special investigations and examinations

Exceptions:

V72.4   Pregnancy examination or test

V72.5   Radiological examination, NEC

V72.6   Laboratory examination

V72.86 Encounter for blood typing

FIRST OR ADDITIONAL: V code categories/subcategories which may be either principal/first listed or additional codes

Codes:

V15.88   History of fall

V43.22   Fully implantable artificial heart status

V46.14   Mechanical complication of respirator [ventilator]

V49.81   Asymptomatic postmenopausal status (age-related) (natural)

V49.84   Bed confinement status

<u>V49.89</u>   <u>Other specified conditions influencing health status</u>

V70.7   Examination of participant in clinical trial

<u>V72.5</u>   <u>Radiological examination, NEC</u>

<u>V72.6</u>   <u>Laboratory examination</u>

V72.86   Encounter for blood typing

Categories/Subcategories:

V01   Contact with or exposure to communicable diseases

V02   Carrier or suspected carrier of infectious diseases

V03-06   Need for prophylactic vaccination and inoculations

V07   Need for isolation and other prophylactic measures

V08   Asymptomatic HIV infection status

V10   Personal history of malignant neoplasm

V12   Personal history of certain other diseases

V13   Personal history of other diseases

    Exception:

    V13.4 Personal history of arthritis

    V13.69 Personal history of other congenital malformations

V16-V19   Family history of disease

V23   Supervision of high-risk pregnancy

V25   Encounter for contraceptive management

V26   Procreative management

    Exception: V26.5 Sterilization status

V28   Antenatal screening

V45.7   Acquired absence of organ

V49.6x	Upper limb amputation status
V49.7x	Lower limb amputation status
V50	Elective surgery for purposes other than remedying health states
V52	Fitting and adjustment of prosthetic device and implant
V53	Fitting and adjustment of other device
V54	Other orthopedic aftercare
V55	Attention to artificial openings
V56	Encounter for dialysis and dialysis catheter care
	Exception: V56.0 Extracorporeal dialysis
~~V57~~	~~Care involving use of rehabilitation procedures~~
V58.3	Attention to surgical dressings and sutures
V58.4	Other aftercare following surgery
~~V58.6~~	~~Long-term (current) drug use~~
V58.7	Aftercare following surgery to specified body systems, not elsewhere classified
V58.8	Other specified procedures and aftercare
V61	Other family circumstances
V63	Unavailability of other medical facilities for care
V65	Other persons seeking consultation without complaint or sickness
V67	Follow-up examination
V69	Problems related to lifestyle
V72.4	**Pregnancy examination or test**
V73-V82	Special screening examinations
V83	Genetic carrier status

ADDITIONAL ONLY: V code categories/subcategories which may only be used as additional codes, not principal/first listed

Codes:

V13.61	Personal history of hypospadias
V22.2	Pregnancy state, incidental
V46.11	**Dependence on respirator, status**
V49.82	Dental sealant status
V49.83	Awaiting organ transplant status
V66.7	Palliative care

Categories/Subcategories:

V09	Infection with drug-resistant microorganisms
V14	Personal history of allergy to medicinal agents

V15   Other personal history presenting hazards to health

        Exception:

        V15.7 Personal history of contraception

        V15.88 History of fall

V21   Constitutional states in development

V26.5   Sterilization status

V27   Outcome of delivery

V42   Organ or tissue replaced by transplant

V43   Organ or tissue replaced by other means

        Exception: V43.22 Fully implantable artificial heart status

V44   Artificial opening status

V45   Other postsurgical states

        Exception: Subcategory V45.7 Acquired absence of organ

V46   Other dependence on machines

        **Exception: V46.12 Encounter for respirator dependence
during power failure**

        V46.13 Encounter for weaning from respirator [ventilator]

V49.6x   Upper limb amputation status

V49.7x   Lower limb amputation status

<u>V58.6</u>   <u>Long-term current drug use</u>

V60   Housing, household, and economic circumstances

V62   Other psychosocial circumstances

V64   Persons encountering health services for specified procedure, not carried out

V84   Genetic susceptibility to disease

V85   **Body Mass Index**

NONSPECIFIC CODES AND CATEGORIES:

V11   Personal history of mental disorder

V13.4   Personal history of arthritis

V13.69   Personal history of congenital malformations

V15.7   Personal history of contraception

V40   Mental and behavioral problems

V41   Problems with special senses and other special functions

V47   Other problems with internal organs

V48   Problems with head, neck, and trunk

V49.0   **Deficiencies of limbs**

V49.1   **Mechanical problems with limbs**

V49.2	**Motor problems with limbs**
V49.3	**Sensory problems with limbs**
V49.4	**Disfigurements in limbs**
V49.5	**Other problems with limbs**
V49.9	**Unspecified condition influencing health status**
~~V49~~	~~Problems with limbs and other problems~~

Exceptions:

~~V49.6 Upper limb amputation status~~

~~V49.7 Lower limb amputation status~~

~~V49.81 Postmenopausal status (age-related) (natural)~~

~~V49.82 Dental sealant status~~

~~V49.83 Awaiting organ transplant status~~

V51	Aftercare involving the use of plastic surgery
V58.2	Blood transfusion, without reported diagnosis
V58.5	Orthodontics
V58.9	Unspecified aftercare
V72.5	Radiological examination, NEC
V72.6	Laboratory examination

19. Supplemental Classification of External Causes of Injury and Poisoning (E-codes, E800-E999)

Introduction: These guidelines are provided for those who are currently collecting E codes in order that there will be standardization in the process. If your institution plans to begin collecting E codes, these guidelines are to be applied. The use of E codes is supplemental to the application of ICD-9-CM diagnosis codes. E codes are never to be recorded as principal diagnoses (first-listed in non-inpatient setting) and are not required for reporting to CMS.

External causes of injury and poisoning codes (E codes) are intended to provide data for injury research and evaluation of injury prevention strategies. E codes capture how the injury or poisoning happened (cause), the intent (unintentional or accidental; or intentional, such as suicide or assault), and the place where the event occurred.

Some major categories of E codes include:

transport accidents

poisoning and adverse effects of drugs, medicinal substances and biologicals

accidental falls

accidents caused by fire and flames

accidents due to natural and environmental factors

late effects of accidents, assaults or self injury

assaults or purposely inflicted injury

suicide or self inflicted injury

These guidelines apply for the coding and collection of E codes from records in hospitals, outpatient clinics, emergency departments, other ambulatory care settings and provider offices, and nonacute care settings, except when other specific guidelines apply.

a. General E Code Coding Guidelines

1) Used with any code in the range of 001-V84.8

An E code may be used with any code in the range of 001-V84.8, which indicates an injury, poisoning, or adverse effect due to an external cause.

2) Assign the appropriate E code for all initial treatments

Assign the appropriate E code for the initial encounter of an injury, poisoning, or adverse effect of drugs, **not for subsequent treatment.**

3) Use the full range of E codes

Use the full range of E codes to completely describe the cause, the intent and the place of occurrence, if applicable, for all injuries, poisonings, and adverse effects of drugs.

4) Assign as many E codes as necessary

Assign as many E codes as necessary to fully explain each cause. If only one E code can be recorded, assign the E code most related to the principal diagnosis.

5) The selection of the appropriate E code

The selection of the appropriate E code is guided by the Index to External Causes, which is located after the alphabetical index to diseases and by Inclusion and Exclusion notes in the Tabular List.

6) E code can never be a principal diagnosis

An E code can never be a principal (first listed) diagnosis.

7) External cause code(s) with systemic inflammatory response syndrome (SIRS)

An external cause code(s) may be used with codes 995.93, Systemic inflammatory response syndrome due to noninfectious process without organ dysfunction, and 995.94, Systemic inflammatory response syndrome due to noninfectious process with organ dysfunction, if trauma was the initiating insult that precipitated the SIRS. The external cause(s) code should correspond to the most serious injury resulting from the trauma. The external cause code(s) should only be assigned if the trauma necessitated the admission in which the patient also developed SIRS. If a patient is admitted with SIRS but the trauma has been treated previously, the external cause codes should not be used.

b. Place of Occurrence Guideline

Use an additional code from category E849 to indicate the Place of Occurrence for injuries and poisonings. The Place of Occurrence describes the place where the event occurred and not the patient's activity at the time of the event.

Do not use E849.9 if the place of occurrence is not stated.

c. Adverse Effects of Drugs, Medicinal and Biological Substances Guidelines

1) Do not code directly from the Table of Drugs

Do not code directly from the Table of Drugs and Chemicals.

Always refer back to the Tabular List.

2) Use as many codes as necessary to describe

Use as many codes as necessary to describe completely all drugs, medicinal or biological substances.

3) If the same E code would describe the causative agent

If the same E code would describe the causative agent for more than one adverse reaction, assign the code only once.

4) If two or more drugs, medicinal or biological substances

If two or more drugs, medicinal or biological substances are reported, code each individually unless the combination code is listed in the Table of Drugs and Chemicals. In that case, assign the E code for the combination.

5) When a reaction results from the interaction of a drug(s)

When a reaction results from the interaction of a drug(s) and alcohol, use poisoning codes and E codes for both.

6) If the reporting format limits the number of E codes

If the reporting format limits the number of E codes that can be used in reporting clinical data, code the one most related to the principal diagnosis. Include at least one from each category (cause, intent, place) if possible.

If there are different fourth digit codes in the same three digit category, use the code for "Other specified" of that category. If there is no "Other specified" code in that category, use the appropriate "Unspecified" code in that category.

If the codes are in different three digit categories, assign the appropriate E code for other multiple drugs and medicinal substances.

7) Codes from the E930-E949 series

Codes from the E930-E949 series must be used to identify the causative substance for an adverse effect of drug, medicinal and biological substances, correctly prescribed and properly administered. The effect, such as tachycardia, delirium, gastrointestinal hemorrhaging, vomiting, hypokalemia, hepatitis, renal failure, or respiratory failure, is coded and followed by the appropriate code from the E930-E949 series.

d. Multiple Cause E Code Coding Guidelines

If two or more events cause separate injuries, an E code should be assigned for each cause. The first listed E code will be selected in the following order:

E codes for child and adult abuse take priority over all other E codes. See Section I.C.19.e, Child and Adult abuse guidelines

E codes for terrorism events take priority over all other E codes except child and adult abuse

E codes for cataclysmic events take priority over all other E codes except child and adult abuse and terrorism.

E codes for transport accidents take priority over all other E codes except cataclysmic events and child and adult abuse and terrorism.

The first-listed E code should correspond to the cause of the most serious diagnosis due to an assault, accident, or self-harm, following the order of hierarchy listed above.

e. Child and Adult Abuse Guideline

1) Intentional injury

When the cause of an injury or neglect is intentional child or adult abuse, the first listed E code should be assigned from categories E960-E968, Homicide and injury purposely inflicted by other persons, (except category E967). An E code from category E967, Child and adult battering and other maltreatment, should be added as an additional code to identify the perpetrator, if known.

2) Accidental intent

In cases of neglect when the intent is determined to be accidental E code E904.0, Abandonment or neglect of infant and helpless person, should be the first listed E code.

f. Unknown or Suspected Intent Guideline

1) If the intent (accident, self-harm, assault) of the cause of an injury or poisoning is unknown

If the intent (accident, self-harm, assault) of the cause of an injury or poisoning is unknown or unspecified, code the intent as undetermined E980-E989.

2) If the intent (accident, self-harm, assault) of the cause of an injury or poisoning is questionable

If the intent (accident, self-harm, assault) of the cause of an injury or poisoning is questionable, probable or suspected, code the intent as undetermined E980-E989.

g. Undetermined Cause

When the intent of an injury or poisoning is known, but the cause is unknown, use codes: E928.9, Unspecified accident, E958.9, Suicide and self-inflicted injury by unspecified means, and E968.9, Assault by unspecified means.

These E codes should rarely be used, as the documentation in the medical record, in both the inpatient outpatient and other settings, should normally provide sufficient detail to determine the cause of the injury.

h. Late Effects of External Cause Guidelines

1) Late effect E codes

Late effect E codes exist for injuries and poisonings but not for adverse effects of drugs, misadventures and surgical complications.

2) Late effect E codes (E929, E959, E969, E977, E989, or E999.1)

A late effect E code (E929, E959, E969, E977, E989, or E999.1) should be used with any report of a late effect or sequela resulting from a previous injury or poisoning (905-909).

3) Late effect E code with a related current injury

A late effect E code should never be used with a related current nature of injury code.

4) Use of late effect E codes for subsequent visits

Use a late effect E code for subsequent visits when a late effect of the initial injury or poisoning is being treated. There is no late effect E code for adverse effects of drugs.

Do not use a late effect E code for subsequent visits for follow-up care (e.g., to assess healing, to receive rehabilitative therapy) of the injury or poisoning when no late effect of the injury has been documented.

i. Misadventures and Complications of Care Guidelines

1) Code range E870-E876

Assign a code in the range of E870-E876 if misadventures are stated by the provider.

2) Code range E878-E879

Assign a code in the range of E878-E879 if the provider attributes an abnormal reaction or later complication to a surgical or medical procedure, but does not mention misadventure at the time of the procedure as the cause of the reaction.

j. Terrorism Guidelines

1) Cause of injury identified by the Federal Government (FBI) as terrorism

When the cause of an injury is identified by the Federal Government (FBI) as terrorism, the first-listed E-code should be a code from category E979, Terrorism. The definition of terrorism employed by the FBI is found at the inclusion note at E979. The terrorism E-code is the only E-code that should be assigned. Additional E codes from the assault categories should not be assigned.

2) Cause of an injury is suspected to be the result of terrorism

When the cause of an injury is suspected to be the result of terrorism a code from category E979 should not be assigned. Assign a code in the range of E codes based circumstances on the documentation of intent and mechanism.

3) Code E979.9, Terrorism, secondary effects

Assign code E979.9, Terrorism, secondary effects, for conditions occurring subsequent to the terrorist event. This code should not be assigned for conditions that are due to the initial terrorist act.

4) Statistical tabulation of terrorism codes

For statistical purposes these codes will be tabulated within the category for assault, expanding the current category from E960-E969 to include E979 and E999.1.

SECTION II. SELECTION OF PRINCIPAL DIAGNOSIS

The circumstances of inpatient admission always govern the selection of principal diagnosis. The principal diagnosis is defined in the Uniform Hospital Discharge Data Set (UHDDS) as "that condition established after study to be chiefly responsible for occasioning the admission of the patient to the hospital for care."

The UHDDS definitions are used by hospitals to report inpatient data elements in a standardized manner. These data elements and their definitions can be found in the July 31, 1985, Federal Register (Vol. 50, No, 147), pp. 31038-40.

Since that time the application of the UHDDS definitions has been expanded to include all non-outpatient settings (acute care, short term, long term care and psychiatric hospitals; home health agencies; rehab facilities; nursing homes, etc).

In determining principal diagnosis the coding conventions in the ICD-9-CM, Volumes I and II take precedence over these official coding guidelines. (See Section I.A, Conventions for the ICD-9-CM).

The importance of consistent, complete documentation in the medical record cannot be overemphasized. Without such documentation the application of all coding guidelines is a difficult, if not impossible, task.

A. Codes for symptoms, signs, and ill-defined conditions

Codes for symptoms, signs, and ill-defined conditions from Chapter 16 are not to be used as principal diagnosis when a related definitive diagnosis has been established.

B. Two or more interrelated conditions, each potentially meeting the definition for principal diagnosis.

When there are two or more interrelated conditions (such as diseases in the same ICD-9-CM chapter or manifestations characteristically associated with a certain disease) potentially meeting the definition of principal diagnosis, either condition may be sequenced first, unless the circumstances of the admission, the therapy provided, the Tabular List, or the Alphabetic Index indicate otherwise.

C. Two or more diagnoses that equally meet the definition for principal diagnosis

In the unusual instance when two or more diagnoses equally meet the criteria for principal diagnosis as determined by the circumstances of admission, diagnostic workup and/or therapy provided, and the Alphabetic Index, Tabular List, or another coding guidelines does not provide sequencing direction, any one of the diagnoses may be sequenced first.

D. Two or more comparative or contrasting conditions.

In those rare instances when two or more contrasting or comparative diagnoses are documented as "either/or" (or similar terminology), they are coded as if the diagnoses were confirmed and the diagnoses are sequenced according to the circumstances of the admission. If no further determination can be made as to which diagnosis should be principal, either diagnosis may be sequenced first.

E. A symptom(s) followed by contrasting/comparative diagnoses

When a symptom(s) is followed by contrasting/comparative diagnoses, the symptom code is sequenced first. All the contrasting/comparative diagnoses should be coded as additional diagnoses.

F. Original treatment plan not carried out

Sequence as the principal diagnosis the condition, which after study occasioned the admission to the hospital, even though treatment may not have been carried out due to unforeseen circumstances.

G. Complications of surgery and other medical care

When the admission is for treatment of a complication resulting from surgery or other medical care, the complication code is sequenced as the principal diagnosis. If the complication is classified to the 996-999 series and the code lacks the necessary specificity in describing the complication, an additional code for the specific complication should be assigned.

H. Uncertain Diagnosis

If the diagnosis documented at the time of discharge is qualified as "probable", "suspected", "likely", "questionable", "possible", or "still to be ruled out", code the condition as if it existed or was established. The bases for these guidelines are the diagnostic workup, arrangements for further workup or observation, and initial therapeutic approach that correspond most closely with the established diagnosis.

Note: This guideline is applicable only to short-term, acute, long-term care and psychiatric hospitals.

I. Admission from Observation Unit

1. Admission Following Medical Observation

When a patient is admitted to an observation unit for a medical condition, which either worsens or does not improve, and is subsequently admitted as an inpatient of the same hospital for this same medical condition, the principal diagnosis would be the medical condition which led to the hospital admission.

2. Admission Following Post-Operative Observation

When a patient is admitted to an observation unit to monitor a condition (or complication) that develops following outpatient surgery, and then is subsequently admitted as an inpatient of the same hospital, hospitals should apply the Uniform Hospital Discharge Data Set (UHDDS) definition of principal diagnosis as "that condition established after study to be chiefly responsible for occasioning the admission of the patient to the hospital for care."

J. Admission from Outpatient Surgery

When a patient receives surgery in the hospital's outpatient surgery department and is subsequently admitted for continuing inpatient care at the same hospital, the following guidelines should be followed in selecting the principal diagnosis for the inpatient admission:

- **If the reason for the inpatient admission is a complication, assign the complication as the principal diagnosis.**

- **If no complication, or other condition, is documented as the reason for the inpatient admission, assign the reason for the outpatient surgery as the principal diagnosis.**

· **If the reason for the inpatient admission is another condition unrelated to the surgery, assign the unrelated condition as the principal diagnosis.**

SECTION III. REPORTING ADDITIONAL DIAGNOSES

GENERAL RULES FOR OTHER (ADDITIONAL) DIAGNOSES

For reporting purposes the definition for "other diagnoses" is interpreted as additional conditions that affect patient care in terms of requiring:

clinical evaluation; or

therapeutic treatment; or

diagnostic procedures; or

extended length of hospital stay; or

increased nursing care and/or monitoring.

The UHDDS item #11-b defines Other Diagnoses as "all conditions that coexist at the time of admission, that develop subsequently, or that affect the treatment received and/or the length of stay. Diagnoses that relate to an earlier episode which have no bearing on the current hospital stay are to be excluded." UHDDS definitions apply to inpatients in acute care, short-term, long term care and psychiatric hospital setting. The UHDDS definitions are used by acute care short-term hospitals to report inpatient data elements in a standardized manner. These data elements and their definitions can be found in the July 31, 1985, Federal Register (Vol. 50, No, 147), pp. 31038-40.

Since that time the application of the UHDDS definitions has been expanded to include all non-outpatient settings (acute care, short term, long term care and psychiatric hospitals; home health agencies; rehab facilities; nursing homes, etc).

The following guidelines are to be applied in designating "other diagnoses" when neither the Alphabetic Index nor the Tabular List in ICD-9-CM provide direction. The listing of the diagnoses in the patient record is the responsibility of the attending provider.

A. Previous conditions

If the provider has included a diagnosis in the final diagnostic statement, such as the discharge summary or the face sheet, it should ordinarily be coded. Some providers include in the diagnostic statement resolved conditions or diagnoses and status-post procedures from previous admission that have no bearing on the current stay. Such conditions are not to be reported and are coded only if required by hospital policy.

However, history codes (V10-V19) may be used as secondary codes if the historical condition or family history has an impact on current care or influences treatment.

B. Abnormal findings

Abnormal findings (laboratory, x-ray, pathologic, and other diagnostic results) are not coded and reported unless the provider indicates their clinical significance. If the findings are outside the normal range and the attending provider has ordered other tests to evaluate the condition or prescribed treatment, it is appropriate to ask the provider whether the abnormal finding should be added.

Please note: This differs from the coding practices in the outpatient setting for coding encounters for diagnostic tests that have been interpreted by a provider.

C. Uncertain Diagnosis

If the diagnosis documented at the time of discharge is qualified as "probable", "suspected", "likely", "questionable", "possible", or "still to be ruled out", code the condition as if it existed or was established. The bases for these guidelines are the diagnostic workup, arrangements for further workup or observation, and initial therapeutic approach that correspond most closely with the established diagnosis.

Note: This guideline is applicable only to short-term, acute, long-term care and psychiatric hospitals.

SECTION IV. DIAGNOSTIC CODING AND REPORTING GUIDELINES FOR OUTPATIENT SERVICES

These coding guidelines for outpatient diagnoses have been approved for use by hospitals/providers in coding and reporting hospital-based outpatient services and provider-based office visits.

Information about the use of certain abbreviations, punctuation, symbols, and other conventions used in the ICD-9-CM Tabular List (code numbers and titles), can be found in Section IA of these guidelines, under "Conventions Used in the Tabular List." Information about the correct sequence to use in finding a code is also described in Section I.

The terms encounter and visit are often used interchangeably in describing outpatient service contacts and, therefore, appear together in these guidelines without distinguishing one from the other.

Though the conventions and general guidelines apply to all settings, coding guidelines for outpatient and provider reporting of diagnoses will vary in a number of instances from those for inpatient diagnoses, recognizing that:

The Uniform Hospital Discharge Data Set (UHDDS) definition of principal diagnosis applies only to inpatients in acute, short-term, long-term care and psychiatric hospitals.

Coding guidelines for inconclusive diagnoses (probable, suspected, rule out, etc.) were developed for inpatient reporting and do not apply to outpatients.

A. Selection of first-listed condition

In the outpatient setting, the term first-listed diagnosis is used in lieu of principal diagnosis.

In determining the first-listed diagnosis the coding conventions of ICD-9-CM, as well as the general and disease specific guidelines take precedence over the outpatient guidelines.

Diagnoses often are not established at the time of the initial encounter/visit. It may take two or more visits before the diagnosis is confirmed.

The most critical rule involves beginning the search for the correct code assignment through the Alphabetic Index. Never begin searching initially in the Tabular List as this will lead to coding errors.

1. Outpatient Surgery

When a patient presents for outpatient surgery, code the reason for the surgery as the first-listed diagnosis (reason for the encounter), even if the surgery is not performed due to a contraindication.

2. Observation Stay

When a patient is admitted for observation for a medical condition, assign a code for the medical condition as the first-listed diagnosis.

When a patient presents for outpatient surgery and develops complications requiring admission to observation, code the reason for the surgery as the first reported diagnosis (reason for the encounter), followed by codes for the complications as secondary diagnoses.

B. Codes from 001.0 through V84.8

The appropriate code or codes from 001.0 through V84.8 must be used to identify diagnoses, symptoms, conditions, problems, complaints, or other reason(s) for the encounter/visit.

C. Accurate reporting of ICD-9-CM diagnosis codes

For accurate reporting of ICD-9-CM diagnosis codes, the documentation should describe the patient's condition, using terminology which includes specific diagnoses as well as symptoms, problems, or reasons for the encounter. There are ICD-9-CM codes to describe all of these.

D. Selection of codes 001.0 through 999.9

The selection of codes 001.0 through 999.9 will frequently be used to describe the reason for the encounter. These codes are from the section of ICD-9-CM for the classification of diseases and injuries (e.g. infectious and parasitic diseases; neoplasms; symptoms, signs, and ill-defined conditions, etc.).

E. Codes that describe symptoms and signs

Codes that describe symptoms and signs, as opposed to diagnoses, are acceptable for reporting purposes when a diagnosis has not been established (confirmed) by the provider. Chapter 16 of ICD-9-CM, Symptoms, Signs, and Ill-defined conditions (codes 780.0-799.9) contain many, but not all codes for symptoms.

F. Encounters for circumstances other than a disease or injury

ICD-9-CM provides codes to deal with encounters for circumstances other than a disease or injury. The Supplementary Classification of factors Influencing Health Status and Contact with Health Services (V01.0-V84.8) is provided to deal with occasions when circumstances other than a disease or injury are recorded as diagnosis or problems.

G. Level of Detail in Coding

1. ICD-9-CM codes with 3, 4, or 5 digits

ICD-9-CM is composed of codes with either 3, 4, or 5 digits. Codes with three digits are included in ICD-9-CM as the heading of a category of codes that may be further subdivided by the use of fourth and/or fifth digits, which provide greater specificity.

2. Use of full number of digits required for a code

A three-digit code is to be used only if it is not further subdivided. Where fourth-digit subcategories and/or fifth-digit subclassifications are provided, they must be assigned. A code is invalid if it has not been coded to the full number of digits required for that code. See also discussion under Section I.b.3, General Coding Guidelines, Level of Detail in Coding.

H. ICD-9-CM code for the diagnosis, condition, problem, or other reason for encounter/visit

List first the ICD-9-CM code for the diagnosis, condition, problem, or other reason for encounter/visit shown in the medical record to be chiefly responsible for the services provided. List additional codes that describe any coexisting conditions. In some cases the first-listed diagnosis may be a symptom when a diagnosis has not been established (confirmed) by the physician.

I. "Probable", "suspected", "questionable", "rule out", or "working diagnosis"

Do not code diagnoses documented as "probable", "suspected," "questionable," "rule out," or "working diagnosis". Rather, code the condition(s) to the highest degree of certainty for that encounter/visit, such as symptoms, signs, abnormal test results, or other reason for the visit. **Please note:** This differs from the coding practices used by short-term, acute care, long-term care and psychiatric hospitals.

J. Chronic diseases

Chronic diseases treated on an ongoing basis may be coded and reported as many times as the patient receives treatment and care for the condition(s).

K. Code all documented conditions that coexist

Code all documented conditions that coexist at the time of the encounter/visit, and require or affect patient care treatment or management. Do not code conditions that were previously treated and no longer exist. However, history codes (V10-V19) may be used as secondary codes if the historical condition or family history has an impact on current care or influences treatment.

L. Patients receiving diagnostic services only

For patients receiving diagnostic services only during an encounter/visit, sequence first the diagnosis, condition, problem, or other reason for encounter/visit shown in the medical record to be chiefly responsible for the outpatient services provided during the encounter/visit. Codes for other diagnoses (e.g., chronic conditions) may be sequenced as additional diagnoses.

For outpatient encounters for diagnostic tests that have been interpreted by a physician, and the final report is available at the time of coding, code any confirmed or definitive diagnosis(es) documented in the interpretation. Do not code related signs and symptoms as additional diagnoses.

Please note: This differs from the coding practice in the hospital inpatient setting regarding abnormal findings on test results.

M. Patients receiving therapeutic services only

For patients receiving therapeutic services only during an encounter/visit, sequence first the diagnosis, condition, problem, or other reason for encounter/visit shown in the medical record to be chiefly responsible for the outpatient services provided during the encounter/visit. Codes for other diagnoses (e.g., chronic conditions) may be sequenced as additional diagnoses.

The only exception to this rule is that when the primary reason for the admission/encounter is chemotherapy, radiation therapy, or rehabilitation, the appropriate V code for the service is listed first, and the diagnosis or problem for which the service is being performed listed second.

N. Patients receiving preoperative evaluations only

For patients receiving preoperative evaluations only, sequence **first** a code from category V72.8, Other specified examinations, to describe the pre-op consultations. Assign a code for the condition to describe the reason for the surgery as an additional diagnosis. Code also any findings related to the pre-op evaluation.

O. Ambulatorysurgery

For ambulatory surgery, code the diagnosis for which the surgery was performed. If the postoperative diagnosis is known to be different from the preoperative diagnosis at the time the diagnosis is confirmed, select the postoperative diagnosis for coding, since it is the most definitive.

P. Routine outpatient prenatal visits

For routine outpatient prenatal visits when no complications are present, codes V22.0, Supervision of normal first pregnancy, or V22.1, Supervision of other normal pregnancy, should be used as the principal diagnosis. These codes should not be used in conjunction with chapter 11 codes.

Medical Terminology

ablation	removal or destruction by cutting, chemicals, or electrocautery
abortion	termination of pregnancy
absence	without
actinotherapy	treatment of acne using ultraviolet rays
adenoidectomy	removal of adenoids
adipose	fatty
adrenals	glands, located at the top of the kidneys, that produce steroid hormones
albinism	lack of color pigment
allograft	homograft, same species graft
alopecia	condition in which hair falls out
amniocentesis	percutaneous aspiration of amniotic fluid
amniotic sac	sac containing the fetus and amniotic fluid
A-mode	one-dimensional ultrasonic display reflecting the time it takes a sound wave to reach a structure and reflect back; maps the structure's outline
anastomosis	surgical connection of two tubular structures, such as two pieces of the intestine
aneurysm	abnormal dilation of vessels, usually an artery
angina	sudden pain
angiography	radiography of the blood vessels
angioplasty	procedure in a vessel to dilate the vessel opening
anhidrosis	deficiency of sweat
anomaloscope	instrument used to test color vision
anoscopy	procedure that uses a scope to examine the anus
antepartum	before childbirth
anterior (ventral)	in front of
anterior segment	those parts of the eye in the front of and including the lens, orbit, extraocular muscles, and eyelid

anteroposterior	from front to back
antigen	a substance that produces a specific response
aortography	radiographic recording of the aorta
apex cardiography	recording of the movement of the chest wall
aphakia	absence of the lens of the eye
apicectomy	excision of a portion of the temporal bone
apnea	cessation of breathing
arthrocentesis	injection and/or aspiration of joint
arthrodesis	surgical immobilization of joint
arthrography	radiography of joint
arthroplasty	reshaping or reconstruction of joint
arthroscopy	use of scope to view inside joint
arthrotomy	incision into a joint
articular	pertains to joint
asphyxia	lack of oxygen
aspiration	use of a needle and a syringe to withdraw fluid
assignment	Medicare's payment for the service, which participating physicians agree to accept as payment in full
asthma	shortage of breath caused by contraction of bronchi
astigmatism	condition in which the refractive surfaces of the eye are unequal
atelectasis	incomplete expansion of lung, collapse
atherectomy	removal of plaque by percutaneous method
atrophy	wasting away
audiometry	hearing test
aural atresia	congenital absence of the external auditory canal
auscultation	listening to sounds within the body
autograft	from patient's own body
avulsion	ripping or tearing away of part either surgically or accidentally
axillary nodes	lymph nodes located in the armpit
bacilli	plural of bacillus, a rod-shaped bacterium
barium enema	radiographic contrast medium
beneficiary	person who benefits from health or life insurance
bifocal	two focuses in eyeglasses, one usually for close work and the other for improvement of distance vision
bilaminate skin	skin substitute usually made of silicone-covered nylon mesh
bilateral	occurring on two sides
biliary	refers to gallbladder, bile, or bile duct
bilobectomy	surgical removal of two lobes of a lung
biofeedback	process of giving a person self-information

biometry	application of a statistical measure to a biologic fact
biopsy	removal of a small piece of living tissue for diagnostic purposes
block	frozen piece of a sample
brachytherapy	therapy using radioactive sources that are placed inside the body
bronchiole	smaller division of bronchial tree
bronchography	radiographic recording of the lungs
bronchoplasty	surgical repair of the bronchi
bronchoscopy	inspection of the bronchial tree using a bronchoscope
B-scan	two-dimensional display of tissues and organs
bulbocavernosus	muscle that constricts the vagina in a female and the urethra in a male
bulbourethral	gland with duct leading to the urethra
bundle of His	muscular cardiac fibers that provide the heart rhythm to the ventricles; blockage of this rhythm produces heart block
bundled codes	one code that represents a package of services
bunion	hallux valgus, abnormal increase in size of metatarsal head that results in displacement of the great toe
burr	drill used to create an entry into the cranium
bursa	fluid-filled sac that absorbs friction
bursitis	inflammation of bursa (joint sac)
bypass	to go around
calcaneal	pertaining to the heel bone
calculus	concretion of mineral salts, also called a stone
calycoplasty	surgical reconstruction of a recess of the renal pelvis
calyx	recess of the renal pelvis
cancellous	lattice-type structure, usually of bone
cardiopulmonary	refers to the heart and lungs
cardiopulmonary bypass	blood bypasses the heart through a heart-lung machine
cardioversion	electrical shock to the heart to restore normal rhythm
cardioverter-defibrillator	surgically placed device that directs an electrical shock to the heart to restore rhythm
carotid body	located on each side of the common carotid artery, often a site of tumor
cartilage	connective tissue
cataract	opaque covering on or in the lens
catheter	tube placed into the body to put fluid in or take fluid out
caudal	same as inferior; away from the head, or the lower part of the body

causalgia	burning pain
cauterization	destruction of tissue by the use of cautery
cavernosa	connection between the cavity of the penis and a vein
cavernosography	radiographic recording of a cavity, e.g., the pulmonary cavity or the main part of the penis
cavernosometry	measurement of the pressure in a cavity, e.g., the penis
central nervous system	brain and spinal cord
cervical	pertaining to the neck or to the cervix of the uterus
cervix uteri	rounded, cone-shaped neck of the uterus
cesarean	surgical opening through abdominal wall for delivery
cholangiography	radiographic recording of the bile ducts
cholangiopancreatography	ERCP, radiographic recording of the biliary system or pancreas
cholecystectomy	surgical removal of the gallbladder
cholecystoenterostomy	creation of a connection between the gallbladder and intestine
cholecystography	radiographic recording of the gallbladder
cholesteatoma	tumor that forms in middle ear
chondral	referring to the cartilage
chordee	condition resulting in the penis being bent downward
chorionic villus sampling	CVS, biopsy of the outermost part of the placenta
circumflex	a coronary artery that circles the heart
Cloquet's node	also called a gland; it is the highest of the deep groin lymph nodes
closed fracture repair	not surgically opened with/without manipulation and with/without traction
closed treatment	fracture site that is not surgically opened and visualized
coccyx	caudal extremity of vertebral column
collagen	protein substance of skin
Colles' fracture	fracture at lower end of radius that displaces the bone posteriorly
colonoscopy	fiberscopic examination of the entire colon that may include part of the terminal ileum
colostomy	artificial opening between the colon and the abdominal wall
component	part
computed axial tomography	CAT or CT, procedure by which selected planes of tissue are pinpointed through computer enhancement, and images may be reconstructed by analysis of variance in absorption of the tissue
conjunctiva	the lining of the eyelids and the covering of the sclera
contraction	drawn together

contralateral	opposite side
cordectomy	surgical removal of the vocal cord(s)
cordocentesis	procedure to obtain a fetal blood sample; also called a percutaneous umbilical blood sampling
corneosclera	cornea and sclera of the eye
corpectomy	removal of vertebrae
corpora cavernosa	the two cavities of the penis
corpus uteri	uterus
crackle	abnormal sound when breathing (heard on auscultation)
craniectomy	permanent, partial removal of skull
craniotomy	opening of the skull
cranium	that part of the skeleton that encloses the brain
curettage	scraping of a cavity using a spoon-shaped instrument
curette	spoon-shaped instrument used to scrape a cavity
cutdown	incision into a vessel for placement of a catheter
cyanosis	bluish discoloration
cystocele	herniation of the bladder into the vagina
cystography	radiographic recording of the urinary bladder
cystolithectomy	removal of a calculus (stone) from the urinary bladder
cystolithotomy	cystolithectomy
cystometrogram	CMG, measurement of the pressures and capacity of the urinary bladder
cystoplasty	surgical reconstruction of the bladder
cystorrhaphy	suture of the bladder
cystoscopy	use of a scope to view the bladder
cystostomy	surgical creation of an opening into the bladder
cystotomy	incision into the bladder
cystourethroplasty	surgical reconstruction of the bladder and urethra
cystourethroscopy	use of a scope to view the bladder and urethra
dacryocystography	radiographic recording of the lacrimal sac or tear duct sac
dacryostenosis	narrowing of the lacrimal duct
debridement	cleansing of or removal of dead tissue from a wound
deductible	amount the patient is liable for before the payer begins to pay for covered services
delayed flap	pedicle of skin with blood supply that is separated from origin over time
delivery	childbirth
dermabrasion	planing of the skin by means of sander, brush, or sandpaper

dermatologist	physician who treats conditions of the skin
dermatoplasty	surgical repair of skin
dialysis	filtration of blood
dilation	expansion
diskectomy	removal of a vertebral disk
diskography	radiographic recording of an intervertebral joint
dislocation	placement in a location other than the original location
distal	farther from the point of attachment or origin
diverticulum	protrusion in the wall of an organ
Doppler	ultrasonic measure of blood movement
dosimetry	scientific calculation of radiation emitted from various radioactive sources
drainage	free flow or withdrawal of fluids from a wound or cavity
duodenography	radiographic recording of the duodenum or first part of the small intestine
dysphagia	difficulty swallowing
dysphonia	speech impairment
dyspnea	shortness of breath, difficult breathing
dysuria	painful urination
echocardiography	radiographic recording of the heart or heart walls or surrounding tissues
echoencephalography	ultrasound of the brain
echography	ultrasound procedure in which sound waves are bounced off an internal organ and the resulting image is recorded
ectopic	pregnancy outside the uterus (i.e., in the fallopian tube)
edema	swelling due to abnormal fluid collection in the tissue spaces
elective surgery	nonemergency procedure
electrocardiogram	ECG, written record of the electrical action of the heart
electrocautery	cauterization by means of heated instrument
electrocochleography	test to measure the eighth cranial nerve (hearing test)
electrode	lead attached to a generator that carries the electrical current from the generator to the atria or ventricles
electroencephalogram	EEG, written record of the electrical action of the brain
electromyogram	EMG, written record of the electrical activity of the skeletal muscles
electronic claim submission	claims prepared and submitted via a computer
electronic signature	identification system of a computer
electro-oculogram	EOG, written record of the electrical activity of the eye

electrophysiology	study of the electrical system of the heart, including the study of arrhythmias
embolectomy	removal of blockage (embolism) from vessel
emphysema	air accumulated in organ or tissue
encephalography	radiographic recording of the subarachnoid space and ventricles of the brain
endarterectomy	incision into an artery to remove the inner lining so as to eliminate disease or blockage
endomyocardial	pertaining to the inner and middle layers of the heart
endopyelotomy	procedure involving the bladder and ureters, including the insertion of a stent into the renal pelvis
endoscopy	inspection of body organs or cavities using a lighted scope that may be inserted through an existing opening or through a small incision
enterolysis	releasing of adhesions of intestine
enucleation	removal of an organ or organs from a body cavity
epicardial	over the heart
epidermolysis	loosening of the epidermis
epidermomycosis	superficial fungal infection
epididymectomy	surgical removal of the epididymis
epididymis	tube located at the top of the testes that stores sperm
epididymography	radiographic recording of the epididymis
epididymovasostomy	creation of a new connection between the vas deferens and epididymis
epiglottidectomy	excision of the covering of the larynx
episclera	connective covering of sclera
epistaxis	nose bleed
epithelium	surface covering of internal and external organs of the body
erythema	redness of skin
escharotomy	surgical incision into necrotic (dead) tissue
eventration	protrusion of the bowel through an opening in the abdomen
evisceration	pulling the viscera outside of the body through an incision
evocative	tests that are administered to evoke a predetermined response
exenteration	removal of an organ all in one piece
exophthalmos	protrusion of the eyeball
exostosis	bony growth
exstrophy	condition in which an organ is turned inside out
extracorporeal	occurring outside of the body

false aneurysm	sac of clotted blood that has completely destroyed the vessel and is being contained by the tissue that surrounds the vessel
fasciectomy	removal of a band of fibrous tissue
Federal Register	official publication of all "Presidential Documents," "Rules and Regulations," "Proposed Rules," and "Notices"; government-instituted national changes are published in the *Federal Register*
fee schedule	services and payment allowed for each service
femoral	pertaining to the bone from the pelvis to knee
fenestration	creation of a new opening in the inner wall of the middle ear
fissure	cleft or groove
fistula	abnormal opening from one area to another area or to the outside of the body
fluoroscopy	procedure for viewing the interior of the body using x-rays and projecting the image onto a television screen
fracture	break in a bone
free full-thickness graft	graft of epidermis and dermis that is completely removed from donor area
fulguration	use of electrical current to destroy tissue
fundoplasty	repair of the bottom of the bladder
furuncle	nodule in the skin caused by *Staphylococci* entering through hair follicle
ganglion	knot
gastrointestinal	pertaining to the stomach and intestine
gastroplasty	operation on the stomach for repair or reconfiguration
gastrostomy	artificial opening between the stomach and the abdominal wall
gatekeeper	a physician who manages a patient's access to health care
glaucoma	eye diseases that are characterized by an increase of intraocular pressure
globe	eyeball
glottis	true vocal cords
gonioscopy	use of a scope to examine the angles of the eye
Group Practice Model	an organization of physicians who contract with a Health Maintenance Organization to provide services to the enrollees of the HMO
grouper	computer used to input the principal diagnosis and other critical information about a patient and then provide the correct DRG code
Health Maintenance Organization	HMO, a health care delivery system in which an enrollee is assigned a primary care physician who manages all the health care needs of the enrollee

hematoma	mass of blood that forms outside the vessel
hemodialysis	cleansing of the blood outside of the body
hemolysis	breakdown of red blood cells
hemoptysis	bloody sputum
hepatography	radiographic recording of the liver
hernia	organ or tissue protruding through the wall or cavity that usually contains it
histology	study of structure of tissue and cells
homograft	allograft, same species graft
hormone	chemical substance produced by the body's endocrine glands
hydrocele	sac of fluid
hyperopia	farsightedness, eyeball is too short from front to back
hypogastric	lowest middle abdominal area
hyposensitization	decreased sensitivity
hypothermia	low body temperature; sometimes induced during surgical procedures
hypoxemia	low level of oxygen in the blood
hypoxia	low level of oxygen in the tissue
hysterectomy	surgical removal of the uterus
hysterorrhaphy	suturing of the uterus
hysterosalpingography	radiographic recording of the uterine cavity and fallopian tubes
hysteroscopy	visualization of the canal and cavity of the uterus using a scope placed through the vagina
ichthyosis	skin disorder characterized by scaling
ileostomy	artificial opening between the ileum and the abdominal wall
ilium	portion of hip
imbrication	overlapping
immunotherapy	therapy to increase immunity
incarcerated	regarding hernias, a constricted, irreducible hernia that may cause obstruction of an intestine
incise	to cut into
Individual Practice Association	IPA, an organization of physicians who provide services for a set fee; Health Maintenance Organizations often contract with the IPA for services to their enrollees
inferior	away from the head or the lower part of the body; also known as caudalingual
inguinofemoral	referring to the groin and thigh
inofemoral	referring to the groin and thigh

internal/external fixation	application of pins, wires, and/or screws placed externally or internally to immobilize a body part
intracardiac	inside the heart
intramural	within the organ wall
intramuscular	into a muscle
intrauterine	inside the uterus
intravenous	into a vein
intravenous pyelography	IVP, radiographic recording of the urinary system
introitus	opening or entrance to the vagina from the uterus
intubation	insertion of a tube
intussusception	slipping of one part of the intestine into another part
invasive	entering the body, breaking skin
iontophoresis	introduction of ions into the body
ischemia	deficient blood supply due to obstruction of the circulatory system
island pedicle flap	contains a single artery and vein that remains attached to origin temporarily or permanently
isthmus	connection of two regions or structures
isthmus, thyroid	tissue connection between right and left thyroid lobes
isthmusectomy	surgical removal of the isthmus
jejunostomy	artificial opening between the jejunum and the abdominal wall
jugular nodes	lymph nodes located next to the large vein in the neck
keratomalacia	softening of the cornea associated with a deficiency of vitamin A
keratoplasty	surgical repair of the cornea
Kock pouch	surgical creation of a urinary bladder from a segment of the ileum
kyphosis	humpback
labyrinth	inner connecting cavities, such as the internal ear
labyrinthitis	inner ear inflammation
lacrimal	related to tears
lamina	flat plate
laminectomy	surgical excision of the lamina
laparoscopy	exploration of the abdomen and pelvic cavities using a scope placed through a small incision in the abdominal wall
laryngeal web	congenital abnormality of connective tissue between the vocal cords
laryngectomy	surgical removal of the larynx
laryngography	radiographic recording of the larynx

laryngoplasty	surgical repair of the larynx
laryngoscope	fiberoptic scope used to view the inside of the larynx
laryngoscopy	direct visualization and examination of the interior of larynx with a laryngoscope
laryngotomy	incision into the larynx
lateral	away from the midline of the body (to the side)
lavage	washing out
leukoderma	depigmentation of skin
leukoplakia	white patch on mucous membrane
ligament	fibrous band of tissue that connects cartilage or bone
ligation	binding or tying off, as in constricting the blood flow of a vessel or binding fallopian tubes for sterilization
lipocyte	fat cell
lipoma	fatty tumor
lithotomy	incision into an organ or a duct for the purpose of removing a stone
lithotripsy	crushing of a stone by sound waves or force
lobectomy	surgical excision of lobe of the lung
lordosis	anterior curve of spine
lumbodynia	pain in the lumbar area
lunate	one of the wrist (carpal) bones
lymph node	station along the lymphatic system
lymphadenectomy	excision of a lymph node or nodes
lymphadenitis	inflammation of a lymph node
lymphangiography	radiographic recording of the lymphatic vessels and nodes
lymphangiotomy	incision into a lymphatic vessel
lysis	releasing
magnetic resonance imaging	MRI, procedure that uses nonionizing radiation to view the body in a cross-sectional view
Major Diagnostic Categories	MDC, the division of all principal diagnoses into 25 mutually exclusive principal diagnosis areas within the DRG system
mammography	radiographic recording of the breasts
Managed Care Organization	MCO, a group that is responsible for the health care services offered to an enrolled group of persons
manipulation	movement by hand
manipulation or reduction	alignment of a fracture or joint dislocation to its normal position
mastoidectomy	removal of the mastoid bone

Maximum Actual Allowable Charge	MAAC, limitation on the total amount that can be charged by physicians who are not participants in Medicare
meatotomy	surgical enlargement of the opening of the urinary meatus
medial	toward the midline of the body
Medical Volume Performance Standards	MVPS, government's estimate of how much growth is appropriate for nationwide physician expenditures paid by the Part B Medicare program
Medicare Economic Index	MEI, government mandated index that ties increases in the Medicare prevailing charges to economic indicators
Medicare Fee Schedule	MFS, schedule that listed the allowable charges for Medicare services; was replaced by the Medicare reasonable charge payment system
Medicare Risk HMO	a Medicare-funded alternative to the standard Medicare supplemental coverage
melanin	dark pigment of skin
melanoma	tumor of epidermis, malignant and black in color
Ménière's disease	condition that causes dizziness, ringing in the ears, and deafness
M-mode	one-dimensional display of movement of structures
modality	treatment method
Mohs' surgery or Mohs' micrographic surgery	removal of skin cancer in layers by a surgeon who also acts as pathologist during surgery
monofocal	eyeglasses with one vision correction
muscle	organ of contraction for movement
muscle flap	transfer of muscle from origin to recipient site
myasthenia gravis	syndrome characterized by muscle weakness
myelography	radiographic recording of the subarachnoid space of the spine
myopia	nearsightedness, eyeball too long from front to back
myringotomy	incision into tympanic membrane
nasal button	synthetic circular disk used to cover a hole in the nasal septum
nasopharyngoscopy	use of a scope to visualize the nose and pharynx
National Provider Identifier	NPI, a 10-digit number assigned to a physician by Medicare
nephrectomy, paraperitoneal	kidney transplant
nephrocutaneous fistula	a channel from the kidney to the skin
nephrolithotomy	removal of a kidney stone through an incision made into the kidney
nephrorrhaphy	suturing of the kidney
nephrostolithotomy	creation of an artificial channel to the kidney
nephrostolithotomy, percutaneous	procedure to establish an artificial channel between the skin and the kidney

nephrostomy	creation of a channel into the renal pelvis of the kidney
nephrostomy, percutaneous	creation of a channel from the skin to the renal pelvis
nephrotomy	incision into the kidney
neurovascular flap	contains artery, vein, and nerve
noninvasive	not entering the body, not breaking skin
nuclear cardiology	diagnostic specialty that uses radiologic procedures to aid in diagnosis of cardiologic conditions
nystagmus	rapid involuntary eye movements
ocular adnexa	orbit, extraocular muscles, and eyelid
olecranon	elbow bone
Omnibus Budget Reconciliation Act of 1989	OBRA, act that established new rules for Medicare reimbursement
oophorectomy	surgical removal of the ovary(ies)
opacification	area that has become opaque (milky)
open fracture repair	surgical opening (incision) over or remote opening as access to a fracture site
open treatment	fracture site that is surgically opened and visualized
ophthalmodynamometry	test of the blood pressure of the eye
ophthalmology	body of knowledge regarding the eyes
ophthalmoscopy	examination of the interior of the eye by means of a scope, also known as funduscopy
optokinetic	movement of the eyes to objects moving in the visual field
orchiectomy	castration, removal of the testes
orchiopexy	surgical procedure to release undescended testes and fixate them within the scrotum
order	shows subordination of one thing to another; family or class
orthopnea	difficulty in breathing, needing to be in erect position to breathe
orthoptic	corrective; in the correct place
osteoarthritis	degenerative condition of articular cartilage
osteoclast	absorbs or removes bone
osteotomy	cutting into bone
otitis media	noninfectious inflammation of the middle ear; serous otitis media produces liquid drainage (not purulent) and suppurative otitis media produces purulent (pus) matter
otoscope	instrument used to examine the internal and external ear
oviduct	fallopian tube
papilledema	swelling of the optic disk (papilla)
paraesophageal hiatus hernia	hernia that is near the esophagus

parathyroid	produces a hormone to mobilize calcium from the bones to the blood
paronychia	infection around nail
Part A	Medicare's Hospital Insurance; covers hospital/facility care
Part B	Medicare's Supplemental Medical Insurance; covers physician services and durable medical equipment that are not paid for under Part A
participating provider program	Medicare providers who have agreed in advance to accept assignment on all Medicare claims
patella	knee cap
pedicle	growth attached with a stem
Peer Review Organizations	PROs, groups established to review hospital admission and care
pelviolithotomy	pyeloplasty
penoscrotal	referring to the penis and scrotum
percussion	tapping with sharp blows as a diagnostic technique
percutaneous	through the skin
percutaneous fracture repair	repair of a fracture by means of pins and wires inserted through the fracture site
percutaneous skeletal fixation	considered neither open nor closed; the fracture is not visualized, but fixation is placed across the fracture site under x-ray imaging
pericardiocentesis	procedure in which a surgeon withdraws fluid from the pericardial space by means of a needle inserted percutaneously
pericardium	membranous sac enclosing heart and ends of great vessels
perineum	area between the vulva and anus; also known as the pelvic floor
peripheral nerves	12 pairs of cranial nerves, 31 pairs of spinal nerves, and autonomic nervous system; connects peripheral receptors to the brain and spinal cord
peritoneal	within the lining of the abdominal cavity
peritoneoscopy	visualization of the abdominal cavity using one scope placed through a small incision in the abdominal wall and another scope placed in the vagina
pharyngolaryngectomy	surgical removal of the pharynx and larynx
phlebotomy	cutting into a vein
phonocardiogram	recording of heart sounds
photochemotherapy	treatment by means of drugs that react to ultraviolet radiation or sunlight
physics	scientific study of energy
pilosebaceous	pertains to hair follicles and sebaceous glands
placenta	a structure that connects the fetus and mother during pregnancy

plethysmography	determining the changes in volume of an organ part or body
pleura	covers the lungs and lines the thoracic cavity
pleurectomy	surgical excision of the pleura
pleuritis	inflammation of the pleura
pneumonocentesis	surgical puncturing of a lung to withdraw fluid
pneumonolysis	surgical separation of the lung from the chest wall to allow the lung to collapse
pneumonostomy	surgical procedure in which the chest cavity is exposed and the lung is incised
pneumonotomy	incision of the lung
pneumoplethysmography	determining the changes in the volume of the lung
posterior (dorsal)	in back of
posterior segment	those parts of the eye behind the lens
posteroanterior	from back to front
postpartum	after childbirth
Preferred Provider Organization	PPO, a group of providers who form a network and who have agreed to provide services to enrollees at a discounted rate
priapism	painful condition in which the penis is constantly erect
primary care physician	PCP, physician who oversees a patient's care within a managed care organization
primary diagnosis	chief complaint of a patient in outpatient setting
prior approval	also known as a prior authorization, the payer's approval of care
proctosigmoidoscopy	fiberscopic examination of the sigmoid colon and rectum
Professional Standards Review Organization	PSRO, voluntary physicians' organization designed to monitor the necessity of hospital admissions, treatment costs, and medical records of hospitals
prognosis	probable outcome of an illness
prostatotomy	incision into the prostate
Provider Identification Number	PIN, assigned to physicians by payers for use in claims submission
pyelography	radiographic recording of the kidneys, renal pelvis, ureters, and bladder
qualitative	measuring the presence or absence of
quantitative	measuring the presence or absence of and the amount of
rad	radiation-absorbed dose, the energy deposited in patient's tissues
radiation oncology	branch of medicine concerned with the application of radiation to a tumor site for treatment (destruction) of cancerous tumors

radiograph	film on which an image is produced through exposure to x-radiation
radiologist	physician who specializes in the use of radioactive materials in the diagnosis and treatment of disease and illness
radiology	branch of medicine concerned with the use of radioactive substances for diagnosis and therapy
rales	coarse sound on inspiration, also known as crackle (heard on auscultation)
real time	two-dimensional display of both the structures and the motion of tissues and organs, with the length of time also recorded as part of the study
reduction	replacement to normal position
Relative Value Unit	RVU, unit value that has been assigned for each service
Resource-Based Relative Value Scale	RBRVS, scale designed to decrease Medicare expenditures, redistribute physician payment, and ensure quality health care at reasonable rates
resource intensity	refers to the relative volume and type of diagnostic, therapeutic, and bed services used in the management of a particular illness
retrograde	moving backward or against the usual direction of flow
rhinoplasty	surgical repair of nose
rhinorrhea	nasal mucous discharge
salpingectomy	surgical removal of the uterine tube
salpingostomy	creation of a fistula into the uterine tube
scan	mapping of emissions of radioactive substances after they have been introduced into the body; the density can determine normal or abnormal conditions
sclera	outer covering of the eye
scoliosis	lateral curve of the spine
sebaceous gland	secretes sebum
seborrhea	excess sebum secretion
sebum	oily substance
section	slice of a frozen block
segmentectomy	surgical removal of a portion of a lung
septoplasty	surgical repair of the nasal septum
serum	blood from which the fibrinogen has been removed
severity of illness	refers to the levels of loss of function and mortality that may be experienced by patients with a particular disease
shunt	an artificial passage
sialography	radiographic recording of the salivary duct and branches
sialolithotomy	surgical removal of a stone of the salivary gland or duct

sinography	radiographic recording of the sinus or sinus tract
sinusotomy	surgical incision into a sinus
skeletal traction	application of pressure to the bone by means of pins and/or wires inserted into the bone
skin traction	application of pressure to the bone by means of tape applied to the skin
skull	entire skeletal framework of the head
somatic nerve	sensory or motor nerve
specimen	sample of tissue or fluid
spirometry	measurement of breathing capacity
splenectomy	excision of the spleen
splenography	radiographic recording of the spleen
splenoportography	radiographic procedure to allow visualization of the splenic and portal veins of the spleen
split-thickness graft	all epidermis and some of dermis
spondylitis	inflammation of vertebrae
Staff Model	a Health Maintenance Organization that directly employs the physicians who provide services to enrollees
steatoma	fat mass in sebaceous gland
stem cell	immature blood cell
stereotaxis	method of identifying a specific area or point in the brain
strabismus	extraocular muscle deviation resulting in unequal visual axes
stratified	layered
stratum (strata)	layer
subcutaneous	tissue below the dermis, primarily fat cells that insulate the body
subluxation	partial dislocation
subungual	beneath the nail
superior	toward the head or the upper part of the body; also known as cephalic
supination	supine position
supine	lying on the back
Swan Ganz catheter	a catheter that measures pressure in the heart
sympathetic nerve	part of the peripheral nervous system that controls automatic body function and sympathetic nerves activated under stress
symphysis	natural junction
synchondrosis	union between two bones (connected by cartilage)
tachypnea	quick, shallow breathing
tarsorrhaphy	suturing together of the eyelids

Tax Equity and Fiscal Responsibility Act	TEFRA, act that contains language to reward cost-conscious health care providers
tendon	attaches a muscle to a bone
tenodesis	suturing of a tendon to a bone
tenorrhaphy	suture repair of tendon
thermogram	written record of temperature variation
third-party payer	insurance company or entity that is liable for another's health care services
thoracentesis	surgical puncture of the thoracic cavity, usually using a needle, to remove fluids
thoracic duct	collection and distribution point for lymph, and the largest lymph vessel located in the chest
thoracoplasty	surgical procedure that removes rib(s) and thereby allows the collapse of a lung
thoracoscopy	use of a lighted endoscope to view the pleural spaces and thoracic cavity or to perform surgical procedures
thoracostomy	incision into the chest wall and insertion of a chest tube
thoracotomy	surgical incision into the chest wall
thromboendarterectomy	procedure to remove plaque or clot formations from a vessel by percutaneous method
thymectomy	surgical removal of the thymus
thymus	gland that produces hormones important to the immune response
thyroglossal duct	connection between the thyroid and the tongue
thyroid	part of the endocrine system that produces hormones that regulate metabolism
thyroidectomy	surgical removal of the thyroid
tinnitus	ringing in the ears
titer	measure of a laboratory analysis
tocolysis	repression of uterine contractions
tomography	procedure that allows viewing of a single plane of the body by blurring out all but that particular level
tonography	recording of changes in intraocular pressure in response to sustained pressure on the eyeball
tonometry	measurement of pressure or tension
total pneumonectomy	surgical removal of an entire lung
tracheostomy	creation of an opening into trachea
tracheotomy	incision into trachea
traction	application of pressure to maintain normal alignment
transcutaneous	entering by way of the skin

transesophageal echocardiogram	TEE, echocardiogram performed by placing a probe down the esophagus and sending out sound waves to obtain images of the heart and its movement
transmastoid	creates an opening in the mastoid for drainage antrostomy
transplantation	grafting of tissue from one source to another
transseptal	through the septum
transtracheal	across the trachea
transureteroureterostomy	surgical connection of one ureter to the other ureter
transurethral resection, prostate	procedure performed through the urethra by means of a cystoscopy to remove part or all of the prostate
transvenous	through a vein
transvesical ureterolithotomy	removal of a ureter stone (calculus) through the bladder
trephination	surgical removal of a disk of bone
trocar needle	needle with a tube on the end; used to puncture and withdraw fluid from a cavity
tubercle	lesion caused by infection of tuberculosis
tumescence	state of being swollen
tunica vaginalis	covering of the testes
tympanolysis	freeing of adhesions of the tympanic membrane
tympanometry	test of the inner ear using air pressure
tympanostomy	insertion of ventilation tube into tympanum
ultrasound	technique using sound waves to determine the density of the outline of tissue
unbundling	reporting with multiple codes that which can be reported with one code
unilateral	occurring on one side
uptake	absorption of a radioactive substance by body tissues; recorded for diagnostic purposes in conditions such as thyroid disease
ureterectomy	surgical removal of a ureter, either totally or partially
ureterocolon	pertaining to the ureter and colon
ureterocutaneous fistula	channel from the ureter to exterior skin
ureteroenterostomy	creation of a connection between the intestine and the ureter
ureterolithotomy	removal of a stone from the ureter
ureterolysis	freeing of adhesions of the ureter
ureteroneocystostomy	surgical connection of the ureter to a new site on the bladder
ureteropyelography	ureter and bladder radiography
ureterotomy	incision into the ureter
urethrocystography	radiography of the bladder and urethra
urethromeatoplasty	surgical repair of the urethra and meatus

urethropexy	fixation of the urethra by means of surgery
urethroplasty	surgical repair of the urethra
urethrorrhaphy	suturing of the urethra
urethroscopy	use of a scope to view the urethra
urography	same as pyelography; radiographic recording of the kidneys, renal pelvis, ureters, and bladder
uveal	vascular tissue of the choroid, ciliary body, and iris
varices	varicose veins
varicocele	swelling of a scrotal vein
vas deferens	tube that carries sperm from the epididymis to the urethra
vasogram	recording of the flow in the vas deferens
vasotomy	incision in the vas deferens
vasorrhaphy	suturing of the vas deferens
vasovasostomy	reversal of a vasectomy
vectorcardiogram	VCG, continuous recording of electrical direction and magnitude of the heart
venography	radiographic recording of the veins and tributaries
vertebrectomy	removal of vertebra
vertigo	dizziness
vesicostomy	surgical creation of a connection of the viscera of the bladder to the skin
vesicovaginal fistula	creation of a tube between the vagina and the bladder
vesiculectomy	excision of the seminal vesicle
vesiculography	radiographic recording of the seminal vesicles
vesiculotomy	incision into the seminal vesicle
viscera	an organ in one of the large cavities of the body
volvulus	twisted section of the intestine
vomer	flat bones of the nasal septum
xanthoma	tumor composed of cells containing lipid material, yellow in color
xenograft	different species graft
xeroderma	dry, discolored, scaly skin
xeroradiography	photoelectric process of radiographs

Combining Forms

abdomin/o	abdomen
acetabul/o	hip socket
acr/o	height/extremities
aden/o	in relationship to a gland
adenoid/o	adenoids
adip/o	fat
adren/o, adrenal/o	adrenal gland
albin/o	white
albumin/o	albumin
alveol/o	alveolus
ambly/o	dim
amni/o	amnion
an/o	anus
andr/o	male
andren/o	adrenal gland
andrenal/o	adrenal gland
angi/o	vessel
ankyl/o	bent, fused
aort/o	aorta
aponeur/o	tendon type
appendic/o	appendix
aque/o	water
arche/o	first
arter/o, arteri/o	artery
arthr/o	joint
atel/o	incomplete
ather/o	plaque
atri/o	atrium

audi/o	hearing
aut/o	self
axill/o	armpit
azot/o	urea
balan/o	glans penis
bi/o	life
bil/i	bile
bilirubin/o	bile pigment
blephar/o	eyelid
brachi/o	arm
bronch/o	bronchus
bronchi/o	bronchus
bronchiol/o	bronchiole
burs/o	fluid-filled sac in a joint
calc/o, calc/i	calcium
cardi/o	heart
carp/o	carpals (wrist bones)
cauter/o	burn
cec/o	cecum
celi/o	abdomen
cephal/o	head
cerebell/o	cerebellum
cerebr/o	cerebrum
cervic/o	neck/cervix
chol/e	gall/bile
cholangio/o	bile duct
cholecyst/o	gallbladder
choledoch/o	common bile duct
cholester/o	cholesterol
chondr/o	cartilage
chori/o	chorion
clavic/o, clavicul/o	clavicle (collar bone)
col/o	colon
colp/o	vagina
coni/o	dust
conjunctiv/o	conjunctiva

cor/o, core/o	pupil
corne/o	cornea
coron/o	heart
cortic/o	cortex
cost/o	rib
crani/o	cranium (skull)
crin/o	secrete
crypt/o	hidden
culd/o	cul-de-sac
cutane/o	skin
cyan/o	blue
cycl/o	ciliary body
cyst/o	bladder
dacry/o	tear
dacryocyst/o	prefix meaning pertaining to the lacrimal sac
dent/i	tooth
derm/o, dermat/o	skin
diaphragmat/o	diaphragm
dips/o	thirst
disk/o	intervertebral disk
diverticul/o	diverticulum
duoden/o	duodenum
dur/o	dura mater
encephal/o	brain
enter/o	small intestine
eosin/o	rosy
epididym/o	epididymis
epiglott/o	epiglottis
episi/o	vulva
erythr/o, erythem/o	red
esophag/o	esophagus
essi/o, esthesi/o	sensation
estr/o	female
femor/o	thighbone
fet/o	fetus
fibul/o	fibula

galact/o	milk
gangli/o	ganglion
ganglion/o	ganglion
gastr/o	stomach
gingiv/o	gum
glomerul/o	glomerulus
gloss/o	tongue
gluc/o	sugar
glyc/o	sugar
glycos/o	sugar
gonad/o	ovaries and testes
gyn/o	female
gynec/o	female
hepat/o	liver
herni/o	hernia
heter/o	different
hidr/o	sweat
home/o	same
hormon/o	hormone
humer/o	humerus (upper arm bone)
hydr/o	water
hymen/o	hymen
hyster/o	uterus
ichthy/o	dry/scaly
ile/o	ileus
ili/o	ilium (upper pelvic bone)
immun/o	immune
inguin/o	groin
ir/o	iris
irid/o	iris
ischi/o	ischium (posterior pelvic bone)
jaund/o	yellow
jejun/o	jejunum
kal/i	potassium
kerat/o	hard, cornea

kinesi/o	movement
kyph/o	hump
lacrim/o	tear
lact/o	milk
lamin/o	lamina
lapar/o	abdomen
laryng/o	larynx
lingu/o	tongue
lip/o	fat
lith/o	stone
lob/o	lobe
lord/o	curve
lumb/o	lower back
lute/o	yellow
lymph/o	lymph
lymphaden/o	lymph gland
mamm/o	breast
mandibul/o	mandible (lower jawbone)
mast/o	breast
maxill/o	maxilla (upper jawbone)
meat/o	meatus
melan/o	black
men/o	menstruation, month
mening/o, meningi/o	meninges
menisc/o, menisci/o	meniscus
ment/o	mind
metacarp/o	metacarpals (hand)
metatars/o	metatarsals (foot)
metr/o	uterus, measure
metr/i	uterus
mon/o	one
muc/o	mucus
my/o, muscul/o	muscle
myc/o	fungus

myel/o	bone marrow, spinal cord
myring/o	ear drum
myx/o	mucus
nas/o	nose
nat/a, nat/i	birth
natr/o	sodium
necr/o	death
nephr/o	kidney
neur/o	nerve
noct/i	night
ocul/o	eye
olecran/o	olecranon (elbow)
olig/o	scant, few
onych/o	nail
oo/o	egg
oophor/o	ovary
ophthalm/o	eye
opt/o	eye, vision
optic/o	eye
or/o	mouth
orch/i, orch/o, orchi/o, orchid/o	testicle
orth/o	straight
oste/o	bone
ot/o	ear
ov/o	egg
ovari/o	ovary
ovul/o	ovulation
ox/i, ox/o	oxygen
oxy/o	oxygen
pachy/o	thick
palat/o	palate
palpebr/o	eyelid
pancreat/o	pancreas

papill/o	optic nerve
patell/o	patella (kneecap)
pelv/i	pelvis (hip)
pericardi/o	pericardium
perine/o	perineum
peritone/o	peritoneum
petr/o	stone
phac/o	eye lens
phak/o	eye lens
phalang/o	phalanges (finger or toe)
pharyng/o	pharynx
phas/o	speech
phleb/o	vein
phren/o	mind, diaphragm
phys/o	growing
pil/o	hair
pituitar/o	pituitary gland
pleur/o	pleura
pneumat/o	lung/air
pneumon/o	lung/air
poli/o	gray matter
polyp/o	polyp
pont/o	pons
proct/o	rectum
prostat/o	prostate gland
psych/o	mind
pub/o	pubis
pulmon/o	lung
pupill/o	pupil
py/o	pus
pyel/o	renal pelvis
pylor/o	pylorus
quadr/i	four
rachi/o	spine
radi/o	radius (lower arm)
radic/o, radicul/o	nerve root
rect/o	rectum

ren/o	kidney
retin/o	retina
rhin/o	nose
rhiz/o	nerve root
rhytid/o	wrinkle
rube/o	red
sacr/o	sacrum
salping/o	uterine tube, Fallopian tube
scapul/o	scapula (shoulder)
scler/o	sclera
scoli/o	bent
seb/o	sebum/oil
semin/i	semen
sept/o	septum
sial/o	saliva
sigmoid/o	sigmoid colon
sinus/o	sinus
somat/o	body
son/o	sound
sperm/o, spermat/o	sperm
sphygm/o	pulse
spir/o	breath
splen/o	spleen
spondyl/o	vertebra
staped/o	middle ear, stapes
staphyl/o	clusters
steat/o	fat
ster/o, stere/o	solid, having three dimensions
stern/o	sternum (breast bone)
steth/o	chest
stomat/o	mouth
strept/o	twisted chain
synovi/o	synovial joint membrane
tars/o	tarsal (ankle)
ten/o	tendon

tend/o, tendin/o	tendon (connective tissue)
test/o	testicle
thorac/o	thorax
thromb/o	clot
thym/o	thymus gland
thyr/o, thyroid/o	thyroid gland
tibi/o	shin bone
toc/o	childbirth
tonsill/o	tonsil
top/o	place
tox/o, toxic/o	poison
trache/o	trachea
trich/o	hair
tympan/o	ear drum
uln/o	ulna (lower arm bone)
ungu/o	nail
ur/o	urine
ureter/o	ureter
urethr/o	urethra
urin/o	urine
uter/o	uterus
uve/o	uvea
uvul/o	uvula
vagin/o	vagina
valv/o, valvul/o	valve
vas/o, vascul/o	vessel
ven/o	vein
ventricul/o	ventricle
vertebr/o	vertebra
vesic/o	bladder
vesicul/o	seminal vesicles

vitre/o	glass/glassy
vulv/o	vulva
xanth/o	yellow
xer/o	dry

Prefixes

a-	not
an-	not
ante-	before
audi-	hearing
bi-	two
brady-	slow
de-	lack of
dys-	difficult, painful
ecto-	outside
endo-	in
epi-	on/upon
eso-	inward
eu-	good/normal
exo-	outward
extra-	outside
hemi-	half
hyper-	excess, over
hypo-	under
in-	into
inter-	between
intra-	within
meta-	change, after
multi-	many
neo-	new
nulli-, nulti-	none
oxy-	sharp, oxygen
pan-	all
para-	beside

per-	through
peri-	surrounding
poly-	many
post-	after
primi-	first
pseudo-	false
quadri-	four
retro-	behind
sub-	under
supra-	above
sym-	together
syn-	together
tachy-	fast
tetra-	four
tri-	three
tropin-	act upon
uni-	one

Suffixes

-agon	assemble
-algesia	pain sensation
-algia	pain
-ar	pertaining to
-arche	beginning
-ary	pertaining to
-asthenia	weakness
-blast	embryonic
-capnia	carbon dioxide
-cele	hernia
-centesis	puncture to remove (drain)
-chezia	defecation
-clast, -clasia, -clasis	break
-coccus	spherical bacterium
-cyesis	pregnancy
-desis	fusion
-dilation	widening, expanding
-drome	run
-dynia	pain
-eal	pertaining to
-ectasis	stretching
-ectomy	removal
-edema	swelling
-emia	blood
-esthesis	feeling
-gram	record
-graph	recording instrument
-graphy	recording process

-gravida	pregnancy
-ia	condition
-iatrist	physician specialist
-iatry	medical treatment
-ical	pertaining to
-ictal	pertaining to
-in	a substance
-ine	a substance
-itis	inflammation
-listhesis	slipping
-lithiasis	condition of stones
-lysis	separation
-malacia	softening
-megaly	enlargement
-meta	change
-meter	measurement or instrument that measures
-metry	measurement of
-oid	resembling
-oma	tumor
-one	hormone
-opia	vision
-opsy	view of
-orrhexis	rupture
-osis	condition
-oxia	oxygen
-para	woman who has given birth
-paresis	incomplete paralysis
-parous	to bear
-penia	deficient
-pexy	fixation
-phagia	eating
-phonia	sound
-phylaxis	protection
-physis	to grow
-plasty	repair
-plegia	paralysis
-pnea	breathing

-poiesis	production
-poly	many
-porosis	passage
-retro	behind
-rrhagia	bursting of blood
-rrhaphy	suture
-rrhea	discharge
-schisis	split
-sclerosis	hardening
-scopy	to examine
-spasm	contraction of muscle
-steat/o	fat
-stenosis	blockage, narrowing
-stomy	opening
-thorax	chest
-tocia	labor
-tom/o	to cut
-tome	an instrument that cuts
-tomy	cutting, incision
-tripsy	crush
-tropia	to turn
-tropin	act upon
-uria	urine
-version	turning

Abbreviations

ABG	arterial blood gas
ABN	Advanced Beneficiary Notice used by CMS to notify beneficiary of payment of provider services
ACL	anterior cruciate ligament
AD	right ear
AFB	acid-fast bacillus
AFI	amniotic fluid index
AGA	appropriate for gestational age
AGCUS	atypical glandular cells of undetermined significance
AKA	above-knee amputation
ANS	autonomic nervous system
APCs	Ambulatory Payment Classifications, patient classification that provides a payment system for outpatients
ARDS	adult respiratory distress syndrome
ARF	acute renal failure
ARM	artificial rupture of membrane
AS	left ear
ASCUS	atypical squamous cells of undetermined significance
ASCVD	arteriosclerotic cardiovascular disease
ASD	atrial septal defect
ASHD	arteriosclerotic heart disease
AU	both ears
AV	atrioventricular
BCC	benign cellular changes
BiPAP	bi-level positive airway pressure
BKA	below-knee amputation
BP	blood pressure
BPD	biparietal diameter

BPH	benign prostatic hypertrophy
BPP	biophysical profile
BUN	blood urea nitrogen
BV	bacterial vaginosis
bx	biopsy
C1-C7	cervical vertebrae
ca	cancer
CABG	coronary artery bypass graft
CBC	complete blood (cell) count
CF	conversion factor, national dollar amount that is applied to all services paid on the Medicare Fee Schedule basis
CHF	congestive heart failure
CHL	crown-to-heel length
CK	creatine kinase
CMS	Centers for Medicare and Medicaid Services, formerly HCFA, Health Care Financing Administration
CNM	certified nurse midwife
CNS	central nervous system
COB	coordination of benefits, management of payment between two or more third-party payers for a service
COPD	chronic obstructive pulmonary disease
CPAP	continuous positive airway pressure
CPD	cephalopelvic disproportion
CPK	creatine phosphokinase
CPP	chronic pelvic pain
CSF	cerebrospinal fluid
CTS	carpal tunnel syndrome
CVA	stroke/cerebrovascular accident
CVI	cerebrovascular insufficiency
D&C	dilation and curettage
D&E	dilation and evacuation
derm	dermatology
DHHS	Department of Health and Human Services
DLCO	diffuse capacity of lungs for carbon monoxide
DRGs	Diagnosis-Related Groups, disease classification system that relates the type of inpatients a hospital treats (case mix) to the costs incurred by the hospital
DSE	dobutamine stress echocardiography

DUB	dysfunctional uterine bleeding
ECC	endocervical curettage
EDC	estimated date of confinement
EDD	estimated date of delivery
EDI	electronic data interchange, exchange of data between multiple computer terminals
EEG	electroencephalogram
EFM	electronic fetal monitoring
EFW	estimated fetal weight
EGA	estimated gestational age
EGD	esophagogastroduodenoscopy
EGJ	esophagogastric junction
EMC	endometrial curettage
EOB	explanation of benefits, remittance advice
EPO	Exclusive Provider Organization, similar to a Health Maintenance Organization except that the providers of the services are not prepaid, but rather are paid on a fee-for-service basis
EPSDT	Early and Periodic Screening, Diagnosis, and Treatment
ERCP	endoscopic retrograde cholangiopancreatography
ERT	estrogen replacement therapy
ESRD	end-stage renal disease
FAS	fetal alcohol syndrome
FEF	forced expiratory flow
FEV_1	forced expiratory volume in 1 second
FEV_1:FVC	ratio of forced expiratory volume in 1 second to forced vital capacity
FHR	fetal heart rate
FI	fiscal intermediary, financial agent acting on behalf of a third-party payer
FRC	functional residual capacity
FSH	follicle-stimulating hormone
FVC	forced vital capacity
fx	fracture
GERD	gastroesophageal reflux disease
GI	gastrointestinal
H or E	hemorrhage or exudate
HCFA	Health Care Financing Administration, now known as Centers for Medicare and Medicaid Services (CMS)
HCVD	hypertensive cardiovascular disease
HD	hemodialysis

HDL	high-density lipoprotein
HEA	hemorrhage, exudate, aneurysm
HHN	hand-held nebulizer
HJR	hepatojugular reflux
H&P	history and physical
HPV	human papillomavirus
HSG	hysterosalpingogram
HSV	herpes simplex virus
I&D	incision and drainage
IO	intraocular
IOL	intraocular lens
IPAP	inspiratory positive airway pressure
IRDS	infant respiratory distress syndrome
IVF	in vitro fertilization
IVP	intravenous pyelogram
JBP	jugular blood pressure
KUB	kidneys, ureter, bladder
L1-L5	lumbar vertebrae
LBBB	left bundle branch block
LEEP	loop electrosurgical excision procedure
LGA	large for gestational age
LLQ	left lower quadrant
LP	lumbar puncture
LUQ	left upper quadrant
LVH	left ventricular hypertrophy
MAT	multifocal atrial tachycardia
MDI	metered dose inhaler
MI	myocardial infarction
MRI	magnetic resonance imaging
MSLT	multiple sleep latency testing
MVV	maximum voluntary ventilation
NCPAP	nasal continuous positive airway pressure
NSR	normal sinus rhythm
OA	osteoarthritis
OD	right eye
OS	left eye
OU	each eye

PAC	premature atrial contraction
PAT	paroxysmal atrial tachycardia
PAWP	pulmonary artery wedge pressure
PCWP	pulmonary capillary wedge pressure
PEAP	positive end-airway pressure
PEEP	positive end-expiratory pressure
PEG	percutaneous endoscopic gastrostomy
PERL	pupils equal and reactive to light
PERRL	pupils equal, round, and reactive to light
PERRLA	pupils equal, round, and reactive to light and accommodation
PFT	pulmonary function test
pH	symbol for acid/base level
PICC	peripherally inserted central catheter
PID	pelvic inflammatory disease
PND	paroxysmal nocturnal dyspnea
PNS	peripheral nervous system
PROM	premature rupture of membranes
PSA	prostate-specific antigen
PST	paroxysmal supraventricular tachycardia
PSVT	paroxysmal supraventricular tachycardia
PT	prothrombin time
PTCA	percutaneous transluminal coronary angioplasty
PTT	partial thromboplastin time
PVC	premature ventricular contraction
RA	remittance advice, explanation of services
RA	rheumatoid arthritis
RBBB	right bundle branch block
RDS	respiratory distress syndrome
REM	rapid eye movement
RLQ	right lower quadrant
RSR	regular sinus rhythm
RUQ	right upper quadrant
RV	respiratory volume
RVG	*Relative Value Guide*
RVH	right ventricular hypertrophy
RVS	relative value studies, list of procedures with unit values assigned to each
RV:TLC	ratio of respiratory volume to total lung capacity

SHG	sonohysterogram
sp gr	specific gravity
SROM	spontaneous rupture of membranes
subcu, subq, SC, SQ	subcutaneous
SUI	stress urinary incontinence
SVT	supraventricular tachycardia
T1-T12	thoracic vertebrae
TAH	total abdominal hysterectomy
TEE	transesophageal echocardiography
TENS	transcutaneous electrical nerve stimulation
TIA	transient ischemic attack
TLC	total lung capacity
TLV	total lung volume
TM	tympanic membrane
TMJ	temporomandibular joint
TPA	tissue plasminogen activator
TSH	thyroid-stimulating hormone
TST	treadmill stress test
TURBT	transurethral resection of bladder tumor
TURP	transurethral resection of prostate
UA	urinalysis
UCR	usual, customary, and reasonable—third-party payers' assessment of the reimbursement for health care services: usual, that which would ordinarily be charged for the service; customary, the cost of that service in that locale; and reasonable, as assessed by the payer
UPJ	ureteropelvic junction
URI	upper respiratory infection
UTI	urinary tract infection
V/Q	ventilation/perfusion scan
VBAC	vaginal birth after cesarean
WBC	white blood (cell) count

Further Text Resources

ANATOMY AND PHYSIOLOGY

Book Title	Author	Imprint	Publication Date	ISBN-13
The Anatomy and Physiology Learning System, 3rd Edition	Applegate	Saunders	2006	978-1-4160-2586-3
Gray's Anatomy for Students	Drake, Vogl, Mitchell	Churchill Livingstone	2005	978-0-443-06612-2
Anthony's Textbook of Anatomy and Physiology, 18th edition	Thibodeau, Patton	Mosby	2006	978-0-323-03982-6

CODING

Book Title	Author	Imprint	Publication Date	ISBN-13
Step-by-Step Medical Coding, 2007 Edition	Buck	Saunders	2007	978-1-4160-0133-1
Saunders 2007 ICD-9-CM, Volumes 1 & 2	Buck	Saunders	2007	978-1-4160-4037-8
Saunders 2007 ICD-9-CM, Volumes 1, 2, & 3	Buck	Saunders	2007	978-1-4160-4040-8
Saunders 2007 HCPCS Level II	Buck	Saunders	2007	978-1-4160-4039-2
The Next Step: Medical Coding from Classroom to Practice, A Worktext, 2nd edition	Buck	Saunders	2006	978-1-4160-2321-0
The Extra Step: Facility-Based Coding Practice	Buck	Saunders	2006	978-1-4160-3450-6
The Extra Step: Physician-Based Coding Practice	Buck	Saunders	2006	978-1-4160-3451-3
CCS Coding Exam Review 2007: The Certification Step	Buck	Saunders	2007	978-1-4160-3678-4
CCS-P Coding Exam Review 2007: The Certification Step	Buck	Saunders	2007	978-1-4160-3689-0
CPC-H Coding Exam Review 2007: The Certification Step	Buck	Saunders	2007	978-1-4160-3717-0

PATHOPHYSIOLOGY

Book Title	Author	Imprint	Publication Date	ISBN-13
Pathology for the Health Professions, 3rd Edition	Damjanov	Saunders	2006	978-1-4160-0031-0
Essentials of Human Diseases and Conditions, 3rd Edition	Frazier, Drzymkowski	Saunders	2004	978-0-7216-0256-1
Pathophysiology for the Health Related Professions, 3rd Edition	Gould	Saunders	2006	978-1-4160-0210-9
The Human Body in Health and Illness, 3rd Edition	Herlihy	Saunders	2007	978-1-4160-2885-7
The Human Body in Health and Disease, 4th Edition	Thibodeau, Patton	Mosby	2005	978-0-323-03162-2

MEDICAL TERMINOLOGY

Book Title	Author	Imprint	Publication Date	ISBN-13
The Language of Medicine, 8th Edition	Chabner	Saunders	2007	978-1-4160-3492-6
Dictionary of Medical Acronyms & Abbreviations, 5th edition	Jablonski	Hanley & Belfus	2005	978-1-560-53632-1
Exploring Medical Language, 6th Edition	LaFleur, Brooks	Mosby	2005	978-0-323-02805-9
Building a Medical Vocabulary (with Spanish Translations), 6th Edition	Leonard	Saunders	2005	978-0-7216-0464-0
Quick & Easy Medical Terminology, 5th Edition	Leonard	Saunders	2007	978-1-4160-2494-1
Mastering Healthcare Terminology, 2nd Edition	Shiland	Mosby	2006	978-0-323-03572-9
Dorland's Illustrated Medical Dictionary, 31st Edition		Saunders	2007	978-1-4160-2364-7

INTRODUCTION TO COMPUTER

Book Title	Author	Imprint	Publication Date	ISBN-13
Computerized Medical Office Procedures: A Worktext	Larsen	Saunders	2002	978-0-7216-9213-5

BASICS OF WRITING/MEDICAL TRANSCRIPTION

Book Title	Author	Imprint	Publication Date	ISBN-13
Essentials of Medical Transcription: A Modular Approach, 2nd Edition	Destafano, Federman	Saunders	2004	978-0-7216-1015-3
Medical Transcription Guide: Do's and Don'ts, 3rd edition	Diehl	Saunders	2005	978-0-7216-0684-2
Diehl & Fordney's Medical Transcribing: Techniques and Procedures, 6th Edition	Diehl	Saunders	2007	978-1-4160-2347-0

COMPREHENSION BUILDING/STUDY SKILLS

Book Title	Author	Imprint	Publication Date	ISBN-13
Career Development for Health Professionals: Success in School and on the Job 2nd edition	Haroun	Saunders	2006	978-0-7216-0609-5

BASIC MATH

Book Title	Author	Imprint	Publication Date	ISBN-13
Basic Mathematics for the Health-Related Professions	Doucette	Saunders	2000	978-0-7216-7938-9
Using Maths in Health Sciences	Gunn	Churchill Livingstone	2001	978-0-443-07074-7

MEDICAL BILLING/INSURANCE

Book Title	Author	Imprint	Publication Date	ISBN-13
Medical Insurance Made Easy: Understanding the Claim Cycle, 2nd Edition	Brown	Saunders	2006	978-0-7216-0556-2
Quick Guide to HIPAA for the Physician's Office	Burton	Saunders	2004	978-0-7216-3935-2
Insurance Handbook for the Medical Office, 9th Edition	Fordney	Saunders	2006	978-1-4160-0100-3
Medical Insurance Billing and Coding: An Essentials Worktext	French, Fordney	Saunders	2002	978-0-7216-9516-7

Index

Note: *Page numbers followed by* **f** *indicate figure.*

Atrium. *See* Left atrium; Right atrium
Atrophy, 10f, 11
  medical term, 42, A68
Attending physician, 269
Atypical glandular cells of undetermined significance (AGCUS), A102
Atypical squamous cells of undetermined significance (ASCUS), A102
AU. *See* Both ears
Audiometry, medical term, A68
Aural atresia, medical term, 241, A68
Auricle (pinna), 31f
Auscultation, medical term, 59, 77, A68
Autograft, medical term, 5, A68
Autonomic nervous system (ANS), 215, 216, A102
AV. *See* Atrioventricular
Avulsion, medical term, 5, A68
Axial skeleton, 30–33
Axillary artery, 72f
Axillary nodes, 186f
  medical term, 187, A68
Axillary vein, 73f
Axon, 213f. *See also* Myelinated axon

B
Bacilli, medical term, 59, A68
Bacterial impetigo, 19
Bacterial UTI, 144–145
Bacterial vaginosis (BV), 95, A103
Balanitis, causes/symptoms/treatment, 127
Barium enema, medical term, A68
Basal cell carcinoma, 24–25
Basilic vein, 73f
BCC. *See* Benign cellular changes
B cells, acute infection, 193
Below-knee amputation (BKA), 42, A102
Beneficiary, 269
  medical term, A68
Benign cellular changes (BCC), A102
Benign lesions, 105–106

Benign prostatic hypertrophy (BPH), 118, A103
  symptoms/screening/treatment, 129
Benign tumors (keratoses), 24
Biceps, aponeurosis, 38f
Biceps femoris, 37f
Bicuspid valve. *See* Mitral valve
Bifocal, medical term, A68
Bilaminate skin, medical term, A68
Bilateral, medical term, A68
Bi-level positive airway pressure (BiPAP), 58, A102
Biliary, medical term, 158, A68
Bilobectomy, medical term, 60, A68
Biofeedback, medical term, A68
Biological substances, adverse effects (E codes guidelines), A56
Biometry, medical term, A69
Biophysical profile (BPP), 95, A103
Biopsy (bx), A103
  codes, 345
  medical term, 5, A69
BiPAP. *See* Bi-level positive airway pressure
Biparietal diameter (BPD), 95, A102
Birthday rule, 269
BKA. *See* Below-knee amputation
Bladder, 344–345
  carcinoma, 148
Block, medical term, A69
Blood
  carrying function, 71
  component, 71
  diseases, ICD-9-CM coding, 396, A20
  formed part, 71
  liquid component, 71
  pressure, elevation, 399
  protection, 71
  regulation, 71
Blood-forming organs, ICD-9-CM coding, 396, A20
Blood pressure (BP), A102. *See also* Jugular blood pressure
  classification, 82f
Blood urea nitrogen (BUN), 138, A103

Blood vessels, 71–72. *See also* Retinal blood vessels
  function, 71
  obstruction, 84–85
  tumors, 232
  types, 71–72
Boil. *See* Furuncle
Bold type, 383
Bones
  classification, 29
  dislocations, 48
  disorders, 48–49
  improper union, 48
  ligaments, bone anchors, 37
  structure, 30f
  tendons, muscle anchors, 37
  tumors, 51
    origin, 51
Bony wall, 31f
Both ears (AU), 240, A102
BP. *See* Blood pressure
BPD. *See* Biparietal diameter
BPH. *See* Benign prostatic hypertrophy
BPP. *See* Biophysical profile
Brace, usage, 383
Brachial artery, 72f
Brachial vein, 73f
Brachiocephalic artery, 74f
Brachiocephalic trunk, 72f
Brachiocephalic vein, 73f
Brachytherapy, medical term, A69
Brackets
  codes, 389
  usage, 382. *See also* Slanted brackets
Brain, 214f
  abscess, 229
  divisions, 213–215
  tumors, 231–233
Brainstem, 213, 214f
Breast
  carcinoma, 106–107
  risks, increased, 106
  structure, 92f
Breech position, 113f
Broad ligament, 91f
Bronchiectasis, 66
Bronchioles, 56f
  medical term, 60, A69
Bronchiolitis, 66
Bronchitis, ICD-9-CM coding, A24–A25
Bronchography, medical term, A69
Bronchoplasty, medical term, 60, A69

Certified Registered Nurse Anesthetist (CRNA), 270
Cervical, medical term, A70
Cervical dilator, insertion, 351
Cervical malignancies, staging, 107
Cervical vertebrae, 33f, 35f. *See also* Seventh cervical vertebra
  C1-C7, 42, A103
Cervix, 91f
  carcinoma, 108
  risks, increased, 108
  uteri, medical term, A70
Cervix uteri, 348
Cesarean, medical term, 96
CF. *See* Contributing factor; Conversion factor
Chemotherapy, exception, 395
CHF. *See* Congestive heart failure
Chief complaint (CC), 287
Childbirth
  complications, ICD-9-CM coding, 401–402, A26–A30
  HIV infection, ICD-9-CM coding, A27
Children
  abuse, E codes guideline, A57
  V codes, A46
CHL. *See* Crown-to-heel length
Chlamydia, cause/symptoms/treatment, 103
Cholangiography, medical term, 158, A70
Cholangiopancreatography, medical term, A70
Cholangitis, 177
Cholecystectomy, medical term, 158, A70
Cholecystitis, 177
Cholecystoenterostomy, medical term, 158, A70
Cholecystography, medical term, A70
Cholelithiasis, 177–178
Cholesteatoma, medical term, 241, A70
Chondral, medical term, 42, A70
Chondroblastoma, 51
Chondrosarcoma, 51
Chordee, medical term, 118, A70

Chorionic villus sampling (CVS), medical term, 96, A70
Choroid (middle layer), 237, 237f
Chronic atrophic gastritis, 166–167
Chronic conditions, ICD-9-CM coding, 388
Chronic esophagitis, 165
Chronic glaucoma, 248
Chronic kidney disease, ICD-9-CM coding, A25–A26
Chronic leukemia, 194
Chronic obstructive pulmonary disease (COPD), 58, 68, A103
  ICD-9-CM coding, A24
Chronic pelvic pain (CPP), 95, A103
Chronic prostatitis, 130
Chronic pyelonephritis, 146
Chronic renal failure, 143–144
Ciliary body, 237f
Circulatory system
  arteries, 72f
  diseases, ICD-9-CM coding, 397–399, A21–A23
  veins, 73f
Circumflex, medical term, 77, A70
Cirrhosis, 176–177
Cisterna chylia, 186f
CK. *See* Creatine kinase
Clavicle, 35f
Clean claim, 270
Cleft lip, 163
Cleft palate, 163, 163f
Cloquet's node, medical term, 187, A70
Closed fracture, 47
  repair, medical term, 42, A70
Closed treatment, medical term, 42, A70
CMG. *See* Cystometrogram
CMS. *See* Centers for Medicare and Medicaid Services
CNM. *See* Certified nurse midwife
CNS. *See* Central nervous system
COB. *See* Coordination of benefits
Coccyx (tailbone), 33f
  medical term, A70
Cochlea, 31f
Codes. *See* Bundled codes; E codes; V codes

Coding resources, A108
Coinsurance, 270
Cold sores. *See* Viral herpes simplex
Collagen, medical term, 5, A70
Collecting ducts, 136f
Colles' fracture, medical term, 42, A70
Colon, 383. *See also* Ascending colon; Descending colon; Sigmoid colon; Transverse colon
Colonic flexure. *See* Left colonic flexure; Right colonic flexure
Colonoscopy, medical term, 158, A70
Colorectal cancer, 173
Colostomy, medical term, 158, A70
Combination codes, 384, 388
Combining forms, A87–A96
Common carotid artery, 72f
Common iliac artery, 72f
Common iliac vein, 73f
Compact bone. *See* Cortical bone
Complete blood count (CBC), A103
Compliance plan, 270
Component, medical term, A70
Comprehension building, resources, A110
Comprehensive examination, 291
Comprehensive history, 289
Computed axial tomography (CAT, CT), medical term, A70
Computers, introduction (resources), A109
Concurrent care, 271
Concussion, 230
Conduction system. *See* Heart
Conductive hearing loss, 249
Condyloid process, 31f
Congenital anomalies, ICD-9-CM coding, 403, A30–A31. *See also* Newborns
Congenital disorders, 150
Congenital heart defects, 85
Congenital neurologic disorders, 224–226
Congestive heart failure (CHF), 76, 85, A103
Conization, 348

Gigantism, 206, 206f
Glabella, 31f, 32f
Glands, 92f
Glans penis, 117f
Glaucoma, 248. *See also*
  Chronic glaucoma;
  Narrow angle glaucoma
  medical term, 241, A74
Glia, 213
Glioblastoma, 232
Gliomas common type,
  231–232
Global obstetric care, routine,
  352
Global package/delivery, 350
Global routine care, physician
  (impact), 352
Globe, medical term, A74
Glomerular disorders, 146
Glomeruli, 136f
Glottis, medical term, 60,
  A74
Gluteus maximus, 37f
Goiter, 207, 207f
Gonadal artery, 72f
Gonadal stromal tumors,
  symptoms/treatment, 109
Gonadal vein, 73f
Gonads. *See* Testes
Gonioscopy, medical term,
  A74
Gonorrhea, cause/
  symptoms/treatment,
  104
Gout (gouty arthritis), 50
GPO. *See* U.S. Government
  Printing Office
Gracilis, 37f
Granulocytosis, 192
Great saphenous vein, 73f
Grouper, medical term, A74
Group Practice Model,
  medical term, A74
Group Provider Number
  (GPN), 271
Growth plate, 30f
Guillain-Barré syndrome, 224

H

H. *See* Hemorrhage
Hand-held nebulizer (HHN),
  59, A105
Hard palate, 56f, 153f
Haustra, 155f
HAV. *See* Hepatitis A virus
HBV. *See* Hepatitis B virus
HCFA. *See* Health Care
  Financing Administration
HCG. *See* Human chorionic
  gonadotropin

HCPCS. *See* Healthcare
  Common Procedure
  Coding System
HCV. *See* Hepatitis C virus
HCVD. *See* Hypertensive
  cardiovascular disease
HD. *See* Hemodialysis
HDL. *See* High-density
  lipoprotein
HDV. *See* Hepatitis D virus
HEA. *See* Hemorrhage,
  exudate, and aneurysm
Head injury, 230–231
Head muscles, names, 39f
Healthcare Common
  Procedure Coding System
  (HCPCS), 379–380
  level I modifiers, 303
  level II modifiers, 283
Health Care Financing
  Administration (HCFA),
  A103, A104
Health Insurance Portability
  and Accountability Act
  (HIPAA), A1
Health maintenance
  organization (HMO), 269,
  271
  medical term, A74
Health status (factors,
  classification),
  Supplemental V01-V84
  (ICD-9-CM coding),
  A38–A54
Hearing, 238
  loss, 249. *See* Conductive
  hearing loss;
  Sensorineural hearing
  loss
Heart, 72–75
  chambers, 72
  walls, 72–73
  conduction system,
  74–75
  disease, 398. *See also*
  Ischemic heart disease
  disorders, 85–87
  electrical system, 74f
  infection/inflammation,
  86
  internal view, 74f
  valves, 74
  wall, disorders, 87
Heartbeat, phases, 75
Heart muscle. *See* Cardiac/
  heart muscle
Hemangioblastoma, 232
Hematoma, 230
  medical term, 5, 78, A75
Hematopoietic organ, 185

Hemic system, 185, 341–342
  anatomy, 185
  answers, 254
  quiz, 189–190
  combining forms, 185, 187
  medical term, 187–188
  pathophysiology, 191–196
  answers, 258
  quiz, 197–198
  prefixes, 187
  suffixes, 187
  terminology, 185
  answers, 254
  quiz, 189–190
Hemodialysis (HD), 138, A104
  medical term, A75
Hemograft, medical term, 5
Hemolysis, medical term, 78,
  A75
Hemolytic anemia, 192
Hemoptysis, 65
  medical term, 60, A75
Hemorrhage, exudate, and
  aneurysm (HEA), A105
Hemorrhage (H), 240, A104
Hemorrhoidectomy codes,
  343
Hepatic vein, 73f
Hepatitis. *See* Nonviral
  hepatitis; Viral hepatitis
  stages, 175–176
  symptoms, 175–176
Hepatitis A virus (HAV), 174
Hepatitis B virus (HBV),
  174–175
Hepatitis C virus (HCV), 175
Hepatitis D virus (HDV), 175
Hepatitis E virus (HEV), 175
Hepatography, medical term,
  A75
Hepatojugular reflux (HJR),
  158, A105
Hernia. *See* Hiatal hernia;
  Paraesophageal hernia;
  Sliding hernia
  codes, 343
  medical term, 158, A75
Herpes simplex type 1, 164
Herpes simplex virus (HSV),
  96
Herpes zoster (shingles), 22
HEV. *See* Hepatitis E virus
HHN. *See* Hand-held nebulizer
Hiatal hernia, 165–166, 165f
High-complexity MDM, 292
High-density lipoprotein
  (HDL), A105
High-severity presenting
  problem, 295
Hilum, 135f

NCPAP. *See* Nasal continuous positive airway pressure
Neck muscles, names, 39
Negative blood cultures, ICD-9-CM coding, A15
Neoplasms, ICD-9-CM coding, 384, 394–395, A16–A18
Nephrectomy, medical term. *See* Paraperitoneal nephrectomy
Nephrocutaneous fistula, medical term, 139, A78
Nephrolithotomy, medical term, 139, A78
Nephron, 136f
Nephron loss, stages, 144
Nephrorrhaphy, medical term, 139, A78
Nephrosclerosis, 149–150
Nephrostolithotomy, medical term, A78. *See also* Percutaneous nephrostolithotomy
Nephrostomy, medical term, 139, A79. *See also* Percutaneous nephrostomy
Nephrotic syndrome, 146–147
Nephrotomy, medical term, A79
Nerve damage, 406
Nervous system, 213
  anatomy, 213–215
    answers, 255
    quiz, 219–220
  cells, 213–215
  combining forms, 215–216
  diseases, ICD-9-CM coding, 397, A21
  divisions, 213–215
  medical abbreviations, 216–217
  medical term, 217
  pathophysiology, 221–233
    answers, 259
    quiz, 235–236
  prefixes, 216
  suffixes, 216
  surgery, 353–354
  terminology, 213–215
    answers, 255
    quiz, 219–220
Neurons, 213
Neuropathy, presence. *See* Diabetic patient
Neurovascular flap, medical term, 5, A79
Nevi. *See* Moles

Newborn (perinatal) guidelines (760-779), ICD-9-CM coding, A31–A33
Newborns
  congenital anomalies, A32–A33
  sepsis, ICD-9-CM coding, A33
  V codes, A46
Newborn sepsis, ICD-9-CM coding, A15
New patient, 285
NFS. *See* National Fee Schedule
NIDDM. *See* Non-insulin dependent diabetes mellitus
Nipple, 92f
Nociceptors, 239
Nodule, 9, 10f
Nonbacterial UTI, cause/treatment, 145
Noncovered in-hospital expenses, 264
Noncovered services, 271
Non-Hodgkin lymphoma, 196
Non-hospital services, 279
Non-insulin dependent diabetes mellitus (NIDDM), 205
Noninvasive, medical term, 78, A79
Nonmechanical obstruction. *See* Small intestine
Nonobstetric curettage, 351
Nonspecific V codes, A48–A49
Nonviral hepatitis, 176
Normal sinus rhythm (NSR), 77, A105
Nose, 55, 56f
Notes, 384. *See also* Excludes notes; Includes notes
NSR. *See* Normal sinus rhythm
Nuclear cardiology, medical term, 78, A79
Nucleus, 213f
Nutritional degenerative disease, 221–222
Nutritional disorders, ICD-9-CM coding, 395–396, A18–A20
Nystagmus, 245
  medical term, A79

O

OA. *See* Osteoarthritis
Obliquus externus, 37f, 38f

OBRA. *See* Omnibus Budget Reconciliation Act of 1989
Observation, V codes, A43
Obstetrics (OB)
  care, routine. *See* Global obstetric care
  cases (rules), ICD-9-CM coding, A26
  principal/first-listed diagnosis selection, ICD-9-CM coding, A26–A27
  V codes, A46
Obstruction. *See* Small intestine
Occipital bone, 31f
Occurrence guideline, placement. *See* E codes
Ocular adnexa, 237f
  medical term, 241, A79
OD. *See* Right eye
Office of the Inspector General (OIG), 268
Office visit, 381
OIG. *See* Office of the Inspector General
Olecranon, medical term, A79
Olfactory sense receptors, 238
Oligodendrocytoma, 232
Omnibus Budget Reconciliation Act of 1989 (OBRA), medical term, A79
Oophorectomy, medical term, 96, A79
Opacification, medical term, A79
Open fracture, 47
  repair, medical term, 43, A79
Open treatment, medical term, A79
Ophthalmodynamometry, medical term, A79
Ophthalmoscopy, medical term, 241, A79
Optic foramen, 32f
Optic nerve, 237f
Optokinetic, medical term, A79
Oral cavity, 155f
  cancer, 164
  disorders, 163–164
  infections, 163–164
Orchiectomy, medical term, 119, A79
Orchiopexy, medical term, 119, A79
Orchitis, 123

Order, medical term, 78, A79
Oropharynx, 56f
Orthopnea, 65
    medical term, 60, A79
Orthoptic, medical term,
    A79
OS. *See* Left eye
Osteitis deformans (Paget's
    disease), 49
Osteoarthritis (OA), 42, A105
    classifications, 49
    medical term, 43, A79
    symptoms, 49
    treatment, 49
Osteoclast, medical term, 43,
    A79
Osteoma, 51
Osteomalacia, 48
Osteomyelitis, 48
Osteoporosis, 48
Osteosarcoma, 51
Osteotomy, medical term, 43,
    A79
Other codes. *See* International
    Classification of Diseases,
    9th Revision, Clinical
    Modification
Otitis externa (swimmer's ear),
    248
Otitis media, 248
    medical term, 241, A79
Otoscope, medical term, 241,
    A79
Ototoxic hearing loss, 249
OU. *See* Each eye
Outer layer. *See* Sclera
Outpatient, 286
Outpatient services, 279
    diagnostic coding, 390–393
    reporting guidelines,
        390–393
Ovarian malignancies,
    staging, 107
Ovaries, 91, 91f, 199f, 201,
    349
    carcinoma, 108–109
    risk, increased, 108
    surgery, 353
Oviducts, 349. *See* Fallopian
    tubes
    laparoscopy, 349
    medical term, A79
Ovulation, 92

P

P. rosea. *See* Pityriasis rosea
PAC. *See* Premature atrial
    contraction
Paget's disease. *See* Osteitis
    deformans

Palate. *See* Hard palate; Soft
    palate
Palatine tonsil, 154f
Palatoglossal arch, 154f
Palatopharyngeal arch, 154f
Pancreas, 155f, 199f, 200, 353
    disorders, 174, 178
Pancreatic cancer, 178
Pancreatitis, 178
Papilledema, medical term,
    241, A79
Papule, 9, 10f
Papulosquamous disorders,
    15–16
    conditions, 15–16
Paraesophageal hernia, 165f
Paraesophageal hiatus hernia,
    medical term, 159, A79
Paraperitoneal nephrectomy,
    medical term, A78
Paraphimosis, 127, 128
    symptom/treatment, 128
Parasitic disease, ICD-9-CM
    coding, 393–394,
    A12–A16
Parathyroid
    disorders, 208
    medical term, 188, A80
Parathyroid gland, 199f, 200
Parenchyma, 136f
Parentheses, usage, 382
Parietal bone, 31f, 32f
Parkinson's disease, 222
Paronychia, medical term,
    A80
Parotid gland, 154f
Paroxysmal atrial tachycardia
    (PAT), 77, A106
Paroxysmal nocturnal
    dyspnea (PND), 59, A106
Paroxysmal supraventricular
    tachycardia (PST/PSVT),
    77, A106
Part A, medical term, A80
Part B, medical term, A80
Partial epilepsies, 229
Partial placenta previa, 111f
Partial thromboplastin time
    (PTT), A106
Participating providers,
    263–264
    program, medical term,
        A80
Past, Family, and Social
    History (PFSH), 288–289
PAT. *See* Paroxysmal atrial
    tachycardia
Patella, 35f, 38f
    medical term, A80
Patellar tendon, 38f

Pathophysiology, resources,
    A109
Patient type, 285–286
PAWP. *See* Pulmonary artery
    wedge pressure
PCP. *See* Primary care
    physician
PCWP. *See* Pulmonary
    capillary wedge pressure
PEAP. *See* Positive end-airway
    pressure
Pectoralis major, 38f
Pedicle, medical term, 6,
    A80
PEEP. *See* Positive end-
    expiratory pressure
Peer Review Organization
    (PRO), 265, 267
    medical term, A80
    reviews, 265
PEG. *See* Percutaneous
    endoscopic gastrostomy
Pelvic inflammatory disease
    (PID), 96, 103, A106
Pelviolithotomy, medical
    term, A80
Pelvis, 33–34
Penis, 117f, 345
    cancer, 128–129
    disorders, 127–129
Penoscrotal, medical term,
    119, A80
Peptic ulcers, 167–168
Percussion, medical term, 60,
    A80
Percutaneous, medical term,
    43, A80
Percutaneous endoscopic
    gastrostomy (PEG), 158,
    A106
Percutaneous fracture repair,
    medical term, 43, A80
Percutaneous
    nephrostolithotomy,
    medical term, A78
Percutaneous nephrostomy,
    medical term, A79
Percutaneous skeletal fixation,
    medical term, 43, A80
Percutaneous transluminal
    coronary angioplasty
    (PTCA), 77, A106
Performance objectives. *See*
    Course
Pericardial effusion, 87
Pericardiocentesis, medical
    term, 78, A80
Pericarditis, 86. *See also* Acute
    pericarditis; Constrictive
    pericarditis

PPO. *See* Preferred provider organization
PPS. *See* Postpolio syndrome
Pre-examination, S3, 408, 413
Preferred provider organization (PPO), 269, 272
  medical term, A81
Prefixes, A97–A98
Pregnancy, 92–93, 110–114. *See also* Ectopic pregnancy; Female genital system/pregnancy complications
  ICD-9-CM coding, 401–402, A26–A30
  late effect, code 677, A29
  diabetes mellitus, A19
  ICD-9-CM coding, A28
  HIV
    impact, 393–394
    infection, ICD-9-CM coding, A27
  life-threatening rupture, 112f
  malpositions/malpresentations, 112
  relationship. *See* Menstruation
Premature atrial contraction (PAC), 77, A106
Premature rupture of membranes (PROM), 96, A106
Premature ventricular contraction (PVC), 77, A106
Prematurity, ICD-9-CM coding, A33
Premenstrual syndrome (PMS), 102
Premenstruation, 92
Presbyopia, 245
Presenting problem. *See* High-severity presenting problem; Low-severity presenting problem; Minimal presenting problem; Moderate-severity presenting problem; Self-limiting presenting problem
  CF, 294
  levels, 294–295
Pressure ulcer (decubitis ulcer), 11–12
  stages, 12f
Priapism, medical term, 119, A81
Primary amenorrhea, 101

Primary bronchus, 56f
Primary care physician (PCP), medical term, A81
Primary diagnosis
  medical term, A81
  selection, 388–389, 401
Primary dysmenorrhea, 101
Primary fallopian tube tumors, 109
Primary fibromyalgia syndrome, symptoms/appearance, 50
Principal diagnosis, selection. *See* International Classification of Diseases, 9th Revision, Clinical Modification
Prior approval, medical term, A81
Prior authorization, 272
PRO. *See* Peer Review Organization
Problem-focused (PF) examination, 290
Problem-focused (PF) history, 289
Proctosigmoidoscopy, medical term, 159, A81
Professional Standards Review Organization (PSRO), medical term, A81
Prognosis, medical term, A81
Proliferation phase. *See* Menstruation
PROM. *See* Premature rupture of membranes
Proprioceptors, 239
Prostate, 345
  cancer, 130–131
Prostate gland, 117f
  disorders, 129–131
Prostate-specific antigen (PSA), 118, A106
Prostatitis, 129–130. *See also* Acute prostatitis; Chronic prostatitis
Prostatotomy, medical term, 119, A81
Proteases, 21
Prothrombin time (PT), A106
Provider Identification Number (PIN), 272
  medical term, A81
Pruritus (itching), 19
PSA. *See* Prostate-specific antigen
Psoriasis, 16–17
PSRO. *See* Professional Standards Review Organization

PST. *See* Paroxysmal supraventricular tachycardia
PSVT. *See* Paroxysmal supraventricular tachycardia
PT. *See* Prothrombin time
PTCA. *See* Percutaneous transluminal coronary angioplasty
Pterion, 31f
PTT. *See* Partial thromboplastin time
Pubis, 35f
Puerperium
  complications (630-677), ICD-9-CM coding, 401–402, A26–A30
  HIV infection, ICD-9-CM coding, A27
Pulmonary artery, 72f, 74f
Pulmonary artery wedge pressure (PAWP), 59, A106
Pulmonary capillary wedge pressure (PCWP), 59, A106
Pulmonary diseases/disorders, 65–67
Pulmonary edema, 66
Pulmonary embolism, 67
Pulmonary function test (PFT), 59, A106
Pulmonary semilunar valve, 74f
Pulmonary vein. *See* Right pulmonary vein
Pulmonic vein, 74f
Pupils equal, round, and reactive to light and accommodation (PERRLA), 240, A106
Pupils equal, round, and reactive to light (PERRL), 240, A106
Pupils equal and reactive to light (PERL), 240, A106
Purkinje fibers, 74f
Pustule, 9–11, 10f
PVC. *See* Premature ventricular contraction
Pyelography, medical term, A81
Pyelonephritis. *See* Acute pyelonephritis; Chronic pyelonephritis
Pyloric stenosis, 168

Q

Qualitative, medical term, A81

Spontaneous abortion, 352
Spontaneous rupture of
   membranes (SROM),
   A107
Sprains/strains, 48
SQ. *See* Subcutaneous
Squamous cell carcinoma,
   24
Squamous suture, 31f
SROM. *See* Spontaneous
   rupture of membranes
Staff Model, medical term,
   A83
Stand-alone code description,
   282
Stasis dermatitis, 14–15
State license number, 272
Status, V code, A39–A42
STDs. *See* Sexually transmitted
   diseases
Steatoma, medical term, 6,
   A83
Stem cell, 341–342
   medical term, 188, A83
Stenosis, 86–87. *See also* Aortic
   stenosis; Mitral stenosis
Stereotaxis, medical term,
   217, A83
Sternal angle, 34f
Sternochondral joint, 34f
Sternoclavicular joint, 34f
Sternocleidomastoideus, 37f,
   38f
Sternum, 35f
   body, 34f
   manubrium, 34f
Stomach, 155, 155f, 165f
   disorders, 166–168
Strabismus, 245
   medical term, 241, A83
Straightforward MDM, 292
Strangulated hernia, 343
Stratified, medical term, 6,
   A83
Stratum (strata), medical
   term, 6, A83
Stress urinary incontinence
   (SUI), 96, A107
Stroke. *See* Cerebrovascular
   accident
Student calendar, C1
Study skills, resources, A110
Stye. *See* Hordeolum
Styloid process, 31f
Subclavian artery, 72f.
   See also Left subclavian
   artery
Subclavian trunk, 186f
Subclavian vein, 73f
Subcutaneous fat, 12f

Subcutaneous (subcu/subq/
   SC/SQ), A107
   medical term, A83
Subcutaneous tissue (680-
   709), ICD-9-CM coding,
   402–403, A30
Sublingual gland, 154f
Subluxation, medical term,
   43, A83
Submandibular gland, 154f
Substances, involvement. *See*
   Drugs
Subungual, medical term, 6,
   A83
Success strategies, S1
Suffixes, A99–A101
SUI. *See* Stress urinary
   incontinence
Sulcus. *See* Median sulcus;
   Terminal sulcus
Superficial inguinal nodes,
   186f
Superficial palmar arch, 72f
Superficial temporal artery,
   72f
Superficial venous palmar
   arch, 73f
Superior, medical term, A83
Superior extensor
   retinaculum, 38f
Superior mesenteric artery, 72f
Superior peroneal
   retinaculum, 37f
Superior vena cava, 73f, 74f
Supination, medical term, 43,
   A83
Supine, medical term, A83
Supplemental tracking codes,
   283
Supraorbital foramen, 32f
Supraventricular tachycardia
   (SVT), 77, A107
SVT. *See* Supraventricular
   tachycardia
Swan Ganz catheter, medical
   term, 78, A83
Swimmer's ear. *See* Otitis
   externa
Sympathetic nerve, medical
   term, 217, A83
Symphysis, medical term, A83
Synarthrosis, 36
Synchondrosis, medical term,
   A83
Syphilis, 104–105
Systemic inflammatory
   response syndrome (SIRS)
   sepsis, 394
Systemic toxicity,
   development, 21

T

T1-T12. *See* Thoracic
   vertebrae
Table of drugs. *See*
   International
   Classification of Diseases,
   9th Revision, Clinical
   Modification
Tabular abbreviations. *See*
   International
   Classification of Diseases,
   9th Revision, Clinical
   Modification
Tachycardia. *See* Multifocal
   atrial tachycardia;
   Paroxysmal atrial
   tachycardia; Paroxysmal
   supraventricular
   tachycardia;
   Supraventricular
   tachycardia
Tachypnea, 65
   medical term, 61, A83
Taenia coli, 155f
TAH. *See* Total abdominal
   hysterectomy
Tailbone. *See* Coccyx
Talus (ankle bone), 35f
Tarsorrhaphy, medical term,
   242, A83
Taste, 238
Tax Equity and Fiscal
   Responsibility Act
   (TEFRA), medical term,
   A84
TEE. *See* Transesophageal
   echocardiography
Teeth, 153
TEFRA. *See* Tax Equity and
   Fiscal Responsibility
   Act
Temporal bone
   squama, 31f
   zygomatic process, 31f
Temporomandibular joint
   (TMJ), 42, A107
Tendon
   disorders, 50–51
   medical term, 43, A84
Tenodesis, medical term, 43,
   A84
Tenorrhaphy, medical term,
   44, A84
TENS. *See* Transcutaneous
   electrical nerve
   stimulation
Tensor fasciae latae, 38f
Teres major, 37f
Teres minor, 37f
Terminal sulcus, 154f

Variocele, 124–125
  medical term, 119, A86
Vascular dementia, 221
Vascular disorders, 81–85,
  149–150, 226–229
Vas deferens, 117, 117f
  medical term, 119, A86
Vasogram, medical term, 119,
  A86
Vasorrhaphy, medical term,
  119, A86
Vasotomy, medical term, 119,
  A86
Vasovasostomy, medical term,
  119, A86
Vastus lateralis, 38f
Vastus medialis, 38f
VBAC. *See* Vaginal birth after
  cesarean
V codes, 389–390. *See also*
    Health status; Nonspecific
    V codes
  categories, A39–A49. *See
    also* History
  miscellaneous codes, A47
  table, A50–A54
  usage, 389–390, A39
Vectorcardiogram, medical
  term, A86
Veins, 72. *See also* Circulatory
  system
Venography, medical term,
  A86
Ventilation/perfusion scan
  (V/Q), 59, A107
Ventral surface. *See* Mouth
Ventricle, 214f. *See also* Left
  ventricle; Right ventricle
Vermiform appendix, 155f
Vermilion surface. *See* Mouth

Verrucae. *See* Warts
Vertebral artery, 72f
Vertebral column, anterior
  view, 33f
Vertebrectomy, medical term,
  217, A86
Vertex position, 113f
Vertigo, medical term, 242,
  A86
Vesical neck, 345
Vesicle, 9–11, 10f
  development, 22
Vesicostomy, medical term,
  139, A86
Vesicovaginal fistula, medical
  term, 97, A86
Vesiculectomy, medical term,
  119, A86
Vesiculography, medical term,
  A86
Vesiculotomy, medical term,
  119, A86
Vessels. *See* Blood vessels
  damage, 406
Vestibule, 56f, 153f
Viral hepatitis, 174–176
Viral herpes simplex (cold
  sores), 21–22
Viscera, medical term, A86
Visceral muscle. *See*
    Smooth/visceral muscle
Visual disturbances. *See* Eye
Vitreous body, anterior
  surface, 237f
Vitreous humor, 238
Voice box. *See* Larynx
Volvulus, medical term, 159,
  A86
Vomer, 32f
  medical term, A86

V/Q. *See* Ventilation/perfusion
  scan
Vulva, 91, 346
  carcinoma, symptoms/
    treatment, 110
Vulvectomy, 347

W

Warts (verrucae), 22–23
Wheal, 9–11, 10f
White blood count (WBC),
  A107
Whitmore-Jewett stages,
  131f
Wilms' tumor, 150
Windpipe. *See* Trachea
With, 383. *See also* And/with
Wounds, debridement (ICD-9-
  CM coding), A36
Wrist
  extensors, 37f, 38f
  flexors, 38f
Writing basics, resources,
  A109

X

Xanthoma, medical term, 6,
  A86
Xenograft, medical term, 6,
  A86
Xeroderma, medical term, 6,
  A86
Xeroradiography, medical
  term, A86
Xiphoid process, 34f

Z

Zygomatic bone, 31f, 32f
Zygomatic process. *See*
    Temporal bone